THE ESSENTIAL GUIDE TO VITAMINS, MINERALS AND HERBAL SUPPLEMENTS

Dr Sarah Brewer

ROBINSON

ROBINSON

First published in Great Britain by Robinson in 2002

This new, completely revised and updated edition published in 2010 by Robinson

Copyright © Sarah Brewer 2002, 2010

7 9 10 8 6

Important Note:
This book is not intended as a substitute for medical advice or treatment.
Any person with a condition requiring medical attention should consult a
qualified medical practitioner or suitable therapist.

A CIP catalogue record for this book
is available from the British Library.

ISBN 978-0-7160-2216-9

Printed and bound in Great Britain by CPI Group (UK) Ltd, Croydon CR0 4YY

Papers used by Robinson are from well-managed forests and other responsible sources

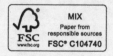

MIX
Paper from
responsible sources
FSC® C104740

Robinson
An imprint of
Little, Brown Book Group
Carmelite House
50 Victoria Embankment
London EC4Y 0DZ

An Hachette UK Company
www.hachette.co.uk

www.improvementzone.co.uk

THE ESSENTIAL GUIDE TO VITAMINS, MINERALS AND HERBAL SUPPLEMENTS

DR SARAH BREWER qualified from Cambridge University with degrees in Natural Sciences, Medicine and Surgery. After working in general practice and sexual health, she now specializes in Nutritional Medicine. Although her first love is medicine, her major passion is writing. She writes regularly for a variety of newspapers and magazines, taking a holistic approach that includes complementary medicine and nutritional medicine. She is the author of 50 popular self-help books, including the Natural Health Guru series. Sarah was voted Health Journalist of the Year in 2002 and is now also a Registered Nutritionist. Her website is www.natural healthguru.co.uk. Follow her nutritional Tweets at www.twitter. com/DrSarahB.

CONTENTS

CONTENTS

DEDICATION

This book is dedicated to my wonderful family, Richard, Saxon, Roman and Sapphire, who willingly provide invaluable back-up and support during those long hours of research and writing

ACKNOWLEDGEMENTS

I would like to thank all the researchers whose work is detailed within this book. Without their active investigation of micro-nutrients, herbal medicines and essential fatty acids, we would have little understanding of the beneficial effects of so many invaluable nutritional supplements.

HOW TO USE THIS BOOK

The first part of this book looks at individual vitamins, minerals, herbs and other supplements. If you want to know more about a particular supplement, most of your questions should be answered here.

The second part of this book looks at a number of common health problems and tells you a little about them, their causes and symptoms plus the main nutritional approaches that are likely to help. Once you have looked up a condition, and selected a few possible remedies, you can then check these out in the first part of the book to choose those that are most likely to suit you.

Doses

The doses given in this book are only meant to be indicative of those in common use. Always follow the manufacturer's instructions as doses will depend on the strength of individual products.

Pregnancy

Never take any supplements during pregnancy or breast-feeding, unless they are especially designed for use at this time (e.g. pregnancy vitamin and mineral blends) or have been recommended by a doctor or qualified medical herbalist.

Health problems

If you have a long-term health problem, always seek advice from a doctor or pharmacist before taking a food supplement or herbal remedy. This is particularly important if you are taking any prescribed drugs, as interactions can occur. It is also important if you have diabetes, as some supplements can affect blood glucose levels.

IMPORTANT NOTES

- This book is not intended to be a substitute for medical advice or treatment. Any person with a condition requiring medical attention should consult a qualified medical practitioner or suitable therapist.

- All suggested doses are for adults only; specialist advice should be sought for supplementation in children.

- Where not otherwise stated, supplements may be taken for an unlimited period, until symptoms improve.

- Where no side effects are mentioned, no serious ones have been reported at standard doses.

- Some herbal supplements may interact with prescribed drugs. Always check with a pharmacist or doctor before combining herbs with drugs.

- Some herbal medicines may cause bleeding, heart problems or low blood sugar in patients undergoing surgery. Always tell your doctor what supplements you are taking as they may need to be stopped before an operation.

INTRODUCTION

A lot of things have changed in the eight years since this book was first published. An extraordinary amount of research has taken place in that time. The evidence to support the use of some supplements for some indications has strengthened, but the evidence to support the use of others has weakened. I've tried to remain as objective as possible when summarizing the use of different vitamins, minerals, herbs and other food supplements. Where possible I've given the results from large analyses (meta-analyses), which pool the data from a number of different trials, to obtain the most reliable overall results. Meta-analyses help to reduce any chance of anomalies that can occur in studies involving low numbers of people. They give a more accurate analysis of the effectiveness of a particular supplement. Where these are not available, I've summarized the results from double-blind, randomized controlled trials in which the outcomes of using a certain supplement are compared with inactive placebo. I have supplied as many references as possible without turning the book into an unwieldy brick. Where references are not given, I guess you'll just have to take my word that I haven't invented the information. Most references can be tracked down by searching for authors and dates via Pub Med (www.ncbi.nlm.nih.gov/sites/entrez).

An almost bewildering range of vitamin, mineral and herbal supplements is available in pharmacies, supermarkets and healthfood stores. In many cases, legislation dictates that full information about the benefits of these supplements cannot be given on their packaging as this would constitute a health claim. This makes it difficult for people wanting to improve particular aspects of their health and well-being to select those supplements most likely to suit them.

The situation is improving for herbal remedies, however, as useful information can now be given for products that have been registered under the Traditional Herbal Registration Scheme. This means the supplements have undergone independent safety and quality assessment by the MHRA (The Medicines and Healthcare products Regulatory Agency www.mhra.gov.uk). These products can be identified by a registration code on their pack starting with the letters THR. Some products have also become Licensed Herbal Medicines as they have been assessed for their safety, quality and – importantly – their effectiveness. These products can be identified by a Product Licence code on their pack starting with the letters PL.

This book aims to tell readers everything they need to know about the main vitamin and mineral supplements and herbal remedies. It provides evidence-based information on the research that supports their use, possible side effects, interactions and key contraindications (who should not take them).

Why take a vitamin and mineral supplement?
In an ideal world, we would get all the vitamins, minerals and essential fatty acids we need from our food. Despite the five-a-day campaign, however, surveys show that only one in eight British adults achieves this. The average intake is just two and a half portions of fruit and vegetables per day. Similarly, over 90 per cent of people do not eat the recommended three servings of wholegrains (rich in B vitamins and trace elements) a day.

Even when we do eat reasonable amounts of healthy foods, their nutritional content is often depleted compared with those eaten just a generation ago. Apart from genetic modification to produce longer-lasting fruit and vegetables with uniform colour and size, intensive farming practices can mean the soils on which crops are grown and livestock reared are deficient in vital trace elements. The most startling example is selenium – intakes in Britain almost halved from 60 mcg in 1974 to just 34 mcg per day in 1994 as a result of using European flour for bread-making in place of selenium-rich flour from the United States[1].

A scientific review of over 150 clinical trials published in the

Journal of the American Medical Association found that lack of many vitamins is a risk factor for heart disease, stroke, some cancers, birth defects, osteoporosis, bone fractures and other major chronic health problems. In an accompanying paper[2], the authors actually state that, 'Pending strong evidence of effectiveness from randomized trials, it appears prudent for all adults to take vitamin supplements.'

Taking an A-to-Z supplement providing around 100 per cent of the recommended daily amount (RDA, see page 16) of as many vitamins and minerals as possible acts as an important, nutritional safety net.

Why take an omega-3 fish oils supplement?

Omega-3 fish oils have a number of beneficial effects in the body (see page 137) and we are advised to eat two to four portions of oily fish per week (with each portion weighing 150 g). Surveys show, however, that the average British adult eats just 50 g of oily fish per week, supplying a meagre 1 g of the most important long-chain omega-3s, EPA and DHA[3]. The dose of long-chain omega-3s required for a demonstrable effect on heart disease risk factors is at least 1.5 g *per day* yet an astonishing 70 per cent of adults eat no oily fish at all. A supplement is therefore an excellent idea.

Effects of age on nutrient needs

As you get older, your need for particular vitamins and minerals will change and the amount of nutrients that can be absorbed from your intestines will decrease. As a result, you tend to need more anti-oxidants (vitamins A, C and E), B vitamins and less iron. It is therefore a good idea to take a vitamin and mineral supplement specially formulated for the over-50 age group. Several studies have now shown that older people who take a multivitamin supplement have better immune function, mount a better response to influenza vaccination, and suffer significantly fewer upper respiratory tract infections than those not taking multivitamin supplements.

1. Rayman MP (1997): Dietary selenium: time to act British Medical Journal 314, 387–88

2. Vitamins for Chronic Disease Prevention in Adults. Clinical applications. Fletcher RH, Fairfield KM, JAMA 2002;287:3127–3129

3. Scientific Advisory Committee on Nutrition. Advice to FSA: on the benefits of oily fish and fish consumption SACN:
www.sacn.gov.uk/news/press_releases/2004_06_24.html

Nutrient	Old EU RDA	New EU RDA	RNI for Men 19–50 years	RNI for Women 19–50 years	EVM 2003 *Upper safe level for long-term use from supplements*
Vitamins					
Vitamin A (retinol equivalents)	800 mcg	800 mcg	700 mcg	600 mcg	1500 mcg[1]
Betacarotene	–	–	–		7 mg
Vitamin B1 (thiamin)	1.4 mg	↓1.1 mg	1 mg	0.8 mg	100 mg
Vitamin B2 (riboflavin)	1.6 mg	↓1.4 mg	1.3 mg	1.1 mg	40 mg
Vitamin B3 (niacin)	18 mg	↓16 mg	17 mg	13 mg	500 mg
Vitamin B5 (pantothenic acid)	6 mg	6 mg	–	–	200 mg
Vitamin B6 (pyridoxine)	2 mg	↓1.4 mg	1.4 mg	1.2 mg	10 mg
Vitamin B12 (cobalamin)	1 mcg	↑2.5 mcg	1.5 mcg	1.5 mcg	2000 mcg
Folic acid) (folate	200 mcg	200 mcg	200 mcg	200 mcg[2]	1000 mcg
Biotin	150 mcg	↓↓50 mcg	10–200 mcg[3]	10–200 mcg[3]	900 mcg
Vitamin C (ascorbic acid)	60 mg	↑80 mg	40 mg	40 mg	1000 mg
Vitamin D (cholecalciferol)	5 mcg	5 mcg	–[4]	–[4]	25 mcg
Vitamin E (tocopherol)	10 mg	↑12 mg	> 4 mg	> 3 mg	540 mg (800 IU)
Vitamin K	–	75 mcg	1 mcg/kg[5]	1 mcg/kg[5]	1000 mcg
Minerals					
Boron	–	–	–[6]	–[6]	6 mg
Calcium	800 mg	800 mg	700 mg	700 mg	1500 mg
Chloride	–	800 mg	2500 mg	2500 mg	–
Chromium	–	40 mcg	–[7]	–[7]	10 mg[1]
Copper	–	1 mg	1.2 mg	1.2 mg	10 mg[1]
Iodine	150 mcg	150 mcg	140 mcg	140 mcg	500 mcg
Iron	14 mg	14 mg	8.7 mg	14.8 mg	17 mg
Magnesium	300 mg	↑375 mg	300 mg	270 mg	400 mg
Manganese	–	2 mg	–[8]	–[8]	4 mg
Phosphorus	800 mg	↓700 mg	550 mg	550 mg	250 mg

Nutrient	Old EU RDA	New EU RDA	RNI for Men 19–50 years	RNI for Women 19–50 years	EVM 2003 Upper safe level for long-term use from supplements
Potassium	–	2000 mg	3500 mg	3500 mg	3700 mg
Selenium	–	55 mcg	75 mcg	60 mcg	350 mcg
Sodium	–	–	1600 mg	1600 mg	–
Zinc	15 mg	↓↓10 mg	9.5 mg	7 mg	25 mg

Table showing EU RDA, UK RNI for adult men and women, and suggested safe intake upper levels of vitamins and minerals

NB: Hyphens (–) indicate no levels set.

1. This upper safe level refers to the total intake from both diet and supplements
2. 400 mcg folic acid for women who could become pregnant
3. Insufficient data to set an RNI but this level is considered adequate
4. For adults confined indoors (no sunlight exposure) and for those aged 65 and over, the RNI for vitamin D is 10 mcg per day
5. Per kilogram of body weight
6. No RNI set, but the World Health Organization suggests that intakes of 1–13 mg boron per day are adequate
7. No RNI set but intakes of trivalent chromium above 25 mcg are thought to be adequate
8. No RNI set but the EU Scientific Committee for Food considers 1–10 mg per day is adequate

The **EU RDA** (Recommended Daily Amount) is based on the highest requirements of any human group and is used for labelling purposes on vitamin and mineral products. This does not take into account the differing needs of men and women.

The **RNI** (Reference Nutrient Intake) values are rather outdated (published by the Department of Health in 1991) but are still the current guidelines for nutrient requirements of adult men and women in the UK. Different values apply for some vitamins and minerals during pregnancy and breast-feeding.

EVM The UK Expert Group on Vitamins and Minerals report on the Safe Upper Limits for Vitamins and Minerals, May 2003. This suggests guidance levels for the maximum daily amounts of each vitamin and mineral that are considered safe for long-term supplementation (in addition to the amounts typically obtained from foods).

Recommended Daily Intakes and Upper Safe Levels

Most supplements supply amounts of vitamins and minerals that contain around the recommended daily intake (RDA, see page 16) of each micronutrient. A few more specialist supplements contain much higher amounts. Check the levels given on the packaging, which will usually state the amount of each vitamin and mineral plus the percentage (%) RDA that represents. The RDA used has been set by the European Union for labelling purposes. This often varies slightly from the Reference Nutrient Intake (RNI, see page 16) which has been set in the UK.

The EU RDAs have recently been updated and new values agreed throughout the European Union. These came into force in October 2009 and are for use on the labels of vitamin and mineral supplements. New supplements will feature these but those in existence before that date do not have to be reformulated or have their labels updated until 2012. You may therefore see different RDAs on different products for the next few years.

The table on page 16 shows the old and new EU RDA, the UK RNI for adult men and women, and the suggested upper level that is safe to take long term within a vitamin and mineral supplement.

How to take supplements

Unless otherwise stated on the packaging, vitamin and mineral supplements should be taken immediately after food. Just four bites of food or a glass of orange juice will do. If you have not eaten for more than 20 minutes, don't take your supplements. Wait until you have a snack/juice and take them then. If taken on an empty stomach, some can cause nausea or indigestion.

Wash supplements down with water or orange juice. Don't take them with coffee or tea, as these may interfere with absorption. Substances found in tea and coffee can inhibit iron absorption by up to 80 per cent if drunk within an hour of a meal or taking a supplement. Grapefruit juice is also known to interact with a number of prescribed and over-the-counter drugs. Although little information is known about the interaction between grapefruit juice and herbal medicines, it is wise not to combine them, just in case.

Fat-soluble substances (e.g. co-enzyme Q10, evening primrose oil, fish oils, vitamins A, D, E, K) should ideally be taken with food containing some fat (e.g. milk). If taking a fish oil supplement that produces fishy 'burps' try emulsifying the oil by shaking your dose with a little milk to increase absorption and reduce after-taste.

If you take a one-a-day vitamin and mineral supplement, it is usually best taken after your evening meal rather than with break-fast. This is because repair processes and mineral movements in your body are greatest at night when growth hormone is secreted.

Where you have to take two or more capsules of the same preparation, however, it is a good idea to spread these out over the day in order to maximize absorption and cause less fluctuation in blood levels.

But, a day's dose is better taken at the time you are most likely to remember. Don't feel you have to follow any strict regime if you find difficulty remembering to take supplements at a certain time, or if they do not fit in with your particular lifestyle. It's easier to remember to take supplements if you get into a routine and take them at the same time each day. Keep them by your toothbrush, for example, or by your keyboard if this helps you remember (as long as they are out of the reach of young children).

If taking the lighter, gelatin capsules, look down at the floor as you swallow to help them go down more easily. For heavier tablets, put your head back as you swallow to help the action of gravity.

Don't swallow supplements in a hurry − if you take your time, your throat muscle will be more relaxed and tablets are less likely to lodge in your gullet.

Herbal remedies
Herbalism, or phytotherapy, can have powerful healing actions − between 30 and 40 per cent of prescription drugs are in fact derived from plant origins. In most cases, herbal supplements contain a blend of constituents that have evolved together over thousands of years to achieve a synergistic balance. This tends to produce a more gentle effect than pharmaceutical extracts containing only one, isolated active ingredient. The risk of side effects with traditional herbal remedies is therefore relatively low, but not non-existent.

Herbal extracts are prepared in ways designed to concentrate the active components of the herb, whether found in the bark, leaves, seeds, roots, flowers or stems. Tinctures are made by soaking herbs in an alcoholic base and may be described as, for example, a 1:10

extract, which means that 10 per cent of the tincture is made up of the herbal base, while 90 per cent is solvent. Traditional herbalists tend to prefer tinctures. Personally, I prefer standardized, solid extracts which are easier to use and which contain consistent, therapeutic levels of ingredients.

Solid extracts are prepared by removing the solvent (e.g. alcohol) used to extract the active components from the original herbal base. The residual solids are then dried and powdered to make tablets or capsules. Solid extracts are described according to their concentration so that, for example, a 10:1 extract means that ten parts crude herb was used to make one part of the extract. The more concentrated the extract, theoretically the stronger it is, although more volatile components may have become lost so that the concentration does not accurately reflect its activity. Because of this, it is best to use a standardized preparation.

Standardization measures the levels of active ingredients present in the extracts and adjusts the concentration to ensure each tablet delivers the same amount – just as with pharmaceutical drugs. This reassures both prescriber and consumer that their selected product delivers an effective dose. Standardized remedies are also more likely to be backed by good quality, randomized, double-blind, placebo-controlled trials.

People often ask me what supplements they should take. My only rule is that you should have a valid reason for each supplement you use. Everyone has different needs and it is difficult to generalize. However, in my view, most people would benefit from taking: a multivitamin and mineral supplement as a nutritional safety net, an omega-3 fish oil supplement for anti-inflammatory, cardiovascular protection and a probiotic for digestive and immune health.

I hope you find this book invaluable and I wish all readers a future that is as healthy and natural as possible.

Sarah Brewer
email: DrSarah@naturalhealthguru.co.uk
www.naturalhealthguru.co.uk

NB: Do not take any vitamin, mineral, herbal or other supplements, except under medical advice, if you:

• Have a long-term medical condition.

• Are taking any prescribed or over-the-counter medications.

• Are pregnant, or planning to be.

• Are breast-feeding.

Doses

A milligram (mg) is one thousandth of a gram, while a microgram (mcg or μg) is one millionth of a gram.

1 g (one gram) therefore equals 1000 mg, and 1 mg equals 1000 mcg.

This can lead to some confusion, as a product containing (for example) 1 g vitamin C contains the same amount as one claiming 1000 mg vitamin C, while a product containing 400 mcg folic acid provides the same amount as one listing 0.4 mg folic acid, although one value may sound more than another.

International units (IU) were used to measure biological activity of vitamins A, D and E before the pure compounds were isolated and quantified. Although these are considered obsolete, they are still occasionally used on packs – especially for vitamin E.

For vitamin A, 1 mcg retinol is equivalent to 3 IU.
For vitamin D, 1 mcg is equivalent to 40 IU.
For vitamin E, 1 mg (or 1000 mcg) is approximately equivalent to 1.5 IU.

For the EU recommended daily amounts (RDAs) of each of these three vitamins, the equivalents are therefore:

Vitamin A: 800 mcg = 2400 IU
Vitamin D: 5 mcg = 200 IU
Vitamin E: old EU RDA 10 mg = 15 IU; new EU RDA 12 mg = 18 IU

PART 1

A–Z
OF
SUPPLEMENTS

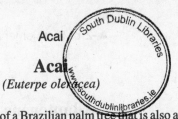

Acai
(Euterpe oleracea)

Acai berries are the fruit of a Brazilian palm tree that is also a source of 'hearts of palm' – the soft, inner shoot tips that are popular in salads.

Acai berries are small and round with a similar size and appearance to grapes, but with an oily coating, less pulp and a single, large seed. As the berries ripen, they turn from green to a dark, purple-black. Bunches of ripe fruit can weight up to 5 kg or more. As a food, they are used to make smoothies, juices, ice-cream and are also added to breakfast cereals.

Acai extracts are now available in tablet form and as freeze-dried powder. They are a good source of fibre, omega-3 essential fatty acids and oleic acid – the same monounsaturated fat as that found in olive oil. Acai also contain calcium, iron, manganese, plant sterols (mainly beta-sitosterol), antioxidant procyanidins (polyphenols) and lignans (a type of phytoestrogen).

South American herbalists use acai fruit to treat diarrhoea, skin ulcers and fever.

Antioxidant: The antioxidant capacity of fresh acai juice is ranked below that of pomegranate, blueberry and black grape juice, is similar to that of cranberry and black cherry juice, but is greater than orange juice, apple juice and iced tea[1]. However, the antioxidant capacity of freeze-dried acai pulp/skin powder is amongst the highest for any food tested, at 161,400 ORAC units (micro TE/100 g) which is even higher than for dark chocolate (103,971 ORAC units), and higher than for Goji berries (25,300 ORAC units)[2]. Consumption of acai pulp has been shown to increase the antioxidant capacity of human volunteers' blood plasma by two- to three-fold[3].

Anti-inflammatory: Acai can inhibit COX-1 and COX-2 enzymes in the body to produce an anti-inflammatory, painkilling effect in a similar way to non-steroidal anti-inflammatory drugs (NSAIDs) though the effect is weaker.

1. Seeram NP et al. J Agric Food Chem 2008; 56(4):1415–22
2. www.oracvalues.com
3. Mertens-Talcott SU et al. J Agric Food Chem 2008; 56(17):7796–802

Dose

500 mg–1 g.

Adaptogens

The concept of plant adaptogens was developed by Soviet scientists during the 1950s. They defined an adaptogen as a substance that exerts effects on both sick and healthy individuals to correct any dysfunction without unwanted side effects. Adaptogens are now recognized as herbal tonics that strengthen, normalize and regulate body functions, especially those involved in the stress response. They increase our ability to adapt to environmental factors and to reduce any associated damage. Single doses of an adaptogen mainly affect the sympathetic nervous system and adrenal glands to provide a rapid response to acute stress, improving mental and physical performance. Repeated doses mainly work through an effect on the hypothalamus-pituitary-adrenal gland group of hormones to improve our response to chronic stress.[1]

Benefits

Adaptogens have wide-ranging benefits and boost immunity through several different actions rather than one specific effect. Some adaptogens have been shown to bring blood pressure and blood glucose, cholesterol and hormone levels back into the normal range, and to counter the fatigue and other symptoms associated with stress and disrupted biorhythms.

Research suggests that adaptogens work by boosting the uptake of oxygen and production of energy within cells. This improves cell function, encourages cell growth and increases cell survival. These effects are believed to improve the function of the adrenal glands, which can become depleted during times of prolonged stress.

Adaptogens are especially helpful for boosting energy levels when fatigue is not directly due to excess physical exertion but to an underlying problem such as poor or irregular diet, hormone imbalance, stress or excess consumption of coffee, nicotine or alcohol. Lifestyle changes to redress the balance (e.g. stopping smoking, getting enough sleep) are also important.

---

1. Panossian A, Wagner H. Phytother Res 2005;19(10):819–38

Adaptogens are often used together with vitamins C (500 mg daily) and B complex (50–100 mg daily in divided doses).

Important herbal adaptogens include:
Ashwagandha
Astragalus
Black cohosh
Dong quai
Korean and American ginsengs
Maca
Maitake
Panax ginseng (Korean and American ginsengs)
Pfaffia
Reishi
Rhodiola
Schisandra
Siberian ginseng
Yerba maté

African prune
(Pygeum africanum; Prunus africanum)

An extract from the bark of the evergreen African plum tree is used to treat male lower urinary tract symptoms in many European countries.

There is good scientific evidence that extracts of *Pygeum africanum* bark can improve lower urinary tract symptoms due to benign prostatic hyperplasia (BPH, see page 559) which is an increasingly common problem in men over the age of 45. It is believed to work by damping down over reactivity of bladder muscle fibres, to improve urinary hesitancy, frequency and the need to get up at night to pass urine.

Research
Prostatism: A Cochrane review looked at 18 randomized controlled trials involving 1,562 men which compared the effects of *Pygeum africanum* against inactive placebo over periods of time that ranged from 30 to 122 days[1]. Compared to placebo, *Pygeum africanum* provided a moderately large improvement in urinary symptoms and

1. Wilt T et al. Cochrane Database Syst Rev 2002;(1):CD001044

measurements of urinary flow. Those using *Pygeum africanum* were more than twice as likely to report an improvement in overall symptoms, with night time voiding reduced by 19 per cent, the amount of urine left in the bladder after voiding (residual volume) reduced by 24 per cent and peak urine flow increased by 23 per cent. The reviewers concluded that *Pygeum africanum* may be a useful treatment option for men with lower urinary symptoms due to BPH, although more studies are needed.

Some evidence suggests that *Pygeum africanum* extracts may inhibit the growth of prostate cancer cells.

Dose
50–200 mg a day.

Side effects that have been reported are generally mild and include nausea, constipation or diarrhoea. The Cochrane review found that the incidence of side effects was comparable to placebo.

Do not take, except under medical advice, if you have diabetes, alcohol dependence or liver disease.

Pygeum africanum is often used together with saw palmetto or stinging nettle extracts.

Pygeum africanum is not recommended for use in women.

Agnus castus
(Vitex agnus castus)

Agnus castus – also known as the chaste tree – is native to the Mediterranean and west Asia. Its fruits were traditionally used by monks to reduce sex drive and help them to remain celibate, hence its name. Among women, it is traditionally used to treat a number of gynaecological conditions, including lack of periods, painful periods, premenstrual syndrome, infertility, lactation problems and menopausal symptoms.

Agnus castus contains a number of substances (diterpenes and clerodadienols) that bind to dopamine receptors in the brain. In low doses, it increases secretion of prolactin hormone from the pituitary gland, which accounts for its traditional use as a celibacy aid. In high doses, however, agnus castus suppresses prolactin hormone secretion (by blocking the receptors) to produce the opposite effect. In a group of 20 healthy males, for example, a dose of 120 mg agnus castus increased prolactin levels by 16 per cent, but at a dose of 480 mg, prolactin levels fell by around 10 per cent.

Other substances present within agnus castus, such as apigenin, have been shown to stimulate oestrogen receptors.

Prolactin hormone lowers sex drive, stimulates production of breast milk and reduces the metabolism of body fat. It is also believed to play a role in premenstrual syndrome (PMS). Levels of prolactin are naturally raised during breast-feeding, stress, and in the presence of a prolactinoma (benign tumour consisting of prolactin-secreting cells).

Research

PMS: There is good evidence that agnus castus fruit extracts can improve the symptoms of premenstrual syndrome and cyclical breast pain. A study involving 170 women with PMS showed that agnus castus fruit extracts improved symptoms by 52 per cent, compared with the same improvement in just 24 per cent of those taking a placebo[1]. The greatest improvement was seen in the reduction of irritability, mood alteration, anger, headache and breast fullness. Other studies have found agnus castus to be effective in relieving physical symptoms such as headaches, sore breasts, bloating and fatigue as well as increased appetite, sweet cravings, nervousness/restlessness, anxiety, depression, mood swings and lack of concentration.

Infertility: Agnus castus has also been used to increase fertility where difficulty in conceiving is linked with low progesterone levels during the second (luteal) phase of the menstrual cycle (from ovulation to the onset of menstruation). In a study involving 67 women with infertility linked with infrequent or absent periods, some took agnus castus for three months, and some took inactive placebo. Spontaneous menstruation, improved progesterone levels in the luteal phase, ovulation and pregnancy were achieved more often in women taking agnus castus (85 per cent) than on placebo (45 per cent)[2]. During the therapy and for six months after, the baby

1. Schellenberg R. BMJ 2001;322(7279):134–7
2. Bergmann J et al. Forsch Komplementarmed Klass Naturheilkd 2000;7(4):190–9

take-home rate was 18.7 per cent for those taking agnus castus and 6.4 per cent for those on placebo although this was not statistically significant. Agnus castus should only be used to treat infertility under medical supervision, however, and is usually stopped as soon as pregnancy is suspected. The safety of agnus castus during pregnancy has not been confirmed.

Breast-feeding: Traditionally agnus castus has been used to promote breast milk flow, even though it reduces levels of the milk-stimulating hormone, prolactin. This is because, although prolactin stimulates the initial production of breast milk after childbirth, levels naturally return to normal pre-pregnancy levels within eight days of delivery. While continued suckling maintains levels at first, they do still decline, so that by three months after the birth, milk secretion in breast-feeding mothers continues despite prolactin levels being within the normal range. Some studies suggest that agnus castus extracts increase milk flow and ease of milk release but results are conflicting. Effects take several weeks to develop and it should only be used under medical supervision if you are breast-feeding.

Agnus castus berries are often used to help improve symptoms of PCOS (polycystic ovary syndrome) but so far there has been little research into their effectiveness, and their use is based on anecdotal and traditional evidence.

Dose
Tablets: 20–600 mg or more a day.

Select products standardized for their agnuside or casticin content.

Agnus castus is slow acting. It takes an average of 25 days for symptoms to start improving and up to six months to achieve its full effects.

Reported side effects are mild, the most common including nausea, headache, gastrointestinal disturbances, menstrual disorders, acne, itching and skin rash. Excess agnus castus may cause a crawling sensation on the skin (like ants) known as formication.

Contraindications
Agnus castus is not recommended during pregnancy or breast-feeding, except under medical supervision. It should not be taken at

the same time as other hormone treatments, such as HRT and hormonal methods of contraception.

As agnus castus is thought to have an anti-androgen effect in men, it is not recommended for use in males, although traditionally it has been given to treat male impotence, premature ejaculation, prostatitis and lack of sexual sensations.

Aloe vera

Native to Africa, aloe vera is a succulent plant with lance shaped, fleshy leaves. There are over 200 different species, of which only three or four are used medicinally, the most useful being Aloe vera Barbadensis. From its fleshy leaves a gel containing a unique mix of vitamins, amino acids, enzymes and minerals may be squeezed, valued for its healing properties for over 6,000 years.

Aloe vera juice can be made from fresh liquid extract (gel) or from powdered aloe. The fresh gel has to be stabilized within hours of harvesting to prevent oxidation and inactivation.

Aloe vera may be taken internally or used externally. The juice contains vitamins, minerals and 20 amino acids (including seven essential amino acids) so it has excellent nutritional properties. The gel also contains substances that:

- Have useful anti-inflammatory and anti-itching properties (anthraquinones and natural plant steroids)
- Hasten wound healing (fibroblast growth factor)
- Are powerful antioxidants (vitamins C, E, carotenoids)
- Are cleansing and antiseptic with certain antibacterial, anti-viral and anti-fungal properties (saponins and anthraquinones)
- Are soothing and analgesic (salicylic acid, bradykinase and the anthraquinones aloin and emodin).

Research
Internal use
Aloe vera juice appears to boost immunity, and is helpful for people with chronic fatigue syndrome and rheumatoid arthritis. It is also used for a variety of intestinal problems, including indigestion, constipation, irritable bowel syndrome (IBS), diverticulosis and for

inflammatory conditions such as ulcerative colitis and Crohn's disease. Little research is available to confirm its effectiveness in treating IBS but there is preliminary evidence of a benefit in treating ulcerative colitis.

Some aloe vera products contain the bitter aloe 'latex' extracted from the inner yellow leaves of the plant. This can cause a brisk, laxative response due to the presence of chemicals known as anthraquinones (e.g. aloin which has a bitter taste). These stimulate contraction of smooth muscle fibres lining the bowel and it usually works within 8–12 hours.

Some evidence suggests that aloe vera can improve glucose control in people with Type 2 diabetes and may contain a blood glucose lowering agent whose identity and mode of action is currently uncertain. An analysis of ten controlled clinical trials involving people with Type 2 diabetes suggests that it can produce significant reductions in glucose and triglyceride levels[1].

External use

Aloe vera gel is used to help treat a number of skin conditions, including sunburn, cracked or sore lips, cold sores, eczema, psoriasis, rosacea, acne, shingles, ulcers, burns, scars, rashes, bites and stings. It may even interfere with the formation of age spots and help those that are already present to fade. As it stimulates dilation of blood capillaries, it improves local circulation, reaches the site of inflammation more quickly and stimulates tissue regeneration when wounds are shallow. By coating the skin in a moisture-rich film, it also prevents damaged skin from drying out.

Lichen planus is a long-term inflammatory disease affecting mucus membranes such as those in the mouth and around the genitals. Applying aloe vera gel has been shown to improve symptoms by at least 50 per cent (a good response) in two out of three people with oral lichen planus, and in women with vulval lichen planus. Burning pain disappeared in one in three people treated, and complete remission occurred in a 7 per cent – significantly better than with placebo.

A double-blind study of 60 adults with psoriasis found that a cream containing aloe vera gel (surprisingly, just 0.5 per cent,

1. Vogler BK, Ernst E. Br J Gen Pract. 1999;49(447):823–8

although 100 per cent gel could be used) applied three times a day healed over 80 per cent of plaques within four weeks as compared with only 8 per cent using a placebo[1].

It is helpful for treating gum disease (gingivitis and periodontitis) when applied as a dental paste, and some dentists use it to help flush mercury from the body during planned mercury amalgam removal. Research involving people with inflamed, bleeding gums (gingivitis) shows that brushing teeth with a dental aloe vera product three times a day is as effective in reducing plaque and gingivitis as a fluoridated toothpaste.

In a laboratory study, human skin cells involved in wound healing (fibroblasts) were obtained from people with Type 2 diabetes and normal controls and cultured with or without aloe vera extracts. Aloe vera extracts were found to increase communication between cells, and to increase the proliferation of cells derived from people with diabetes. The researchers suggest that aloe vera may improve wound healing in people with diabetes[2].

NB: Aloe vera gel should not be applied to infected or deep (e.g. surgical) wounds as some evidence suggests it may increase the time taken for wounds to heal.

Dose

If taking the aloe latex for its laxative effect, start with a small dose of gel (e.g. 1 teaspoon) and work up to around 1–2 tablespoons per day to find the dose that suits you best.

Aloe vera juice may be taken more liberally (e.g. 50–100 ml, three times daily).

When selecting a product, aim for one made from 100 per cent pure aloe vera. Its strength needs to be at least 40 per cent by volume to be effective and should ideally approach 95–100 per cent. You may find it more palatable to choose a product containing a little natural fruit juice (e.g. grape, apple) to improve the flavour.

Side effects

Many products claim to be aloin- and emodin-free, which means they should not produce a laxative effect. However, independent laboratory tests on leading brands in the USA found high levels of

1. Syed TA et al. Trop Med Int Health 1996;1(4):505–9
2. Abdullah KM et al. J Altern Complement Med 2003;9(5):711–8

aloin in juices claimed to be aloin-free. If you do not want the laxative effect, select a product that is stamped with an IASC-certified seal (from the International Aloe Science Council); this shows that it has been produced according to recommended guidelines.

Some women using aloe vera notice that it increases their menstrual flow, but no serious side effects have been reported at standard doses. Some people develop a mild itching rash due to allergy when applying aloe vera gel on the skin; if this occurs, then discontinue treatment.

A few cases of liver inflammation (hepatitis) have been reported in people taking aloe vera products, including an aloe vera leaf tea.

Contraindications

Do not take aloe vera by mouth during pregnancy, as the anthraquinones it may contain can stimulate uterine contractions which could result in miscarriage.

Do not use aloe vera when breast-feeding. If aloin enters breast milk it can trigger stomach cramps and diarrhoea in infants.

Alpha-lipoic acid

Alpha-lipoic acid (ALA – also known as thioctic acid) is a vitamin-like substance that is made in the body in small amounts. It is also obtained from the diet in foods such as carrots, yams, sweet potatoes, beets and red meat. ALA acts as a co-enzyme with B group vitamins to speed up certain metabolic reactions needed for energy production in cells. This has the potential to improve cell function within the nervous system and in important organs such as the pancreas and kidneys. ALA is also a powerful antioxidant that helps to regenerate other important antioxidants such as vitamins C and E, enhancing their effectiveness.

Research

Diabetic neuropathy: Alpha-lipoic acid is used to improve nerve function in people with diabetic neuropathy, who experience symptoms of tingling, numbness, burning and pain. ALA appears to reduce oxidation of the fatty myelin sheath surrounding nerve fibres, which is vital for transmission of nerve signals. Studies suggest that high dose ALA can improve symptoms of diabetic neuropathy by 47 per cent – twice the reduction seen in those taking inactive placebo (24 per cent)[1]. No significant adverse reactions have been reported.

Dementia: The protective effect of ALA on nerve sheaths may also be helpful for people with dementia. Some evidence suggests that it may slow the progression of symptoms in people with mild rather than moderate Alzheimer's disease, and needs further investigation.

Glucose control: By improving cell function, ALA also seems to improve the body's use of insulin and to improve diabetic control. This is partly through its ability to increase insulin sensitivity and assist removal of glucose from the circulation. It has been shown to boost uptake of glucose into skeletal muscle cells by as much as 50 per cent[2]. This, in turn, may reduce glucose uptake by fat cells to reduce weight gain in people with Type 2 diabetes, although this requires further investigation. ALA should only be taken by people with diabetes under medical supervision as blood glucose levels may need frequent monitoring, and the dosage of anti-diabetic drugs adjusted, to prevent hypoglycaemia.

Diabetic kidney disease: Oxidative stress plays a major part in the development of kidney damage in people with diabetes. Research suggests that, as an antioxidant, ALA can reduce oxidative stress and urinary albumin protein excretion – an important indicator of kidney damage. In a trial involving 84 people with either Type 1 or Type 2 diabetes, those who took 600 mg ALA per day had no significant deterioration in kidney function or urinary albumin concentration, compared with those taking placebo in whom significant deterioration was found. This suggests that taking ALA may help to preserve kidney function[3].

Alpha-lipoic acid also improves liver cell function, and has been used to help treat hepatitis, cirrhosis and other liver diseases

1. Ruhnau KJ et al. Diabet Med. 1999; 16(12):1040–3
2. Jacob S et al. Arzneimittel-Forschung 1995; 45: 872–4
3. Morcos M et al. Diabetes Res Clin Pract. 2001; 52(3):175-83

including toxic damage, e.g. due to mushroom poisoning. It is also used to boost energy levels, and may be helpful for people with chronic fatigue.

Dose
As an antioxidant, alpha-lipoic acid is usually taken in doses of 50–100 mg a day. In clinical trials, high doses of 200–600 mg, three times a day, have been used for therapeutic effects, under medical supervision.

Side effects
Mild skin rashes or gastrointestinal side effects have occurred, but are rare.

Seek advice before taking ALA if you have heart, liver or kidney problems.

Monitor blood glucose levels carefully when taking it as it can stimulate uptake of glucose into muscle cells to improve glucose control. This is good news, but you need to know how to adjust your anti-diabetes medication accordingly to avoid a hypoglycaemic episode.

Amino acids

Amino acids are the basic building blocks that are linked together within cells to make proteins. Chains containing between two and ten amino acids are known as peptides; those with 10–100 amino acids are called polypeptides, while chains of over 100 amino acids, which fold into complex three-dimensional shapes, are referred to as proteins.

How does the body use proteins?
Over 50 per cent of the body's dry weight is made up of protein. Some proteins play a structural role (e.g. collagen), some regulate metabolic reactions (enzymes) while others are vital for immune defences (antibodies).

Body proteins are constantly being broken down and re-formed – mostly during sleep under the control of growth hormone. Every day, around 80–100 g protein in your body is broken down and replaced. Most muscle protein is renewed every six months – 98 per cent of the body's proteins are renewed within one year.

The breakdown of protein releases its constituent amino acids, which are metabolized in the liver to produce a poisonous by-product, ammonia. This is detoxified by converting it into urea and releasing it into the circulation, where it is transported to the kidneys for excretion in urine.

There are 21 amino acids that are important for human health. Your cells can make 12 of these from other materials, but the remaining nine must come from your diet and are known as the nutritionally essential amino acids.

The Essential Amino Acids	The Amino Acids you can make
Histidine	Alanine
Isoleucine	Arginine
Leucine	Asparagine
Lysine	Aspartate
Methionine	Cysteine
Phenylalanine	Glutamate
Threonine	Glutamine
Tryptophan	Glycine
Valine	Proline
	Selenocysteine
	Serine
	Tyrosine

Protein in the diet

Dietary protein can be divided into two groups: first-class proteins, which contain significant quantities of all the essential amino acids (e.g. animal meat, fish, eggs, dairy products) and second-class proteins, which contain some essential amino acids but not all (e.g. vegetables, rice, beans, nuts).

Second-class proteins need to be mixed and matched by eating as wide a variety of foods as possible. For example, the essential amino acid missing from haricot beans is found in bread. Hence, combining cereals with pulses or seeds and nuts provides a balanced amino acid intake. Vegetarians can also obtain a balanced protein intake by eating a combination of five parts rice to one part beans.

When digested, dietary proteins are broken down to release their amino acid building blocks. This process starts in the stomach, where an enzyme (pepsin) divides the bonds between certain amino acid chains to form short peptide chains. Once in the small intestine, these are further attacked by enzymes released from the intestinal wall and pancreas. Chains of double and triple amino acids are absorbed into cells lining the gut and cleaved to release single amino acids into the bloodstream. These are then used as building blocks to make over 50,000 different proteins and polypeptides needed by the human body.

Dose
You need a daily intake of around 1 g per 1 kg of body weight, so someone weighing 70 kg needs around 70 g protein per day in their diet. This represents about 15 per cent of daily energy intake. Those taking part in competitive sports will need more than this. For example, an athlete training for two hours a day needs to obtain 1.1–1.4 g protein per kilogram of body weight per day, depending on the intensity of exercise. Weight-lifters in training may need as much as 2–3.5 g protein per kilogram of body weight a day.

Most people obtain more than enough protein in their diet. Protein supplements are available for athletes as intact proteins, partially digested (hydrolysed) peptides or free amino acids. Some research suggests that the hydrolysates (dipeptides and tripeptides) may be the best options for bulking up muscle as they are most readily absorbed and utilized in the body.

Amino acid supplements are absorbed most effectively if taken between meals (two hours before or after eating). If using an individual amino acid for more than two weeks, it is best taken with a mixed amino acid complex to guard against amino acid imbalances. Individual amino acid supplements should not normally be taken for more than 12 weeks except under medical supervision.

Anthocyanins

Anthocyanins (from the Greek: anthos = flower, kyáneos = purple) are the most abundant flavonoids in fruits and vegetables. They are water-soluble pigments with a red, blue or purple colour depending on the level of acidity – they are often used as pH indicators (red = acid, blue = alkali). They act as a plant 'sunscreen' by absorbing blue-green and UV light.

Anthocyanins are present in blue-red fruit and vegetables, e.g. blueberries, cranberries, bilberries, raspberries, blackberries, black-currants, black cherries, black grapes, acai berries, blood oranges, figs, beetroot, red cabbage, black soybeans and aubergines. They are also responsible for the red coloration of autumn leaves.

Anthocyanins are produced in low amounts in other fruit and vegetables such as bananas, fennel, potatoes and red tomatoes. Recently, a genetically modified purple tomato was developed, which had two Snapdragon genes inserted. These switched on the natural tomato gene that regulates synthesis of tomato anthocyanins to super-boost their production. The purple colour is therefore 'natural' to the tomato plant and not, for example, due to a flower pigment that is not normally present in tomatoes.

There are over 550 different anthocyanins. These can be divided into sugar-free anthocyanidin aglycones and anthocyanin glycosides. Colourless precursors are known as proanthocyanidins and are found, for example, in grapeseed extracts.

Anthocyanins are considered secondary metabolites and allowed as a food additive with E-number 163. The daily intake of anthocyanins in Western populations is estimated at about 200 mg.

Research
Laboratory evidence suggests they have the following potential health benefits:

- Antioxidant to protect against premature ageing and cancer
- Improve circulation and protect against heart disease
  - Decrease blood pressure
  - Increase HDL-cholesterol
  - Reduce blood stickiness
- Increase insulin sensitivity to protect against diabetes
- Antimicrobial
  - Viruses
  - Bacteria
  - Yeasts

- Improve eye health, protecting against retinopathy and cataracts
- Anti-inflammatory by reducing production of cytokines such as TNF-alpha.

They appear to work by 'switching off' genes involved in abnormal cell proliferation, cell death (apoptosis) and growth of abnormal blood vessels (angiogenesis) – for example into tumours and the retinae.

Different plants contain different anthocyanins (e.g. cyanidin, delphinidin, malvidin, pelargonidin, peonidin, petunidin, myrtilin) so research relating to one source (e.g. blackcurrant anthocyanins) is not automatically applicable to another source (bilberry anthocyanins or, indeed, purple tomatoes).

Lifespan: Cancer-prone mice fed a diet supplemented with high-anthocyanin (purple) tomato powder showed a significant extension of life span (182 days versus 142 days)[1].

Eyes: Bilberry extract is used to treat several eye disorders including macular degeneration, cataracts, night-blindness, glaucoma, retinitis pigmentosa and diabetic retinopathy. Its effectiveness in treating visual problems results from a number of actions. Its anthocyanin blue-red pigments protect the membranes of light sensitive and other cells in the eyes, reduce hardening and furring up of blood vessels, stabilize tear production, increase blood flow to the retina, regenerate the light sensitive pigment, rhodopsin, as well as increasing the strength of collagen fibres in capillaries and supportive connective tissues. Those with diabetic retinopathy, in which haemorrhages form within the retina of the eye, especially benefit from these actions.

The antioxidant effects of bilberries may help to prevent the development and progression of cataracts, especially when combined with vitamin E. In one study of 50 patients with age-related cataracts, bilberry extract plus vitamin E stopped cataracts progressing in 97 per cent of cases[2]. In another study, 40 patients (all but three of whom had diabetic retinopathy) took 160 mg bilberry extracts or placebo twice a day for one month[3]. Those taking placebo

1. Butelli E et al. Nat Biotechnol. 2008 26(11):1301–8
2. Bravetti G. nn Ottalmol Clin Ocul 1989;115:109
3. Perossini M et al. Ann Ottalmol Clin Ocul 1987;113:1173

then crossed over to take bilberry for one month. While taking bilberry extracts, 79 per cent with visible retinal abnormalities on ophthalmologic examination showed improvement compared with no improvements when taking placebo. Similar results were found in a similar trial involving 31 people, of whom 20 had diabetic retinopathy[1]. Some researchers suggest that taking bilberry extracts can reduce short-sightedness after five months of regular use, perhaps by improving the reactivity and focusing ability of the eye lens.

Circulation: Bilberry extracts strengthen blood vessels and the collagen-containing connective tissue that supports them. These actions are used to treat easy bruising syndrome, thread veins (telangiectasis), varicose veins and haemorrhoids. In one study of almost 50 people with varicose veins, the taking of 480 mg bilberry extracts per day increased local circulation to reduce fluid retention, feelings of heaviness, pins and needles, pain, and improved the appearance of overlying skin. In addition, bilberry reduces the risk of stroke and inhibits unwanted clot formation. Because of its beneficial effects on the circulation, bilberry extract is prescribed in some parts of Europe for patients due to undergo surgery as it has been shown to reduce excessive bleeding by over 70 per cent. Anthocyanins from black chokeberry lowered blood pressure and cholesterol and triglycerides in 22 healthy people and 25 with metabolic syndrome[2].

Gout: The anthocyanins found in dark blue-red pigmented fruits (e.g. bilberries, cherries, grapes, blueberries) can lower uric acid levels and prevent gout attacks.

Antioxidants

Antioxidants are protective substances that help to neutralize damaging oxidation reactions in the body. These reactions are triggered by chemicals known as free radicals.

A free radical is a molecular fragment that carries a minute,

1. Scharrer A, Ober M. Kiln Monatsbl Augenheikld Beih 1981;178:386–9
2. Broncel M et al. Pol Merkur Lekarski 2007 23(134):116–9

negative electrical charge in the form of a spare electron. This charge makes it highly unstable, so it naturally tries to lose the charge by passing on its spare electron during collisions with other molecules and cell structures. This process is known chemically as an oxidation reaction. Oxidation automatically produces another unstable free radical from the molecule that takes the negatively-charged electron on board and this, in turn, needs to pass on the charge. As a result, oxidation usually triggers chain reactions in which electrons are rapidly passed from one molecule to another with damaging results. Body proteins, fats, cell membranes and genetic material (DNA) are constantly under attack from free radicals, with each cell undergoing an estimated 10,000 free radical oxidations per day.

When genetic material is damaged, mutations can occur and this is thought to be the main mechanism that triggers cancer. Oxidation of harmful LDL-cholesterol in the circulation creates changes that cause scavenger cells (macrophages) to recognize the fat as foreign. These cells try to remove the oxidized fat by engulfing it, and quickly become over-laden to form bloated 'foam' cells. These leave the circulation by squeezing between cells lining the artery wall where they become trapped and accumulate to form fatty plaques known as atheroma. Lack of antioxidants is now thought by many researchers to be an underlying cause of hardening and furring up of the arteries (atherosclerosis).

Free radical damage has been linked with a number of conditions, including:

- Coronary heart disease and stroke
- Deteriorating vision due to cataracts and macular degeneration
- Premature ageing of the skin
- Chronic inflammatory diseases such as arthritis
- Alzheimer's disease
- Parkinson's disease
- Impaired immunity
- Poor sperm count and quality
- Congenital birth defects
- Cancer.

Free radicals are continuously produced in the body as a result of:

- Normal and abnormal metabolic reactions
- Muscle contraction during exercise
- Smoking cigarettes
- Drinking excessive amounts of alcohol
- Exposure to environmental pollutants
- Exposure to X-rays
- Exposure to UVA sunlight, especially if sunburned
- Taking some drugs – especially antibiotics or paracetamol.

The generation of a certain number of free radicals is unavoidable, and even desirable as they are involved in some important reactions, including fighting infections. Antioxidant protection against excessive free radical attack does appear to provide health benefits, however. This is especially true for people with diabetes, who are exposed to significantly increased levels of oxidative stress due to oxidation reactions involving glucose.

Antioxidants are our main defence against excessive free radical attack and work by quickly neutralizing free radicals before they can damage our cells. Several essential vitamins and minerals act as antioxidants. Of these, the most important are vitamins A, C, E and selenium.

Fruit, vegetables and nuts are the main dietary source of antioxidants, and the evidence supporting their consumption is overwhelming. In addition to antioxidant vitamins and minerals, they contain thousands of other substances with powerful antioxidant actions, including carotenoids (see page 86), isoflavones (see page 197), tannins, lignans and flavonoids such as catechins (found in green tea) and anthocyanins (see page 38). These antioxidants have a beneficial effect on cholesterol balance, blood pressure, glucose control and circulatory health. Polyphenols in red wine, blueberries and green tea, for example, have an effect on nitric oxide, a chemical released in blood vessel linings which promotes blood vessel dilation.

People with the highest intake of fruit and vegetables have the lowest blood pressure, lowest total and LDL-cholesterol levels, and the lowest risk of developing diabetes, coronary heart disease and stroke. Research involving over 126,000 people, for example, shows that, even after taking other heart disease risk factors into account, those with the highest intake of fruit and vegetables were 20 per cent less likely to experience a heart attack over the next ten years compared with those eating the least. Each additional serving of fruit or vegetables eaten per day reduces the risk of coronary heart disease by 4 per cent[1]. Green leafy vegetables appeared to be the most beneficial, closely followed by vitamin C-rich fruits such as citrus, berries and capsicum bell peppers. A meta-analysis of seven studies involving almost a quarter of a million people showed that the risk of a stroke fell by 11 per cent for each portion of fruit eaten per day, and by 3 per cent for each portion of vegetables[2].

> Aim to eat at least five, and preferably 8–10, servings of different fruit and vegetables per day. Eating fruit and vegetables raw (where appropriate) or only lightly steamed provides the greatest nutritional benefit.

The ORAC score

The antioxidant potential of fruit and vegetables is assessed by measuring their ORAC (Oxygen Radical Absorbance Capacity) score. Researchers have estimated that the average person following a Western diet obtains around 5,700 ORAC units per day. Ideally, you need at least 7,000 ORAC units for health and the optimum level to aim for is 20,000 ORAC units per day, or more.

The following table shows which fruit and vegetables have the highest ORAC score to help maximum your antioxidant intake. Interestingly, dark chocolate (at least 70 per cent cocoa solids) which is obtained from the cocoa bean contains the highest level of antioxidants found in any common food item.

Fruit/Vegetable	ORAC score* per 100 g
Acai pulp/skin powder	161,400
Dark chocolate	103,971
Goji berries	25,300
Pecan nuts	17,940
Red kidney beans	14,413
Walnuts	13,541
Pinto beans	12,359
Pomegranate	10,500
Red lentils	9,766

1. Joshipura KJ et al. Ann Intern Med 2001; 134:1106–1114
2. Dauchet L et al. Neurology 2005;65(8):E17–8

Hazelnuts	9,645
Cranberries	9,456
Blueberries	9,260
Prunes	8,578
Black beans	8,040
Pistachios	7,983
Black plums	7,339
Globe artichoke	6,552
Red plums	6,239
Blackberries	5,348
Raspberries	4,925
Almonds	4,454
Red Delicious apple	4,275
Green peas	4,039
Chickpeas (garbanzo)	4,030
Dates	3,895
Strawberries	3,577
Figs	3,383
Cherries	3,361
Peanuts	3,166
Red cabbage	3,146
Raisins	3,037
Gala apple	2,828
Beetroot	2,774
Golden Delicious apple	2,670
Spinach	2,640
Aubergine (eggplant)	2,533
Lemons/Limes	2,412
Avocado	1,933
Pears (green varieties)	1,911
Oranges (navel)	1,814
Peaches	1,863
Red leaf lettuce	1,785
Pears (Red Anjou)	1,773
Macadamias	1,695
Tangerines	1,620
Russet potatoes (cooked)	1,555
Red grapefruit	1,548
Green cabbage	1,359

Red potatoes (cooked)	1,326
Red grapes	1,260
Broccoli (cooked)	1,259
Onions (yellow)	1,220
Carrots (raw)	1,215
Green grapes	1,118
Mangoes	1,002
Kiwi	918
Cauliflower	647
Iceberg lettuce	451
Tomatoes	337
Watermelon	142
Cucumber	115

*Derived from Wu X et al. J Agric Food Chem 2004;52:4026–4037

If you select five average servings made up of: blueberries, plums, red kidney beans, spinach and red peppers you can rack up an astonishing 33,000 ORAC units in a single day. On the other hand, if your five servings comprise a kiwi, slice of watermelon, a mixed salad, cauliflower and carrots you would obtain less than 2,000 ORAC units – even though you have achieved the recommended five servings a day.

By balancing your intake of foods with high, medium and low ORAC scores you can maximum the antioxidant potential of your diet on a daily basis. The higher a fruit or vegetable's ORAC score, the higher its ability to neutralize free radicals – the molecular fragments that damage cells through a chemical process known as oxidation.

As well as supplying antioxidants, fruit and vegetables provide other important phytochemicals and nutrients, including vitamins, minerals, trace elements and fibre. Because of this, the majority of the five to ten servings of fruit and vegetables you eat per day (e.g. three out of five, or seven out of ten) should ideally be in the form of vegetables rather than fruit, even though vegetables tend to have a lower ORAC score. This is because vegetables tend to contain less water (so are a more concentrated source of nutrients) and less sugar as well as more fibre.

Supplements

Antioxidant supplements are among the most popular types of supplement available. Those containing extracts of fruit and vegetables are most 'natural' and supply a known ORAC score. They tend to contain extracts from high ORAC plants such as cranberry, bilberry, raspberry, plum, wild cherry, spinach, tea and other dark green leaves.

Individual antioxidant supplements are also available, including alpha-lipoic acid, pine bark extracts (Pycnogenol®), co-enzyme Q10, carotenoids such as lutein and lycopene, cat's claw, bilberry, ginkgo, glutathione, grapeseed extracts, green tea, reishi, all of which have their own entries. See also vitamins A, C, E and mineral selenium.

The evidence supporting the use of antioxidant supplements is contradictory. Some studies have even found an increased risk of lung cancer in long-term smokers taking vitamin E and betacarotene supplements. However, in order for antioxidants to have a beneficial effect, they need to be consumed on a regular basis over many years. Taking them for a short period of time after having smoked for many years is unlikely to reverse the damage that has already occurred. In addition, these trials did not include vitamin C which is important to regenerate vitamin E which becomes a free radical itself after performing its antioxidant function. These studies underline the importance of taking a blend of antioxidants – preferably natural ones present in fruit and vegetables – rather than using certain antioxidants in isolation.

Arginine

L-arginine is an amino acid that can be synthesized in the body but may become essential for adults under stress or for those who are recovering from injury or surgery. It must then come from the diet, and can be found in many protein foods such as nuts, seeds, pulses, beetroot, onions, grapes, rice, egg yolk and red meat. Lack of arginine has been linked with poor wound healing, hair loss, rashes, constipation and fatty liver changes.

L-arginine plays an important role in the metabolism of dietary protein and the formation of urea in the liver. It is also used to produce nitric oxide (NO), which is essential for blood vessel dilation. NO is involved in a number of physiological processes, including the regulation of blood pressure, circulatory tone and normal erectile function in males. It is involved in the production of insulin, glucagon growth hormone and antidiuretic hormone (vasopressin). It also plays a role in collagen synthesis and wound healing and is therefore needed during recovery from surgery, injuries and burns. Arginine is used to make creatine phosphate – a substance well known to sports people who take creatine as an energy-inducing supplement to boost muscle strength, especially during weight-lifting.

Research

Heart failure: L-arginine may improve congestive heart failure by promoting blood vessel dilation, increasing arterial blood flow, prolonging exercise duration and increasing the distance that can be walked[1,2,3]. It is also used to reduce an abnormally raised cholesterol level, hardening and furring up of the arteries (atherosclerosis), coronary heart disease and angina. In one study, people with angina who took L-arginine three times a day increased the amount of exercise they could take at moderate intensity without having to stop because of chest pain.

Blood pressure: By promoting blood vessel dilation, L-arginine can lower blood pressure. In those with borderline hypertension, reductions of 11/4.9 mmHg have been recorded, together with a 23 per cent improvement in arterial compliance (elasticity)[4]. In those with normal blood pressure, non-significant changes occurred.

Erectile dysfunction: Some researchers believe that L-arginine is one of the best all-round prosexual supplements for men. By boosting blood flow to the penis, it improves erectile function. A few small trials have found that significantly more men reported improvement in erectile difficulties when taking L-arginine

1. Bednarz B et al. Kardiol Pol 2004;60(4):348–53
2. Rector TS et al. Circulation 1996;93(12):2135–41
3. Hambrecht R et al. J Am Coll Cardiol 2000;35(3):706–13
4. Miller AL. Altern Med Rev 2006;11(1):23–9

compared with placebo. It is often combined with Pycnogenol® (pine bark extracts) for a synergistic effect[1].

Sperm health: The protein in seminal fluids consists of as much as 25 per cent arginine which helps to improve the quality and motility of sperm. Sperm count can sometimes be increased in men with an unexplained low sperm count by taking L-arginine supplements.

Dose

2–3 g, one to three times daily. When taken for its beneficial sexual actions, it should ideally be taken one hour before sex.

Doses of above 20 g daily are not recommended.

It can take between two and six weeks for L-arginine to achieve its optimum effect.

Side effects

Side effects are uncommon, but high doses may lead to diarrhoea. Reversible thickening and coarsening of the skin has been reported with long-term use.

Some evidence has suggested that L-arginine helps replication of herpes viruses and may stimulate a recurrence of *Herpes simplex* infections (cold sores) although this is not proven.

Contraindications

Do not take L-arginine if :

- You are pregnant or breast-feeding.
- Have diabetes (may increase blood glucose levels).
- Have reduced kidney or liver function.
- Have an auto-immune condition (e.g. rheumatoid arthritis, glomerulonephritis) except under medical supervision (studies in rats have suggested that a low-arginine diet is more beneficial for immune function in these cases).
- Have schizophrenia (may make symptoms worse).

1. Stanislavov R et al. In J Impot Res 2008;20(2):173–80

Artichoke

(Cynara scolymus)

Globe artichoke is a perennial herb native to the Mediterranean. Its leaves contain several unique substances such as cynarin, luteolin, cynardoside, scolymoside and chlorogenic acid. Although the fleshy flower is eaten as a delicacy, it is the leaves that contain the most active ingredients.

Globe artichoke is antioxidant and has similar liver regenerating properties to milk thistle. It is used to:

- Increase bile secretion and improve digestion of dietary fats
- Reduce blood cholesterol levels
- Protect liver cells from toxins – especially alcohol
- Improve digestive symptoms such as bloating, flatulence, nausea and abdominal pain related to poor fat digestion, hangover or irritable bowel syndrome
- Promote growth of probiotic bacteria in the bowel.

Artichoke extracts promote the secretion of bile. Bile is a yellow-green fluid which is made in the liver and stored in the gall bladder until needed. When food leaves the stomach and enters the first section of the small intestines (duodenum) this triggers a reflex contraction of the gall bladder which squirts bile into the duodenum where it mixes with food. Bile contains salts and acids that break down fat globules into smaller particles (emulsification) so they can be absorbed and processed more easily.

Artichoke supplements can improve symptoms related to dyspepsia, irritable bowel syndrome (IBS) and hangover, such as bloating, abdominal pain, nausea, vomiting, constipation and fat intolerance. Much of this benefit is related to improved bile secretion. Artichoke also contains inulin, a prebiotic fibre that stimulates growth of 'friendly' probiotic bacteria in the bowel.

Research

Liver function: A randomized, placebo-controlled trial involving 20 men with acute or chronic digestive symptoms found that 320 mg artichoke extracts increased bile secretion by over 127 per cent after 30 minutes, 151 per cent after 60 minutes and by 94 per cent after

90 minutes[1]. Artichoke has also been shown to reduce fatty infiltration of the liver and to reduce cholesterol synthesis.

Irritable Bowel Syndrome: Over 550 people with dyspepsia and 279 with irritable bowel syndrome took 640 mg artichoke leaf extracts three times a day with meals. Symptoms of abdominal pain, bloating, flatulence, abdominal pain and constipation significantly improved over a six week period. Good benefits were noticed within ten days and 84 per cent of patients and physicians rated the overall effect as good or excellent[2].

Cholesterol: Increasing evidence suggests that, by improving bile flow, artichoke extracts can lower 'bad' LDL-cholesterol levels and triglyceride levels while raising 'good' HDL-cholesterol. This effect is due to cynaroside and luteolin blocking synthesis of excess cholesterol in the liver. Studies suggest that taking artichoke extract for six to 12 weeks can lower total cholesterol levels by between 4.2 per cent[3] and 18.5 per cent[4].

Dose
Extracts: 320–1,800 mg daily, with food.

Side effects
Usually well tolerated. Side effects of hunger and transient increase in flatulence have been reported. Rarely, allergic reactions may occur.

Contraindications
Do not use globe artichoke if there is obstruction of bile ducts or jaundice.

In case of gallstones, use only after consulting a physician.

1. Kirchoff R et al. Phytomed 1994;1:107
2. Walker AF et al. Phytother Res 2001; 15:58–61
3. Bundy R et al. Phytomed 2008;15(9):668–75
4. Englisch W et al. Arzneimittelforschung 2000;50(3):260–5

Ashwagandha
(Withania somnifera)

Ashwagandha – also known as winter cherry or Indian ginseng – is a small evergreen shrub native to India, the Mediterranean and the Middle East. Its dried root contains iron and a series of unique steroidal lactones known as withanolides.

Ashwagandha has antioxidant, anti-inflammatory, anti-fungal and antibiotic activity. It is used as a restorative tonic in Ayurvedic medicine to improve resistance to stress. It is a powerful adaptogen with effects similar to Korean ginseng and may improve mental acuity, reaction time and physical performance.

Studies suggest, for example, that ashwagandha can prevent the depletion of vitamin C and cortisol (an adrenal hormone) during times of stress, as well as preventing stress-related gastrointestinal ulcers. It reduces anxiety and promotes serenity and deep sleep, especially in those suffering from overwork or nervous exhaustion.

It is traditionally used as an aphrodisiac to improve libido (especially during convalescence) and is sometimes used to treat impotence.

It may also lower cholesterol and triglyceride levels, and improve glucose control.

Benefits
Immune function: Ashwagandha taken by mouth, twice daily for four days significantly increased activation of T lymphocytes and Natural Killer cells (which fight abnormal cells)[1].

Dose
Capsules standardized to contain 2–5 mg withanolides: 150–300 mg. Because ashwagandha is somewhat difficult to digest, it is often taken in powder form with ginger, warm milk, honey or hot water.

Side effects
Some reports suggest that high doses of ashwagandha can increase levels of thyroid hormones and may produce symptoms of thyrotoxicosis (overactive thyroid gland).

---

1. Mikolai J et al. J Altern Complement Med 2009;15(4):423–30

Astaxanthin

Astaxanthin is a pink-red carotenoid produced by some red yeasts and microalgae. When these microalgae are consumed by Antarctic krill, prawns, salmon, rainbow trout and crabs, it becomes concentrated in their flesh, roes or shells which acquire a pink colour. Crustaceans turn pink/red when cooked, for example, because astaxanthin is released from the proteins to which it is bound. Astaxanthin provides the pink feather colour of flamingos when present in their diet. It is also included in animal feeds to impart colour to farm-raised salmon, roe and to colour the yolk of hens' eggs.

Astaxanthin is produced by microalgae to provide protection against ultraviolet light. The highest concentrations are found in a tropical alga, *Haematococcus pluvialis,* which remains green until exposed to strong sunlight. It then rapidly produces astaxanthin and turns red. This is the source of most natural astaxanthin that is available commercially. Astaxanthin can also be produced synthetically.

Unlike some carotenoids, astaxanthin cannot be converted into vitamin A in the body. It does, however, have an antioxidant potential that is around ten times greater than most other carotenoids, such as betacarotene, and as much as 500 times greater than vitamin E.

Research

Cholesterol: A study involving 24 volunteers suggests that astaxanthin can inhibit oxidation of circulating LDL-cholesterol[1]. It may therefore provide some protection against the development of atherosclerosis, but this hypothesis needs to be confirmed in large trials.

A number of studies suggest that astaxanthin can protect human nerve and brain cell cultures from degenerative changes, but whether or not it has protective effects against neurodegenerative disease in the body is uncertain.

Dose
6 mg daily.

---

1. Iwamoto T et al. J Atheroscler Thromb 2000; 7(4):216-22

Astragalus
(Astragalus membranaceus)

Astragalus (also known as Chinese milkvetch) is a herbaceous perennial native to northern China, Japan, Korea and Tibet. Its root has been used as a traditional Chinese herbal tonic for over 2,000 years. The medicinal creamy-white root is harvested from plants that are four to seven years old and has a sweet taste, similar to liquorice, that is used as a thickening sweetener in cooking.

Astragalus is classed as an adaptogen, helping to support adrenal gland function during times of physical stress, to improve physical endurance as well as being an immune enhancer. It contains a variety of unique substances such as astragalosides, and unique isoflavones, that have a beneficial effect on immune function. It appears to increase proliferation of T-lymphocytes (cells that regulate immune responses), boost the activity of phagocytic (cell-eating) white blood cells, increase the activity of natural killer cells (which wipe out infected or abnormal body cells) and improve antibody synthesis. It also stimulates production of the powerful anti-viral substance interferon and has anti-viral as well as antibacterial and anti-fungal actions. It is widely used to improve recovery from respiratory infections (colds, flu, bronchitis, sinusitis) and urinary tract infections. It also has mild diuretic properties and can lower blood pressure.

As astragalus also increases production of red blood cells (to improve oxygen carriage in the circulation) it is used in the Ayurvedic treatment of anaemia. In people undergoing treatment for cancer, astragalus is sometimes used to improve tolerance to chemotherapy, protect adrenal gland function, reduce bone marrow suppression and to minimize any gastrointestinal side effects. It is also helpful in protecting against the free radicals generated during both chemotherapy and radiotherapy.

Other uses include stimulating sperm motility, improving healing of wounds and peptic ulcers and reducing excessive perspiration (including night sweats). It is also used for its protective actions in inflammation of the liver (e.g. chronic hepatitis) or kidneys (nephritis).

Benefits

Coronary heart disease: Astragalus has been used to reduce platelet aggregation, strengthen heart muscle contraction, correct abnormal cardiac electrical activity, dilate blood vessels and reduce angina pain. Early Chinese studies suggest it is as effective as a commonly prescribed drug (nifedipine). More research is needed to confirm this, however.

Diabetes: Astragalus is often recommended to people with diabetes to improve the effectiveness of medical therapy, and to reduce complications such as high blood pressure and poor wound healing. Some research suggests that it reduces insulin resistance and improves glucose tolerance[1].

Dose

For general use, 250–500 mg a day.

It is best used under the supervision of a medical herbalist. Astragalus is usually taken for two to three weeks and then alternated with another immune booster such as Echinacea or cat's claw. If taken for a respiratory or urinary infection, the dose is usually increased to four times a day.

Choose extracts that are standardized to 0.5 per cent glucosides and 70 per cent polysaccharides. It is often used together with Korean ginseng or Echinacea.

Side effects

The most common side effects are mild stomach upsets and allergic reactions.

Contraindications

- Traditionally, astragalus is best avoided if you have a fever or if you suffer from skin disorders.
- Avoid during pregnancy and breast-feeding except under specialist advice.

---

1. Mai XQ et al. Phytomedicine 2009;16(5):416–25

Bee products

The four main bee products used as health supplements are:

- Bee pollen
- Royal jelly
- Propolis
- Medicinal honey.

Bee pollen

Pollen is an ultra-fine dust made up of sex cells produced on the anthers of male flowers. When foraging for nectar, bees visit as many as 1,500 blossoms during their life. The collected pollen is compressed into granules – known as bee pollen – and transported back to the hive. Each granule contains as many as 5 million live pollen grains and is stored in honeycomb cells as 'beebread', to feed young, developing bees.

Bee pollen is rich in B-complex vitamins, essential fatty acids, and also contains 28 minerals, 22 amino acids and thousands of enzymes and co-enzymes. Bee pollen needs to be freeze-dried to preserve its nutrients intact.

Benefits

Unfortunately, little research has been carried out into the beneficial effects of bee pollen although it is widely used as a nutritious tonic. Some evidence suggests it is helpful for reducing hay fever allergic symptoms such as sneezing, runny nose, watering eyes and nasal congestion. This may act by desensitizing the immune system, and bee pollen collected from your local environment seems to be most effective in this respect. However, bee pollen retains its allergenic potential and may trigger allergic reactions in some people.

Dose

If you have allergies, only take bee pollen under medical supervision. If taking it for general nutritional health, and you do not have any known allergies, start with a few granules daily, and if no allergic symptoms develop (e.g. wheezing, rash, headache, itching), increase the dose to 250 mg–2 g daily for at least one month.

Contraindications
Bee pollen should be avoided if you are allergic to bee products or to pollen, especially if you have asthma or are allergic to bee stings. Do not take if you have liver disease or bleeding disorders.

Royal jelly

Royal jelly is a milky-white substance – also known as bee's milk – secreted in the salivary glands of worker honey bees. It is a highly concentrated food given to all larvae for the first three days of their lives. After that, they're nourished on a diet of honey, pollen, and water except for the larva destined to become a queen bee which continues to receive royal jelly. It is such a nutritious and potent energy source that the queen bee grows to be 50 per cent larger than other genetically identical female bees and lives for nearly 40 times longer.

Royal jelly is one of the richest natural sources of vitamin B5 (pantothenic acid), and also contains other B vitamins as well as vitamins A, C, D and E, 20 amino acids, essential fatty acids, minerals such as potassium, calcium, zinc, iron and manganese plus acetylcholine – a neurotransmitter needed to transmit messages from one nerve cell to another. It also contains antioxidant flavonoids and a powerful antibiotic that has been named royalisin. It is effective against gram-positive bacteria (e.g. *Staphylococci, Streptococci*) and may be effective when applied to skin although it is largely inactivated by stomach enzymes when taken by mouth.

Benefits
In the laboratory, royal jelly seems to have an anti-tumour effect against a type of cancer cell known as sarcoma. Royal jelly is traditionally taken to boost energy levels and mental alertness, and to combat stress, fatigue and insomnia. As a tonic, it boosts feelings of well-being, increases vitality, improves the complexion and helps to maintain healthy skin, hair and nails.

Royal jelly may help to protect against hardening and furring up of the arteries (atherosclerosis) by lowering total blood fats and abnormal cholesterol levels. In studies, doses of 50–100 mg royal jelly per day decreased total serum cholesterol levels by 14 per cent and total serum lipids by 10 per cent – possibly by increasing cholesterol excretion in the bile and decreasing its reabsorption in the gastrointestinal tract so that less enters the circulation[1].

Researchers have recently identified a substance called dipeptide YY in royal jelly which appears to inhibit renin, a hormone involved in blood pressure control. It is being investigated as a possible treatment for high blood pressure.

Royal jelly is used traditionally to improve menopausal symptoms. Researchers have now confirmed that it contains substances with oestrogenic activity. It also contains substances that promote collagen production in skin fibroblasts which might have a beneficial effect against skin ageing.

Dose
Typically 50–100 mg a day.

Royal jelly must be blended with honey or freeze-dried to preserve its active ingredients. It is best kept refrigerated and taken on an empty stomach.

Contraindications
Royal jelly has been known to trigger severe asthma attacks in some people so do not take if you are allergic to bee products, or if you suffer from asthma or other allergic conditions.

Propolis

Propolis is a yellow-brown sticky resin – sometimes known as bee glue – that is made by some species of bees from wax mixed with the resinous sap of a variety of trees (e.g. beech, birch, chestnut, conifers). More than 180 compounds have been identified in propolis, many of which have anti-inflammatory, antioxidant and immune-stimulating properties.

Bees use propolis as a cement to repair cracks and crevices in the hive and in honeycombs. It is also placed around hive entrances to help keep infections at bay. Given that a typical hive contains 50,000

1. Vittek J. Experientia 1995;51(9–10):927–35

bees, has a temperature of up to 95° Fahrenheit and 90 per cent humidity – perfect conditions for the growth of moulds, mildew and bacteria – it is remarkably effective.

Propolis is a rich source of B group vitamins and also contains flavonoids – at a concentration 500 times greater than that in oranges – that help to improve the absorption and action of vitamin C.

Benefits

Propolis works against bacteria by preventing bacterial cell division and by breaking down bacterial walls and cytoplasm. It is especially active against the bacteria that cause upper respiratory tract and skin infections, including strains that are resistant to penicillin.

Propolis has been used for over 2,000 years as an antiseptic salve to hasten wound healing, to overcome sore throats and as a supplement to boost energy levels and treat stomach ulcers. It helps to overcome infections of the skin, ear, nose, mouth and sinuses, and is frequently taken to boost immunity against colds and flu in winter.

One constituent of propolis, caffeic acid phenethyl ester, has been shown to have anti-cancer, anti-inflammatory and immune-boosting properties. It has also been shown to increase regeneration of tissues, including bone. It may also prevent unwanted blood clots and can help to lower high blood pressure.

Research is currently focusing on the immune-boosting properties of propolis, which has been found to regulate the activity of immune cells such as macrophages which fight infections, B lymphocytes which produce antibodies, natural killer cells which destroy abnormal cancerous or virus-infected cells, and leucocytes involved in inflammatory responses.

Dose

250–500 mg a day. For acute infections, higher doses may be taken (e.g. four to eight 400–600 mg capsules a day for two weeks).

As propolis is not water-soluble, it is usually extracted in alcohol and made into a tincture. It is also available as chewing gum, chips, lozenges, and powdered in capsules.

Contraindications

Propolis should not be taken by anyone who has an allergy to bee products. It causes allergic reactions in between 1 and 7 per cent of those taking it, including contact dermatitis in people with eczema.

Medicinal honey

Honey has been used for centuries to promote the healing of wounds and leg ulcers. Its high concentration of natural sugars absorbs fluid and creates a strong, osmotic environment in which bacteria cannot thrive. Many honeys also release low levels of anti-septics, such as hydrogen peroxide and gluconic acid, which inhibit the growth of skin bacteria. In addition, some honeys – especially those derived from the nectar of medicinal plants native to New Zealand and Australia – contain natural substances with a more powerful, antimicrobial action. Of these, the best known is Manuka honey, made by bees feeding on nectar from the flower of the Manuka, or New Zealand tea tree (*Leptospermum scoparium*) or from the closely related Australian *Leptospermum polygalifolium*. Some but not all Manuka honeys contain an antibacterial agent known as the Unique Manuka Factor or UMF which can be tested for and given a UMF rating. The rating shows which percentage of phenol (a strong, carbolic disinfectant) the honey is equivalent to in activity against the skin bacterium *Staphylococcus aureus*. A level of 10 indicates antibacterial activity equivalent to a 10 per cent phenol solution, and is the minimum level at which a UMF rating is awarded. Manuka honey with a minimum UMF rating of 10 is said to be 'Active'.

Benefits
Medicinal honeys have an exceptional, antibacterial activity against more than 250 types of bacteria – including antibiotic-resistant strains such as MRSA (methicillin resistant *Staphylococcus aureus*), MSSA (methicillin sensitive *Staphylococcus aureus*), vancomycin-resistant enterococci (VRE), *Pseudomonas aeruginosa*, *Acineto-bacter calcoaceticus* and *Klebsiella pneumoniae*.

Medicinal honeys also reduce inflammation and contain growth factors that promote wound healing. Those developed for clinical use (e.g. Medihoney Wound Gel from pharmacies) have been shown to:

- Rapidly clear infection and reduce the inflammatory response
- Provide a protective, antibacterial barrier against cross infection and re-colonization
- Promote natural debridement of wounds and the removal of slough and necrotic tissue (autolysis)
- Create a moist, healing environment in which new cells can flourish
- Allow easy removal of dressings, so disturbance of healing tissues is minimal
- Rapidly neutralize unpleasant wound odours (within 12 to 24 hours).

NB: It is important that you do not apply to wounds medicinal honey from a jar which is designed for oral consumption. Some honeys contain spores from Clostridium bacteria, and only medicinal honey designed for topical use must be used.

Helicobacter: Taken orally, Manuka honey with a high UMF rating has been used as a natural treatment to help eradicate *Helicobacter pylori*, a bacterium which infects the stomachs and is associated with peptic ulceration. Early studies showed some promise in this area, but a small follow-up study involving six people taking Manuka honey, and six people taking normal honey plus an antacid drug, found that none responded to treatment and all remained positive for *H. pylori*.

Chemotherapy: Eating a honey called Life Mel can help maintain levels of infection-fighting white blood cells (neutrophils) when undergoing chemotherapy[1]. This helps to protect against a condition called neutropenia, in which the level of white blood cells fall. The honey is produced by bees which are fed a special diet of immune-enhancing herbs such as Siberian ginseng, Echinacea and cat's claw.

Dose
To help eradicate *H. pylori*: usually taken on an empty stomach at a dose of four teaspoons, four times a day, for eight weeks. This provides around 80 kcals per dose. There are no guarantees it will work.

1. Zidan J et al. Med Oncol 2006;23(4):549–52

Betacarotene

Betacarotene is a carotenoid that consists of two molecules of vitamin A joined together. These can be split in the liver, and in the cells lining the small intestine, to produce retinol vitamin A when needed. However, the conversion is inefficient, especially where intakes of other micro-nutrients such as zinc are low. It is estimated that 6 mcg betacarotene is needed to produce 1 mcg of pre-formed retinol.

Research

Coronary heart disease: Several studies suggest that natural dietary intakes of betacarotene and vitamin A are important in reducing the risk of coronary heart disease. A meta-analysis of the results of 15 trials suggests that people with the highest intake of betacarotene, from both diet and supplements, have a 22 per cent lower risk of coronary heart disease than those with the lowest intakes[1].

Dose

Not recommended on its own, especially not for smokers. Some studies have found that high dose betacarotene may increase the risk of lung cancer in smokers. A meta-analysis of the results from four studies, involving over 109,000 people, found that long-term use of high dose betacarotene supplements increased the risk of lung cancer by 24 per cent among current smokers. There was no significant increased risk among former smokers[2].

It is prudent for smokers to avoid taking betacarotene on its own. In fact, there is little benefit in anyone taking betacarotene supplements on their own. It is more beneficial to take a mixed carotenoid supplement, providing a blend of different nutrients. This balance is naturally obtained when consuming red-yellow-orange-green fruit and vegetables.

1. Ye Z, Song H. Eur J Cardiovasc Prev Rehabil 2008; 15(1):26–34
2. Tanvetyanon T, Bepler G. Cancer 2008;113(1):150–7

Bilberry
(Vaccinium myrtillus)

Bilberry is a small deciduous shrub native to central and northern Europe, northern Asia, and North America. It is related to the blueberry, blackcurrant and grape. While the American blueberry has creamy or white coloured flesh, that of the bilberry is purple so its content of antioxidant pigments is considerably higher. Bilberries are a rich source of tannins, anthocyanins (see page 38) and flavonoid glycosides that have antioxidant and anti-inflammatory actions.

Bilberry has been used medicinally for over a thousand years. The dried berries were traditionally used for their astringent qualities in the treatment of diarrhoea, and have also been used to treat scurvy, cystitis, kidney stones and inflammation of the mucous membranes of mouth and throat.

Extracts are used to strengthen blood vessels and the collagen-containing connective tissue that supports them, as well as improving circulation. These actions are helpful in the treatment of easy-bruising syndrome, thread veins (telangiectasis), phlebitis, varicose veins and haemorrhoids, for which they are particularly suited for use in pregnancy.

Research

Circulation: In a study of almost 50 people with varicose veins, taking 480 mg bilberry extracts per day increased local circulation to reduce fluid retention, feelings of heaviness, pins and needles and pain, as well as improving the appearance of overlying skin. In addition, bilberry reduces the risk of stroke and inhibits unwanted clot formation. Because of their beneficial effects on the circulation, bilberry extracts are prescribed in some parts of Europe for patients due to undergo surgery as their use has been shown to reduce excessive bleeding.

Eye health: Bilberry extracts are also used to treat many eye disorders including macular degeneration, cataracts, night-blindness, glaucoma, retinitis pigmentosa and diabetic retinopathy. Bilberry's effectiveness in treating visual problems results from a number of actions. Its antioxidant blue-red pigments protect the membranes of light-sensitive and other cells in the eyes, reduce hardening and furring up of blood vessels, stabilize tear production, increase blood flow to the retina, regenerate the light-sensitive pigment rhodopsin, as well as increasing the strength of collagen fibres in capillaries and supportive connective tissues.

Bilberry is helpful for people with diabetic retinopathy, in whom haemorrhages form within the retina of the eye. In a trial involving 40 people, all but three of whom had diabetic retinopathy, participants either took 160 mg bilberry extracts twice a day for one month, or inactive placebo[1]. They then crossed over into the other group for another month. While taking bilberry extracts, almost 80 per cent showed improvement in visible retinal abnormalities on ophthalmologic examination, compared with none of those taking placebo. Similar results were found in a trial involving 31 people, of whom 20 had diabetic retinopathy[2].

The antioxidant effects also help to prevent the development and progression of cataracts. In a study of 50 people with age-related cataracts, bilberry extract plus vitamin E stopped cataract progression in 97 per cent of cases[3]. Some researchers have also suggested that taking bilberry extracts can reduce short-sightedness after five months of regular use, perhaps by improving the reactivity and focusing ability of the eye lens.

The antioxidant anthocyanins found in bilberries and other dark, blue-red pigmented fruits can lower uric acid levels and are said to prevent gout attacks when around 250 g of the fruits are eaten daily. They have also been used to improve breast pain due to benign fibrocystic disease and to reduce painful periods through their muscle relaxing action. There is little research in these areas, however.

Bilberry extracts are under further investigation for their potentially beneficial effects on glucose tolerance, cholesterol balance, blood pressure regulation and ability to protect against peptic ulceration.

1. Perossini M et al. Ann Ottalmol Clin Ocul 1987;113:1173
2. Scharrer A, Ober M. Kiln Monatsbl Augenheikld Beih 1981;178:386–9
3. Bravetti G. Ann Ottalmol Clin Ocul 1989;115:109

Dose

10–60 g dried ripe fruit a day.

Dry extract (25 per cent anthocyanins): 80–160 mg, one to three times a day. Higher doses may be used to treat diabetes.

Excess

No toxicity has been found even at high doses, as bilberry extract is water-soluble and excess is quickly excreted through the urine and bile.

Biotin

Biotin is a water-soluble member of the vitamin B group. It is an essential co-factor for four carboxylase enzymes involved in the synthesis and metabolism of glucose, fatty acids, amino acids, genetic material and stress hormones. It plays an important role in glucose balance, and in the growth and repair of skin, hair and nails. Biotin is widespread in the diet and good sources include meat, liver, oily fish, wholegrains, rice, nuts, cauliflower, egg yolk and yeast extracts. It is also produced by probiotic bacteria in the bowel, from which it can be absorbed.

Research

Glucose control: Biotin is needed for the proper function of an enzyme, glucokinase, which plays a role in the metabolism of glucose. Biotin has the potential to improve glucose metabolism by stimulating insulin secretion from pancreatic beta-cells, by increasing the breakdown of glucose (glycolysis) in the liver by stimulating the conversion of glucose to fats and/or glycogen (a starchy, energy storage molecule). It may also have an effect on the glucose receptors (known as GLUT 4) that are needed to transport glucose into cells under the influence of insulin.

Blood levels of biotin are lower in people with Type 2 diabetes than in those without, and taking supplements has been shown to increase the activity of carboxylase enzymes within the white blood cells of people with diabetes. Biotin supplements have also been shown to improve the results of oral glucose tolerance tests in some people with diabetes. The few trials that have used biotin alone have involved small numbers of people, but suggest biotin supplements have the potential to produce significant improvements in fasting blood glucose levels. Average reductions were 45 per cent compared with those taking placebo[1].

A recent study involving 447 people with poorly controlled Type 2 diabetes showed significant improvements in fasting glucose levels (and HbA1c – a measure of short-term glucose control) in those taking both chromium picolinate (600 mcg) and biotin (2 mg) daily[2].

Biotin therapy has also been shown to improve symptoms of diabetic peripheral neuropathy, but although significant improvements were reported within four to eight weeks of treatment, only three patients were involved. More research is needed in this area.

Deficiency

Lack of biotin affects the function of some metabolic enzymes and may result in hypoglycaemia between meals and raised blood levels of ammonia. It has also been associated with dry, flaky skin, a rash around the nose and mouth, brittle hair, patches of hair loss, reversible baldness, tiredness, loss of appetite, nausea, depression, muscle pains and wasting, as well as reduced immunity – especially against fungal yeast infections.

Dietary deficiency of biotin is unusual, however, except in those following very low-calorie weight loss diets and in those eating large amounts of raw egg white over a long period (e.g. body builders who eat a dozen raw eggs a day). Raw egg white contains a protein, avidin, which binds to biotin in the gut and prevents its absorption. Cooked egg white does not have this effect.

People on long-term antibiotic treatment (e.g. for acne) may also be at risk of deficiency due to loss of the normal probiotic bowel bacteria that make biotin. When taking antibiotics, taking a probiotic supplement (see page 258) will help to overcome this effect.

It is estimated that one in every 123 people has an inherited inborn error of biotin metabolism. This is believed to affect their immunity against yeast infections and may be linked with recurrent vaginal thrush infections. In such cases high-dose biotin supplements will solve the problem if biotin deficiency is to blame.

1. Maebashi M et al. J Clin Biochem Nutr. 1993; 14:211–218
2. Albarracin CA et al. Diabetes Metab Res Rev 2008;24(1):41–51

Nails: Veterinarians use biotin supplements to strengthen the hooves of horses and the claws of swine. In women with brittle nails, taking biotin supplements has been shown to increase nail plate thickness by 25 per cent as determined by scanning electron microscopy[1]. Splitting of nails was reduced by improved regularity of the cell arangement on the back surface of the nails. In one study, 22 out of 35 people showed clinical improvement but 13 (37 per cent) showed no change[2].

Dose

The old EU RDA for biotin was 150 mcg per day. The new RDA has been significantly reduced to 50 mcg daily. There is no UK RNI, but intakes of 10–200 mcg are believed to be adequate. The upper safe level for long-term use from supplements is suggested as 900 mcg.

For maintaining healthy skin, hair and nails, intakes of around 1000 mcg (1 mg) a day may be taken short term. Two out of three people respond, with nails growing significantly thicker.

Bitter melon
(Momordica charantia)

Bitter melon (also known as balsam pear, Ampalaya, Karela or Karolla) is the unripened fruit of an Asian vine. It is used in Ayurvedic and Chinese medicine to improve glucose tolerance. Its main active component, charantin, contains a mixture of steroidal compounds that have a glucose-lowering action. A protein chain known as polypeptide-p is also present, which slows glucose absorption and reduces the production of glucose in the liver (gluco-neogenesis). This protein chain has structural similarities to animal insulin[3] and bitter melon is often referred to as plant insulin.

Benefits

Glucose control: In people with Type 2 diabetes, eating the fruit or drinking the juice has been shown to have significant effects on glucose tolerance and glycosylated haemoglobin A1c levels with no increase in insulin levels[4]. In a trial involving 40 people with poorly controlled

1. Colombo VE et al. J Am Acad Dermatol 1990;23(6 Pt 1):1127–32
2. Hochman LG et al. Cutis 1003;51(4):303–5
3. Basch E et al. Am J Health Syst Pharm. 2003;60(4):356–9
4. Leatherdale BA et al. BMJ 1981;282(6279):1823–4

Type 2 diabetes, one group took Mormordica capsules three times a day after meals, for three months, while another group took placebo. The level of glycosylated haemoglobin (HbA1c) improved more in those taking Momordica than in controls[1]. Although the improvement was small (0.24 per cent), any improvement in HbA1c is beneficial; every percentage point above normal increases the chance of developing diabetes-related complications by 20 per cent.

Dose

3 g per day (1 g after each meal).

50–100 ml juice daily under medical supervision only.

High doses can cause abdominal pain and diarrhoea.

May interact with other glucose-lowering agents. People taking hypoglycaemic drugs should use bitter melon with caution, under medical supervision, to avoid hypoglycaemia.

Black cohosh
(Cimicifuga racemosa)

Black cohosh – also known as squaw root or black snakeroot – is native to Canada and eastern parts of the USA. It is classed as an adaptogen (see page 26) that helps to balance female hormones. It is mainly used to help relieve menopausal hot flushes and night sweats, but is also used to help relax menstrual cramps, treat painful or irregular periods, low libido, hormone imbalances and pre-menstrual syndrome. It is especially helpful in reducing feelings of depression, anxiety, tension, and mood swings.

Its dried roots contain a number of oestrogen-like plant hormones (phytoestrogens) of which formononetin is thought to be the most important. Rather than having an overt oestrogen-like action, however, it is believed to reduce menopausal symptoms through a direct action on the brain. It has been shown to lower levels of LH produced by the pituitary gland by as much as 20 per cent. This in turn decreases ovarian output of progesterone hormone to normalize oestrogen-progesterone balance. Interestingly, it seems to enhance blood circulation in the genitals, and some evidence suggests that it causes a significant

---

1. Dans AM et al. J Clin Epidemiol 2007;60(6):554–9

increase in weight of the uterus and ovaries as a result.

As black cohosh has a normalizing effect on female sex hormones, it may be used to improve low sex drive where this is linked with hormonal imbalances, such as after childbirth, irregular menstruation and around the time of the menopause. It is also used to help relieve symptoms of endometriosis.

It also has an effect on dilation of blood vessels, and reduces menopausal hot flushes and sweating.

Benefits

Menopause: Black cohosh is one of the most widely used and studied natural alternatives to hormone replacement therapy (HRT). Several comparison studies have found that standardized extracts produced better results in relieving hot flushes, vaginal thinning and dryness, depression and anxiety compared to standard HRT (conjugated oestrogens). A German trial has shown that black cohosh plus St John's Wort was effective in treating 78 per cent of women with hot flushes and other menopausal problems. Most women experienced significant improvement in symptoms within two to four weeks. In another study, black cohosh out-performed diazepam and oestrogen HRT in relieving depressive moods and anxiety. However, a meta-analysis of data from 16 studies found that results were conflicting and that more research is needed to support its use[1]. A beneficial effect cannot be excluded however[2]!

Dose

Usually 40–200 mg standardized extracts daily.

Side effects

Some people experience headaches behind the eyes, nausea, or indigestion if they have taken too much black cohosh.

A few cases of abnormal vaginal bleeding and miscarriage have been reported but it is not clear if black cohosh was responsible.

Some reports suggest that black cohosh may have an adverse effect on liver function in some people. Inflammation of the liver (hepatitis) has also occurred.

A review of side effects from 13 clinical trials suggests that black

1. Palacio C et al. Drugs Aging 2009 26(1):23–36
2. Berrelli F, Ernst E. Pharmacol Res 2008;58(1):8–14

cohosh is safe, and that in most case reports of liver problems it is not possible to definitely cite black cohosh as the cause[1,2]. Further investigation is undoubtedly needed. It should therefore be used with caution in people with risk factors for liver disease (e.g. regular use of drugs such as paracetamol, or high alcohol intake). Regular liver function tests may be advised in some cases.

Black cohosh does not have an oestrogen-like effect on the breast[3] and actually appears to decrease local oestrogen formation in normal human breast tissue[4]. Because its action does not stimulate oestrogen-sensitive tumours (and may, in fact, inhibit them) black cohosh extracts have been used in women with a history of breast cancer. A study involving over 1,100 women with breast cancer concluded that taking black cohosh extracts was unlikely to increase the risk of breast cancer recurrence. A systematic review of evidence from five clinical and 21 preclinical studies suggests that the use of black cohosh appears to be safe in breast cancer patients without risk for liver disease although, as always, further research is needed[5]. It should only be used in women with a history of breast cancer under medical supervision.

Contraindications
Black cohosh should not be taken during pregnancy (may stimulate uterine contractions) or when breast-feeding.

Blue-green algae

Blue-green algae are classed as cyanobacteria. They evolved over 3.5 billion years ago as the first successful life form on earth and now flourish in warm, alkaline lakes. Those available in supplement form include Spirulina and Aphanizomenon flos-aquae. A similar supplement, Chlorella, is classed as a green algae. As it is difficult to cultivate and loses much of its nutritional value during processing, it is now less widely used.

Blue-green algae are a rich wholefood source of over 100

1. Berrelli F, Ernst E. Am J Obstet Gynecol 2008;199(5):455–66
2. Mahady GB et al. Menopause 2008;15(4 Pt 1):628–38
3. Ruhlen RL et al. Nutr Cancer 2007;59(2):269–77
4. Stute P et al. Maturitas 2007;57(4):382-91
5. Walji R et al. Support Care Cancer 2007;15(8):913–21

synergistic and easily assimilated nutrients including antioxidants, vitamins, minerals, enzymes, gammalinolenic acid, essential and non-essential amino acids, iron, chlorophyll, protein and other bioactive substances. Although it is a vegetarian source of vitamin B12, there is some controversy other whether it is present in a reliably absorbable form.

As the basis for the development of life on earth, algae are one of the most easily assimilable foods for the human body. They consist of up to 70 per cent protein which is present in the easily absorbed form of glyco-proteins, rather than as lipoproteins which are found in most other protein food sources.

Gram for gram, blue-green algae are the richest natural source of carotenoids, containing more natural betacarotene than carrots.

Substances extracted from blue-green algae have effects in laboratory cells that suggest they may have beneficial effects against cancer, diabetes, coronary heart disease, degenerative disease, heavy metal toxicity and radiation poisoning. They have recently been shown to have an immunosuppressant effect against abnormal cell proliferation. They also promote the growth of probiotic intestinal bacteria.

Algae have a chelating effect, helping to bind harmful toxins in the digestive tract (e.g. heavy metals) and remove them from the body. The blue phytochemical, phycocyanin, found in Spirulina for example, has a powerful detoxifying action helping to reduce kidney damage due to heavy metals such as mercury.

Blue-green algae are widely taken to improve bad breath (halitosis), aid digestion and to detox.

Benefits

Cholesterol: Recent human trials suggest that taking Spirulina supplements can significantly improve markers of immune function and antioxidant status, lower levels of 'bad' LDL-cholesterol and raise 'good' HDL-cholesterol, compared with placebo[1].

Allergic rhinitis: Spirulina can produce significant improvements in symptoms of allergic rhinitis such as nasal discharge, sneezing, congestions and itching, compared with placebo[2].

1. Park HJ et al. Ann Nutr Metab 2008;52(4):322–8
2. Cinkgi C et al. Eur Arch Otorhinolaryngol 2008;265(10):1219–23

Leukoplakia: A trial involving 44 people with precancerous lesions of the mouth (oral leukoplakia) who took 1 g Spirulina per day for one year, found that over half the lesions vanished in 45 per cent of those taking Spirulina compared with only 7 per cent of those taking placebo[1].

Dose

Varies from product to product, but typically 3–6 g a day. Large amounts may be consumed as a food without apparent harm.

Best taken with food.

Side effects

A few mild side effects such as headache, flushing and sweating have been reported.

Blue-green algae contain the amino acid, phenylalanine, which can cause adverse effects in people with a genetic metabolic abnormality called phenylketonuria.

Algae harvested from the wild rather than grown under controlled conditions may, potentially, be contaminated with toxic algae or pollutants such as heavy metals, which have been associated with diarrhoea, vomiting and liver damage. Select a recognized, mainstream brand – preferably one that is certified organic, meaning it has grown in unpolluted waters.

Boron

Boron is a trace element obtained from fruit and vegetables, especially apples, grapes, pears, plums, prunes, strawberries, avocado and broccoli.

Boron has several complex actions that depend on its ability to inhibit or stimulate a variety of enzymes. It is thought to be involved in normal brain function by affecting the movement of chemicals across the membrane of brain cells. It is also important for bone health through its ability to boost production of active vitamin D (needed for absorption of calcium from the intestines) and to reduce excretion of calcium and magnesium.

1. Mathew B et al. Nutr Cancer 1995;24(12):197–202

Benefits

Osteoporosis: Some researchers have suggested that osteoporosis is a boron-deficiency disease, though there is no clear evidence that supplements can prevent or treat osteoporosis. Benefits were suggested by a small study in which 12 post-menopausal women followed a low-boron diet for 17 weeks and then took boron supplements (3 mg a day) for seven weeks. After just eight days on boron, they excreted 44 per cent less calcium and 33 per cent less magnesium than before. Their production of both oestrogen and testosterone hormones also doubled[1]. However, a later, similar study lasting three weeks found no effect on minerals or hormone levels, although improvements in calcium balance were observed[2].

Dose

There is no EU RDA or UK RNI. The World Health Organization suggests that intakes of between 1–13 mg per day are adequate. The upper safe level for long-term use from supplements is suggested as 6 mg daily.

A higher than average intake of boron in vegetarians (around 10 mg a day compared with 0.5–1 mg in non-vegetarians) may account for their lower risk of osteoporosis.

Excess

Toxicity can occur at intakes of 100 mg a day or more, causing symptoms such as headache, muscle pain, nausea, vomiting, red eyes, rash and peeling skin plus reduced fertility.

Boswellia

Boswellia is an Ayurvedic gum resin derived from the tree, Boswellia serrata. The resin is also known as frankincense. It contains a number of anti-inflammatory substances, including boswellic acids, which appear to be as effective as some non-

1. Nielsen FH et al. FASEB J 1987;1(5):394–7
2. Beattie JH, Peace HS. Br J Nutr 1993;69(3):871–84

steroidal, anti-inflammatory drugs, but without the adverse effects of gastric irritation. Boswellic acids have recently been shown to work by inhibiting the production of inflammatory immune chemicals such as 5-lipoxygenase, interleukins and TNF-alpha.

Boswellia has been used to treat chronic inflammatory conditions such as osteoarthritis, rheumatoid arthritis, asthma, ulcerative colitis, eczema and psoriasis.

Benefits
Rheumatoid arthritis: In people with rheumatoid arthritis, boswellia resin has produced significant reductions in pain, duration of morning stiffness and disability compared with placebo.

Osteoarthritis: In a cross-over trial involving 30 people with knee OA, boswellia significantly improved pain, increased knee flexion and increased walking distance compared with placebo, as well as decreasing the frequency of knee swelling[1]. Another trial involving 66 people with osteoarthritis compared the effects of boswellia against the non-steroidal anti-inflammatory drug, valdecoxib, for six months. In those taking boswellia, pain, stiffness and ability to perform daily activities improved within two months, with benefits lasting for one month after stopping treatment. In those taking a non-steroidal anti-inflammatory drug, benefits were seen within one month but lasted for only as long as the drug was taken[2]. So, although boswellia showed a slower onset of action, the benefits persisted after treatment stopped.

Ulcerative colitis: In 30 patients with colitis who were given either boswellia or the standard drug treatment, sulfasalazine, 18 out of 20 taking boswellia showed improvement and 14 went into remission; of those taking sulfasalazine, 6 out of 10 showed similar improve-ment, with 4 out of 10 going into remission. This suggests that boswellia can be at least as effective as standard drug treatment[3]. In another trial, 82 per cent of those with ulcerative colitis taking

1. Kimmatkar N et al. Phytomedicine 2003;10(1):3–7
2. Sontakke S et al. Indian J Pharmacol 2007;39:27–29
3. Gupta I et al. Planta Med 2001;67(5):391–5

boswellia went into remission compared with 75 per cent taking the usual anti-inflammatory or steroidal drug treatments[1]. This again suggests it is at least as effective as standard medical treatment. Benefits have also been found in people with collagenous colitis[2].

Crohn's disease: In a study involving 87 people with Crohn's disease, 44 were treated with boswellia and 39 with the drug mesalazine. The symptoms score for those taking boswellia reduced by 90 points, compared with an average reduction of 53 points in those taking standard drug therapy. This suggests that boswellia can be at least as effective as standard drug treatment[3].

Asthma: In a study involving 40 people with asthma, 70 per cent showed improvement of symptoms and lung function within six weeks, compared with 27 per cent of those on placebo[4].

Dose

150–400 mg, one to three times per day. Select products standardized to contain at least 37.5 per cent boswellic acids.

Brewer's yeast
(Saccharomyces cerevisiae)

Brewer's yeast may be classed as a probiotic organism. It is traditionally used as a protein supplement, energy booster and immune enhancer. It is a particularly rich source of B vitamins and trace minerals such as chromium. Medicinally, it has been used to treat acute diarrhoea, acne, pre-menstrual symptoms and to prevent candida proliferation.

Benefits

Diarrhoea: In Germany, brewer's yeast strain Hansen CBS 5926 is used for treating acute diarrhoea, and for preventing and treating traveller's diarrhoea. Oral intake of fermentable yeast can cause flatulence, however, so although it may be helpful in reducing

1. Gupta I et al. Eur J Med Res 1997;2(1):37–43
2. Madisch A et al. Int J Colorectal Dis 2007;22(12):1445–51
3. Gerhardt H et al. Z Gastroenterol 2001;39(1):11–7
4. Gupta I et al. Eur J Med Res 1998;3(11):511–4

diarrhoea in some people, in others it may make symptoms such as bloating worse, especially in those with IBS.

Immune function: Brewer's yeast has been used to prevent colds and influenza, and appears to reduce the incidence and duration of these viral infections compared with placebo[1].

Diabetes: High chromium brewer's yeast supplements have been shown to improve glucose control, triglycerides, total and HDL-cholesterol in people with Type 2 diabetes[2,3].

Cholesterol: High chromium brewer's yeast extracts have been shown to significantly reduce total cholesterol and increase HDL cholesterol, although there was no placebo group for comparison[4].

Dose
250–750 mg a day.

Side effects
Skin prick testing suggests that some people with allergic conditions such as atopic eczema, rhinitis and asthma have reactions against brewer's yeast. Cross reaction can also occur with other yeasts, including *Candida albicans* and *Pityrosporum ovale* (which is linked with seborrhoeic dermatitis/dandruff).

Bromelain

Bromelain is the name given to a group of sulphur-containing protease (protein-digesting) enzymes derived from the stem of the pineapple plant (*Ananas sativus*). It may be taken with meals to aid the digestion of protein, but as it is absorbed intact into the circulation from the intestines, it is mainly used for its systemic effects.

Bromelain reduces the production of inflammatory chemicals (cytokines) and reduces the migration of inflammatory immune cells

1. Moyad MA et al. Urol Nurs 2008;28(1):50–5
2. Li YC. Biol Trace Elem Res 1994;41(3):341–7
3. Bahijiri SM et al. Saudi Med J 2000;21(9):831–7
4. Elwood JC et al. J Am Coll Nutr 1982;1(3):263–74

to sites of inflammation. As a result, it can damp down pain, stiffness and swelling in conditions such as arthritis, sinusitis, ulcerative colitis, urinary tract infection and immune skin conditions. It has also been shown to reduce platelet clotting in laboratory tests and may have a similar blood-thinning action to aspirin.

Bromelain has an anti-inflammatory action and is used to reduce pain, swelling and inflammation associated with exercise, bruising, sprains, wounds, minor operations, burns, osteoarthritis and skin rashes. It is sometimes recommended before minor surgery and liposuction, to reduce post-operative swelling and bruising, and as a supplement to take after childbirth to boost healing. It also has a useful mucus-thinning action and can help to reduce phlegm in respiratory conditions such as sinusitis, bronchitis and asthma.

Benefits

Knee pain: Bromelain was shown to reduce pain and swelling in adults with mild acute knee pain of less than three months' duration[1]. However, in a follow-up double-blind placebo controlled trial involving 31 people with moderate to severe knee OA, taking 800 mg per day bromelain for four weeks was no more effective than placebo[2].

However, bromelain in combination with another enzyme, trypsin, and an antioxidant, rutin, appears to be at least as effective in reducing symptoms due to osteoarthritis of the hip and knee as the non-steroidal anti-inflammatory drug, diclofenac, after three to six weeks of treatment[3,4,5].

Sinusitis: A trial involving 116 children under the age of 11 years found that bromelain was helpful in reducing symptoms of sinusitis, with those receiving bromelain recovering significantly more quickly than those on placebo (6.6 days versus 8 days)[6].

Colitis: Bromelain decreases production of inflammatory cytokines produced by human white blood cells. Anecdotal reports and

1. Walker AF et al. Phytomedicine 2002;9(8):681–6
2. Brien S et al. QJM 2006;99(12):841–50
3. Klein G et al, Clin Exp Rheumatol 2006;24(1):25–30
4. Akhtar NM et al. Clin Rheumatol 2004;23(5):410–5
5. Tilwe GH et al. J Assoc Physicians India 2001;49:617–21
6. Braun JM et al. In Vivo 2005;19(2):417–21

laboratory evidence suggests that it may be helpful in treating ulcerative colitis[1].

Blood clotting: Bromelain has been used to complement the treatment of angina. It has a useful blood-thinning action, and may work by reducing platelet clumping[2]. In one study, people with angina who took 1000–1400 mg bromelain found that their symptoms either improved or disappeared within three months.

Dose

250–500 mg, three times a day.

Select supplements containing at least 2000 milk clotting units.

Side effects

Some people are allergic to pineapple products, including bromelain. Those with industrial exposure to bromelain may develop contact dermatitis and/or asthma from inhalation of bromelain.

Note: Before undergoing liposuction, or any other surgery, it is important to consult your surgeon/anaesthetist before taking bromelain as it has a blood-thinning action.

Butterbur
(Petasites hybridus)

Butterbur grows in damp, marshy areas and is sometimes known as bog rhubarb. It contains a number of substances such as petasin, and isopetasin, which have analgesic and antispasmodic actions. It reduces inflammation by reducing secretion of histamine and leukotrienes by immune cells.

Benefits

Migraine: A study involving 58 children with migraine gave one group butterbur extracts, one group music therapy, and another group placebo for eight weeks. The researchers found that both

---

1. Onken JE et al. Clin Immunol 2008;126(3):345–52
2. Glaser D, Hilberg T. Platelets 2006;17(1):37–41

butterbur and music therapy were helpful[1]. In a study involving 245 people with migraine, butterbur extracts (65 mg twice daily) were significantly more effective than placebo and, over four months of treatment, reduced the frequency of migraine attacks by 36 per cent (compared with 26 per cent for placebo)[2]. Other studies have found reductions in migraine frequency of up to 60 per cent.

Hay fever: A study involving 330 people with allergic rhinitis found that butterbur extracts were as effective as the prescribed anti-histamine fexofenadine[3]. Another study involving 125 people with seasonal allergic rhinitis found that butterbur was as effective as the antihistamine, cetirizine[4]. It is less likely to cause sedation, drowsiness and fatigue than drug treatment.

Asthma: Taking butterbur can improve the effectiveness of inhaled corticosteroids through an additional anti-inflammatory action[5].

Dose
50–75 mg extract, two or three times daily.

Select products standardized to contain a minimum of 7.5 mg petasin and isopetasin.

Calcium

Calcium is an important structural mineral of which we each contain around 1.2 kg – more than any other mineral. Most of this is stored in the skeleton as hydroxyapatite. Around 99 per cent of calcium absorbed from the diet goes straight into our bones and teeth. The other 1 per cent (around 10 g) plays a crucial role in blood clotting, muscle contraction, nerve conduction, the smooth functioning of the immune system and the production of energy.

Calcium is absorbed in the small intestine, a process that is dependent upon the presence of vitamin D. Lack of calcium at any

1. Oelkers-Ax R et al. Eur J Pain 2008;12(3):301–13
2. Lipton RB et al. Neurology 2004;63(12):2240–4
3. Schapowal A et al. Phytother Res 2005;19(6):530–7
4. Schapowal A et al. BMJ 2002;324(7330):144–6
5. Lee DK et al. Clin Exp Allergy 2004;34(1):110–4

stage in life means that bone stores are raided, greatly increasing the risk of osteoporosis in the future. Good intakes of calcium are therefore vital throughout life, especially during childhood and adolescence when bones are still developing, and in later years when bones are naturally starting to thin down.

Dietary sources of calcium include milk and dairy products, eggs, green leafy vegetables especially broccoli (but not spinach, whose oxalate content reduces its bioavailability), tinned salmon (including the bones), nuts and seeds, pulses and bread made from fortified flour. It is relatively easy to increase calcium intake by drinking an extra pint of skimmed or semi-skimmed milk per day, which contains 720 mg calcium per pint. Skimmed milk provides as much calcium as whole milk but without the additional fat. The calcium found in milk is also in the readily absorbable form of calcium lactate.

Interestingly, the bioavailability of calcium in brassica vegetables is higher than that in dairy products – 61 per cent of calcium found in broccoli is absorbable, compared with only 32 per cent of that in milk. The reason remains unknown. Only 30–40 per cent of the calcium present in other food and drinks is absorbed. Some types of dietary fibre (phytates from wheat in unleavened bread, e.g. chapatti) also bind calcium in the bowel to form an insoluble, non-absorbable salt. High-fibre diets, which speed the passage of food through the bowels, will also reduce the amount of calcium absorbed.

Calcium supplements are effective antacids, helping to reduce symptoms of heartburn and indigestion.

Benefits

Osteoporosis: Taking daily calcium supplements of 1000–1500 mg helps to prevent bone loss in older women, especially during the winter months when vitamin D levels are naturally low due to reduced sun exposure. A meta-analysis of data from 29 trials, involving almost 64,000 adults, found that taking calcium supplements could reduce the rate of bone loss and reduce the risk of all types of fracture by 12 per cent[1]. Where compliance was good, fracture reduction increased to 24 per cent. The most effective doses were 1200 mg calcium plus 800 IU vitamin D.

---

1. Tang BM et al. Lancet 2007;370(9588):657–66

Blood pressure: Low intakes of calcium are linked with high blood pressure and stroke. This is partly because calcium promotes sodium excretion, and partly because calcium plays a role in blood vessel contraction and dilation. A study involving almost 29,000 women aged 45 years or over found that, after adjusting for major hypertension risk factors, those with the highest intakes of calcium from dairy products had the lowest risk of developing hypertension. A meta-analysis of 40 studies involving almost 2,500 adults found that taking 1200 mg calcium per day reduced blood pressure by 1.86/0.99 mmHg. In those with relatively low calcium intakes, the benefit was greater with a reduction in blood pressure of 2.63/1.30 mmHg – a small but significant difference[1]. If taking a calcium channel blocker drug, however, the blood pressure lowering effect of calcium supplements is lost.

Cancer: Good dietary intakes of calcium appear to inhibit the development of a number of cancers – possibly by buffering the effects of bile acids. A meta-analysis of 60 studies, involving over 26,000 people found that those with a high intake of milk and dairy products were 22 per cent less likely to develop colon cancer than those with low intakes[2]. Results were similar for calcium from dietary or supplement sources.

PMS: Alterations in calcium homeostasis are associated with mood disturbances and clinical symptoms similar to those of PMS. Calcium may alleviate PMS by enhancing hormone receptor activity, neuromuscular transmission or through effects on monoamine and serotonin neurotransmitters. A cross-over trial involving 33 women with PMS found that taking 1000 mg calcium improved three PMS symptoms – negative affect, water retention and pain – significantly more than placebo. Overall, 73 per cent reported fewer symptoms during treatment with calcium, 15 per cent preferred placebo, while 12 per cent had no clear preference[3]. In a controlled trial involving 466 women with moderate to severe PMS, taking calcium (1200 mg per day) for three cycles produced a significant 48 per cent reduction in total symptom scores, including

1. Van Mierlo LA et al. J Hum Hypertens 2006;20(8):571–80
2. Huncharek M et al. Nutr Cancer 2009;61(1):47–69
3. Thys-Jacobs S et al. J Gen Intern Med 1989; 4:183–189

negative effect, fluid retention, food cravings and pain compared with a 33 per cent reduction for placebo[1].

Deficiency

Deficiency is widespread with 56 per cent of the fertile, adult female population aged 19–24 years obtaining less than the RNI of 700 mg daily. Low intakes of calcium are linked with muscle problems (aches, pains, twitching, spasm, cramps), palpitations, high blood pressure, osteoporosis, gum disease and loose teeth.

Dose

The EU RDA for calcium is 800 mg per day. The UK RNI for adults aged 19–50 years is 700 mg. The upper safe level for long-term use from supplements is suggested as 1500 mg.

Calcium tablets are best taken with meals. Some evidence suggests that they are better taken with an evening meal rather than breakfast as calcium flux is greatest in the body at night, when growth hormone is secreted. If taking a high dose, however, it is usually best to divide it into two or three smaller doses spread throughout the day to improve absorption. People with a tendency to kidney stones should ideally take calcium supplements together with essential fatty acids (e.g. evening primrose oil) but always seek medical advice first.

Those taking certain tetracycline antibiotics need to ensure they do not eat or drink calcium-containing foods for at least an hour either side of taking their medication. This is because calcium binds with some tetracyclines to reduce their absorption.

Calcium salts that are most easily absorbed are calcium lactate (in milk), calcium gluconate, calcium malate and calcium citrate (which is less likely to cause constipation than calcium carbonate and is also better for those with less stomach acid production, e.g. older people).

The amount of elemental calcium supplied per gram of supplement will affect the recommended dose. Test your calcium supplement by adding it to vinegar at room temperature and stirring every five minutes. If it hasn't dissolved after 30 minutes, it is unlikely to do so in your stomach either and you should switch to another brand. Effervescent tablets or calcium-enriched drinks usually help to improve absorption.

---

1. Thys-Jacobs S et al. Am J Obstet Gynecol 1998; 179: 444–52

Carnitine

L-carnitine is a non-essential amino acid that is made in the liver. Vitamins B3, B6, C and the mineral iron are essential for its conversion. Dietary sources include red meat, especially lamb and beef, offal and dairy products. The main vegetable sources of L-carnitine are avocado and fermented soybean products.

L-carnitine is an antioxidant, but its most important role is in regulating fat metabolism. It is needed to transport long-chain fatty acids into the energy-producing mitochondria found in all body cells where they are burned to produce energy. The more L-carnitine that is available, the more fat can be burned for fuel – especially in heart muscle cells. L-carnitine is also needed to break down the branched-chain amino acids (leucine, isoleucine and valine) so they can be used as an energy source by muscle cells when other sources of energy are in short supply. By helping to mobilize fat stores and boost energy production, it may play a useful role in weight loss.

L-carnitine aids digestion by stimulating the secretion of gastric and pancreatic juices and it has beneficial effects on blood fat levels by raising beneficial HDL (high-density lipoprotein) cholesterol while lowering total cholesterol and triglyceride levels overall. It may therefore be useful for treating hardening and furring up of the arteries (atherosclerosis), poor circulation and coronary heart disease.

Benefits

Heart disease: When heart muscle cells do not receive enough oxygen, metabolism is impaired and free fatty acids build up and may damage heart cells. Research suggests that L-carnitine helps to neutralize these and may quickly become used up. Providing additional supplies may help to minimize heart damage in those at risk of a heart attack. In those with chronic stable angina, L-carnitine can improve exercise tolerance and duration[1], improve cardiac function and reduce exercise-induced angina[2]. Among a group of 44 men with angina, almost 23 per cent who took L-carnitine supple-

1. Iver RN et al. J Assoc Physicians India 2000;48(11):1050–2
2. Cacciatore L et al. Drugs Exp Clin Res 1991;17(4):225–35

ments for four weeks became free of exercise-induced angina compared with only 9 per cent taking inactive placebo[1].

Claudication: L-carnitine has been shown to improve the distance walked without pain in patients with calf pain (intermittent claudication) due to hardening and furring up of the arteries (atherosclerosis). Several studies suggest that taking 1 g to 3 g carnitine per day can significantly improve pain-free walking distance in those with more severe claudication – most likely by improving energy metabolism within muscle cells[2,3].

Diabetic neuropathy: Some studies suggest it can improve symptoms of diabetic neuropathy which can cause pain, burning sensations, pins and needles and numbness. Analysis of data from two clinical trials involving almost 1,700 people with diabetic neuropathy found that taking at least 2 g L-carnitine per day can reduce pain scores and may improve nerve conduction speed[4]. It appears to promote regeneration of nerve fibres, and improve sensitivity of nerve fibres to vibration perception as well as reducing pain. It does not seem to affect insulin sensitivity, and is best taken early in the disease process for maximum benefit.

Athletic performance: L-carnitine is popular among athletes, who take it before exercise in an attempt to increase maximum oxygen uptake and the efficiency of muscle contraction during intensive exercise (e.g. running a marathon). Unfortunately, most studies show that, in healthy athletes, taking L-carnitine does not significantly increase muscle carnitine content, mitochondrial numbers or physical performance[5]. It appears to have no significant effect on aerobic or anaerobic exercise performance[6].

Chronic fatigue: As L-carnitine is needed for production of energy in muscle cells, it may play a role in chronic fatigue syndrome

1. Cherchi A et al. Int J Pharmacol Ther Toxicol 1985;23(10):569–72
2. Brevetti G et al. J Am Coll Cardiol 1999;34(5):1618–24
3. Hiatt WR et al. Am J Med 2001;110(8):616–22
4. Evans JD et al. Ann Pharmacother 2008;42(11):1686–91
5. Wachter S et al. Clin Chim Acta 2002;318(1–2):51–61
6. Smith WA et al. Int J Sport Nutr Exerc Metab 2008;18(1):19–36

(CFS). However, research comparing blood and urinary levels of carnitine in people with chronic fatigue has not shown any differences compared with levels in healthy controls[1]. Even so, a small study comparing the effects of L-carnitine versus an anti-viral drug found statistically significant improvement with the supplement after eight weeks' treatment. It may, however, be beneficial for fatigue in elderly people by increasing total lean muscle mass and increasing physical and cognitive function[2].

Sperm health: L-carnitine is needed for energy production within sperm cells for optimum sperm motility. It may therefore be helpful for some men with infertility due to reduced sperm movements. When 100 men with low fertility were treated with 2 g L-carnitine per day, there was a statistically significant increase in total sperm count and in the proportion of sperm that could swim forwards vigorously[3]. It appears to be effective in improving sperm health in both smokers and non-smokers[4].

Erectile dysfunction: Some studies have found that L-carnitine improved the response to sildenafil (Viagra) in men with diabetes who had not responded to sildenafil on its own.

Peyronie's disease: A study comparing L-carnitine to tamoxifen in 48 men with Peyronie's found it was significantly more effective at reducing pain during intercourse and in minimizing penile curvature[5]. However, another study found that carnitine and/or vitamin E was no more effective than placebo[6].

Dose

500 mg–3 g a day usually in divided doses.

It is often combined with the antioxidant, alpha-lipoic acid (see page 34).

1. Jones MG et al. Clin Chim Acta 2005;360(1–2):173–7
2. Malaquarnera M et al Am J Clin Nutr 2007;86(6):1738–44
3. Lenzi A et al. Fertil Steril 2003;79:292–300
4. Khademi A et al. J Assist Reprod Genet 2005;22(11–12):395–9
5. Biagiotti G, Cavallini G. BJU Int 2001;88(1):63–7
6. Safarinejad MR et al. J Urol 2007;178(4 Pt 1):1398–403

Excess
Diarrhoea may occur at doses in excess of 4 g a day. Increased body odour can also occur at very high doses.

Carotenoids

Over 600 carotenoids are present in fruit and vegetables, but only a few such as alphacarotene, astaxanthin (see page 53), betacarotene (page 62), lycopene (page 213), lutein (page 211) and zeaxanthin are currently recognized as important for human health.

Carotenoids are found in yellow, orange, red and dark green fruits and vegetables, including sweetcorn, carrots, pumpkins, spinach, mangoes, oranges, peaches, guavas, watermelons, spinach and other dark-green leafy vegetables. They are rapidly destroyed by heat and overcooking.

Around 50 of the identified carotenoids can be converted into vitamin A in the body and are said to have pro-vitamin A activity. Of these, the most prevalent in the diet are alphacarotene, betacarotene, gammacarotene and cryptoxanthin. It takes 6 mcg of betacarotene to yield 1 mcg of retinol vitamin A. For other carotenoids with pro-vitamin A activity, it takes 12 mcg to yield 1 mcg of retinol.

Benefits
They have an important antioxidant action in the body, especially in protecting cell membranes from free radical attack, and by reducing oxidation of circulating fats such as cholesterol.

Macular degeneration: Those who eat the most carotenoids have at least a 60 per cent lower risk of developing age-related macular degeneration (AMD) of the eye than those with low intakes. These benefits are mainly related to lutein and zeaxanthin.

Hip fracture: Increased intakes of total carotenoids may lower the risk of hip fracture according to a 17-year study involving almost 1,000 adults with an average age of 75 years. When the effect of individual carotenoids was assessed, lycopene had the greatest protective effect. Carotenoids are believed to protect bone health through their antioxidant activity as oxidation reactions appear to increase bone resorption[1].

Glucose control: A study[2] involving 133 people with diabetes, 155 people with glucose intolerance and 288 matched controls with normal glucose found that those with the highest intake of carotenoids from carrots and pumpkins were 50 per cent less likely to have poor glucose tolerance than those with low intakes. Blood levels of alpha- and beta-carotenes, lycopene, beta-cryptoxanthin, zeaxanthin and lutein all showed a beneficial effect suggesting that intake of vegetables and fruits rich in carotenoids might be a protective factor against developing raised blood glucose levels.

Dose

6–15 mg mixed carotenoids per day, ideally taken together with other antioxidants such as vitamins C, E and selenium.

Carotenodermia, in which the skin acquires an orange colour due to a high intake of carotenoids, is harmless and will quickly resolve once intakes are reduced. In fact, this effect is deliberately sought to protect the skin in certain photosensitivity disorders, and high-dose carotenoids have not shown any significant toxicity.

Contraindications

High doses of carotenoids should be avoided during pregnancy.

Cat's claw
(Uncaria tomentosa)

Cat's claw (also known as *uña de gato*) is derived from a woody South American vine native to the Amazon rainforest. Its root and bark contain potent alkaloids and antioxidants, such as quinic acid, some of which have been found in the laboratory to possess antiviral, antibacterial and anti-cancer activity. In the laboratory, it enhances repair of cell DNA, appears to reduce the proliferation of

1. Sahni S et al. J Bone Miner Res 2009; 24(6):1086–94
2. Suzuki K et al. J Epidemiol 2002;12(5):357–66

cancerous cells and to promote their programmed cell death (apoptosis).

Cat's claw is used to balance and support immune function by prolonging the lifespan of white blood cells (lymphocytes) and boosting their ability to absorb and destroy (phagocytose) micro-organisms, abnormal cells and foreign particles. It has traditionally been used to help treat recurrent infections, including sinusitis, and conditions associated with long-term pain including gout.

Benefits

Rheumatoid arthritis: It has anti-inflammatory actions, especially towards gastrointestinal inflammatory conditions such as gastritis, and joint problems. In a trial involving 40 people with rheumatoid arthritis who were taking anti-inflammatory drugs, cat's claw extracts were added to their treatment regime. In those receiving cat's claw for 24 weeks, there was a 53 per cent reduction in the number of painful joints compared with 24 per cent in those receiving placebo[1]. Only minor side effects were reported.

Osteoarthritis: A trial involving 45 people with osteoarthritis of the knee found that taking cat's claw supplement significantly reduced pain within the first week of therapy[2].

Dose

It is generally advisable to start with a low dose (e.g. 300 mg standardized extracts) and slowly build up to a therapeutic dose (e.g. 750 mg standardized extracts or more). It is best taken under medical supervision.

Side effects

High doses of cat's claw may cause diarrhoea. It may cause reversible worsening of the symptoms of Parkinson's disease.

Contraindications

Cat's claw increases the immune rejection of foreign cells, and should not be used:

1. Mur E et al. J Rheumatol 2002;29(4):678–81
2. Piscoya J et al. Inflamm Res 2001;50(9):442–8

- During pregnancy or breast-feeding
- By anyone who has recently had – or is scheduled to receive – an organ/bone marrow transplant or skin-graft
- By those taking immunosuppressive drugs
- By those with Parkinson's disease (a worsening of symptoms has been reported).

Some researchers also recommend that cat's claw is stopped two days before and after receiving chemotherapy.

Catuaba
(Erythroxylon vacciniifolium; Trichilia catigua)

Catuaba – known as the 'tree of love' – is the name given to several tree species that are native to Brazil. The bark of these trees contains aromatic resins and nonaddictive alkaloids – catuabins – that are distantly related to cocaine.

Benefits
Catuaba bark is traditionally used as an aphrodisiac to stimulate sexual desire and to promote erotic dreams. It is said to boost sexual energy in both men and women. Those using it claim that erotic dreams usually start between five and 21 days of taking extracts regularly, and that these are followed by increased sexual desire. It is also said to improve peripheral blood flow which may be another mechanism for boosting sexual performance, and it has been used to combat extreme exhaustion. None of these attributes appears to have been subjected to published clinical trials.

Interestingly, catuaba extracts appear to have antibacterial and anti-viral properties in the laboratory. They are also under investigation for an antidepressant action.

Dose
1 g on waking, and 1 g on going to bed.

Cayenne

(Capsicum frutescens)

Cayenne, or chilli pepper, is a perennial shrub native to Mexico. The immature (green) and ripe (scarlet) fruits are a popular 'hot' culinary spice. Cayenne peppers contain steroidal saponins known as capsaicinoids, of which around 70 per cent is in the form of capsaicin. Capsaicinoids are especially concentrated in the white tissue supporting the chilli seeds.

Capsaicin is an irritant that produces a burning sensation when in contact with mucus membranes such as those in the mouth. The hotter the pepper, the higher its capsaicin content. The hotness of chilli peppers is measured according to the Scoville Scale, in which a sweet bell pepper has a Scoville rating of Zero (no capsaicin) while the hottest chilli, the habanero, has a rating of 200,000 plus – this means its juice must be diluted more than 200,000 times before its capsaicin becomes undetectable.

Scoville rating	Type of pepper
15,000,000–16,000,000	Pure capsaicin
350,000–577,000	Habanero
100,000–350,000	Scotch Bonnet
100,000–200,000	Jamaican Hot Pepper
50,000–100,000	Thai Pepper
30,000–50,000	Cayenne Pepper, Tabasco Pepper
10,000–23,000	Serrano Pepper
7,000–8,000	Tabasco Sauce
2,500–8,000	Jalapeno Pepper
500–1000	Anaheim Pepper
100–500	Pimento; Pepperoncini
0	Sweet Bell Pepper

Cayenne is traditionally used to stimulate circulation to the hands, feet and genitals, and to promote sweating. It is said to have aphrodisiac properties and to help maintain an erection. It aids digestion, relieves flatulence and reduces the risk of peptic ulcers by stimulating production of protective stomach mucus, and by improving blood flow in the stomach wall.

Capsaicin cream or ointment may be helpful for reducing skin itching, pain due to fibromyalgia, post-herpetic pain, diabetic neuropathy, and for stimulating poor circulation to the digits as occurs in Raynaud's syndrome. It is also included in creams designed to be rubbed into joints to reduce discomfort in osteoarthritis. It provides a dual benefit as capsaicin also blocks the activity of decapeptide substance P (DSP), thereby protecting against cartilage breakdown in osteoarthritis.

Herbalists also use chilli extracts to stimulate the secretion of gastric juices, improve digestion, prevent infection and to treat some types of diarrhoea. However, recent research shows that following a chilli-rich diet decreases gastric acid secretion.

Benefits
Pain: Although it can trigger painful burning sensations, it is used medically as an analgesic. It works by sinking down to nerve endings and reducing their content of a chemical, known as substance P, that is needed to transmit pain impulses to the brain. As a result, its continued presence can numb pain. A meta-analysis of the results from six clinical trials involving over 650 people found that topical capsaicin was significantly more effective than placebo in achieving a 50 per cent or greater reduction in pain[1].

Dose
Usually around 500–1000 mg a day.

Note: Chilli ointment or cream should not be applied to raw skin or to the eyes as this will be excruciatingly painful.

Chamomile
(Matricaria chamomilla or M. recutita)

German chamomile is one of the most important medicinal herbs. It was used by the ancient Egyptians, Greeks and Romans for its soothing and relaxing properties, and also to reduce fevers. It

---

1. Mason L et al. BMJ 2004;328(7446):991

remains a popular herbal remedy today. It is a rich source of anti-oxidant polyphenols, including coumarins and flavonoids which are soluble in water. Drinking chamomile tea is therefore an important nutritional source of antioxidants.

Chamomile contains chamazulene and alpha-bisabolol which have anti-allergic, anti-inflammatory, and antispasmodic actions. It is also a sedative. It helps to relieve intestinal spasm associated with wind, colic and irritable bowel syndrome, and can also relieve menstrual cramps and may improve asthma. Chamomile infusions are often used to help cleanse the skin, mouth, gums and eyes. It has a mild sedative action, helping to reduce anxiety, stress and to promote sleep. Chamomile tea may be given to children and taken during pregnancy.

Chamomile is used externally to help reduce skin and mucous membrane inflammation, including eczema and inflammation of the genital region (baths and irrigation).

Benefits

Diarrhoea: A study involving 255 children (aged six months to six years) with acute diarrhoea found that, compared with placebo, a preparation containing chamomile/apple pectin significantly reduce the duration of symptoms[1].

Diabetes: Recent research suggests that drinking chamomile tea may help to reduce blood glucose levels by inhibiting the break-down of glycogen stores in the liver[2]. It may also reduce the accumulation of sorbitol within cells of diabetic subjects – one of the main causes of diabetes complications. Although these findings need further investigation, there is little harm in enjoying a cup of soothing chamomile tea as a potent source of dietary anti-oxidants.

Dose

1–3 cups chamomile tea a day.

1. Becker B et al. Arzneimittelforschung 2006;56(6):387–93
2. Kato A et al. J Agric Food Chem 2008;56(17):8206–11

Chitosan

Chitosan is a polysaccharide, fibre supplement derived from shell-fish such as crabs and prawns. It can also be obtained from the cell walls of certain fungi.

Benefits
Chitosan is marketed as a 'fat attractor' that is claimed to aid weight loss by absorbing dietary fat in the intestines so more is excreted. When combined with a low-fat diet, this may promote weight loss and reduce circulating blood fat levels.

Weight loss: A number of clinical trials have suggested that volunteers following a low-calorie diet lose more weight when taking chitosan than those not taking it. Significant improvements in blood pressure and blood fat levels have also occurred.

However, a meta-analysis of 14 trials involving over 1,000 participants suggests that the effects of chitosan are small, amounting to an average increase in weight loss of 1.7 kg compared with placebo over an average of eight weeks[1]. When the analysis was restricted to high quality trials, the difference was just 0.6 kg.

Dose
3–6 g a day.

Chloride

Chloride is a negatively charged electrolyte of chlorine. The body contains around 115 g of chloride ions, kept constant by the excretion of excess salts in sweat, urine and faeces.

Chloride, together with sodium (outside the cells) and potassium (inside the cells), regulates the body's fluid, electrolyte and acid/alkaline balance. It also aids digestion through the production of hydrochloric acid in the stomach, and through cleansing body wastes in the liver.

Foods containing chloride include fruits, vegetables, kelp, seafood, table salt and processed foods. As chloride is widespread in foods, deficiency is unlikely except in excessive vomiting.

1. Mhurchu CN et al. Obes Rev 2005; 6(1):35–42

Dose

The newly set EU RDA for chloride is 800 mg. The UK RNI for adults is 2500 mg per day. Dietary supplements are rarely needed and should only be taken under medical supervision.

Choline and phosphatidylcholine (Lecithin)

Choline is an essential substance related to the B vitamins, and to the amino acid, methionine. Until recently, it was thought to be made in the body in adequate amounts to meet our needs. Since 1998, however, this is no longer thought to be the case, especially in later life.

Choline is a component of phosphatidylcholine, which is vital for the structural integrity of cell membranes. It acts as a building block for the production of certain neurotransmitters in the brain, including acetylcholine, noradrenaline and dopamine. It is therefore involved in concentration and alertness. Choline also acts as an emulsifier to help break down dietary fats into smaller particles that can be absorbed and used in the body, and is involved in HDL-cholesterol metabolism. Cholesterol transport in the circulation, and its removal from the tissues, depends on the activity of an enzyme called lecithin cholesterol acyltransferase (LCAT). This enzyme appears to protect against atherosclerosis, and its activity is influenced by the types of fatty acid in our diets. A diet high in saturated fat appears to have a negative effect on LCAT activity.

Most dietary choline is derived from the closely related substance, phosphatidyl-choline (also known as lecithin). Choline is obtained from many food sources, including egg yolk, liver, meat, fish, wheatgerm, peanuts, Brazil nuts, beans and green leafy vegetables. The lecithin found in supplements is usually extracted from soybeans.

If choline is in short supply, cells cannot function properly and enter a process known as apoptosis or programmed cell death. Conditions that have been linked with choline deficiency include fatty liver degeneration, hardening of the arteries, Alzheimer's disease, high blood pressure, nervousness, learning difficulties, depression and stomach ulcers.

Benefits

Memory: Phosphatidylcholine supplements can increase brain levels of acetylcholine and improve memory storage and retrieval. Some studies have shown improvements in memory test scores in people taking lecithin, while others have shown no benefit. A review of 12 clinical trials involving 90 people with Alzheimer's disease, Parkinsonian dementia or subjective memory problems did not show any clear benefits for those with diagnosed dementia, but did find benefits for those with subjective memory problems[1].

Depression: People with depression who failed to respond to prescribed drugs have also benefited from taking phosphatidylcholine supplements.

Cholesterol: In 47 people with Type 2 diabetes, taking a lecithin and soy protein supplement for 12 weeks was shown to significantly reduce total cholesterol by 12 per cent, LDL-cholesterol by 16 per cent and increase beneficial HDL-cholesterol by 11 per cent. In addition, blood triglyceride levels fell by 22 per cent[2].

Liver health: Research suggests that lack of choline is linked with an increased risk of developing liver cancer. If choline is in short supply, liver cells are unable to process and export dietary fats, which build up inside them to produce fatty liver degeneration and liver cell death. Abnormal regeneration of liver tissues then results in a build-up of collagen (fibrosis), cirrhosis and can trigger cancerous changes. Choline also helps to eliminate toxins from the liver and gall bladder and may be recommended for people with gallstones.

Dose

Adequate intakes are believed to be between 425–550 mg per day for adults.

Doses suggested are in the range of 2–4 g daily. Higher doses may be taken under medical supervision.

One tablespoon of lecithin granules provides 1725 mg phosphati-

1. Higgins JP, Flicker L. Cochrane Database Syst Rev 2003;(3):CD001015
2. Ristic MD et al. Nutr Metab Cardiovasc Dis 2006;16(6):395–404

dylcholine and 250 mg choline – a little less than the amount present in a hen's egg. They are best taken with meals to boost absorption.

Lecithin supplements should ideally be taken with vitamin B5 to improve their effect in the body.

Contraindications

Choline and lecithin supplements should not be taken by those with manic depression except under medical supervision in case it worsens the condition.

High doses of choline can cause indigestion, anorexia, sweating and, over time, nerve and cardiovascular distress as well as a strong, fishy body odour. Lecithin supplements are therefore generally preferred.

Chondroitin

Chondroitin sulphate is a natural substance found in the body which stimulates formation of cartilage and joint connective tissues. It is also important for the production of synovial fluid – the joint's oil – making it thicker and more cushioning.

Chondroitin supplements are widely taken by people with osteoarthritis, usually together with glucosamine, as a source of materials needed to boost joint repair. Chondroitin is also believed to suppress the enzymes involved in breaking down cartilage.

Benefits

Osteoarthritis: Chondroitin sulphate has been used alone to treat osteoarthritis in a number of trials. In five meta-analyses of data from these trials, four showed significant beneficial effects against pain, and one showed reduced need for analgesics in people taking the chondroitin supplements. These studies suggest that chondroitin sulphate has a slight to moderate effect on osteoarthritis and a low incidence of side effects[1]. Although some studies have not shown benefit, currently available data does suggest that chondroitin sulphate has structure-modifying effects in osteoarthritic knees[2].

---

1. Monfort J et al. Curr Med Res Opin 2008;24(5), 1303–1308
2. Uebelhart D. Osteoarthritis Cartilage 2008;16 Suppl 3:S19–21

Chondroitin plus Glucosamine: Until recently, most evidence suggested that the combination of glucosamine and chondroitin has a synergistic action that is significantly greater than the effects of the two individual substances added together. This is because glucosamine stimulates production of cartilage building blocks (glycosaminoglycans) while chondroitin sulphate inhibits their breakdown. A meta-analysis of 15 trials looking at the effects of combining glucosamine sulphate with chondroitin sulphate, in 1,775 people with osteoarthritis of the knee, found that, while glucosamine and chondroitin appeared to reduce joint pain and improve mobility in people with OA of the knee, there was not enough data to assess whether or not chondroitin also helped to preserve the knee joint space in the same way as glucosamine[1].

Recently, some researchers have suggested that combining glucosamine sulphate with chondroitin sulphate may decrease the bioavailability of glucosamine to reduce its effectiveness[2]. This is currently under investigation.

Dose

1200 mg per day.

Some chondroitin is synthesized from marine sources (shark cartilage) while others use bovine (cow) cartilage.

Safety

A recent review confirmed the excellent safety profile of chondroitin sulphate.

If taking blood thinning agents, regular blood-clotting checks may be needed when taking chondroitin due to a possible increased bleeding time in some people.

Increased concentrations of chondroitin in prostate cancer tissue have been linked with increased rate of relapse although this does not appear to affect survival outcome[3]. It is important to note that these findings occurred in men who were not taking chondroitin supplements. However, if you have prostate cancer you may be advised to avoid taking chondroitin supplements.

1. Richy F et al. Arch Int Med 2003; 163(13), 1514–22
2. Bruyere O. Osteoarthritis Cartilage 2008;16(2), 254–60
3. Ricciardelli C et al. Prostate 2009;69(7):761–9

Chromium

Chromium exists in several forms in nature. The hexavalent form of chromium (used in industry) is toxic and can cause skin and mucous membrane ulceration, gastro-enteritis, liver and kidney problems and cancer. However, the trivalent form is non-toxic at recommended doses and can produce beneficial effects in the body. Supplements usually contain either chromium picolinate or chromium polynicotinate. Concerns about the safety of chromium picolinate were raised based on research in fruit flies, but after thorough investigation, they have been dismissed by the US Institute of Medicine, the UK Committee on Mutagenicity and the Food Standards Agency (who, since 2004, no longer suggest people avoid this type of chromium).

Foods containing chromium include egg yolk, red meat, cheese, fruit and fruit juice, wholegrains, honey, vegetables and condiments such as black pepper and thyme. As plants do not need chromium, the content of fruit and vegetables depends entirely on the amount and type of chromium present in the soil in which the plants are grown. Processing can reduce the mineral content of foods by up to 80 per cent. Most refined carbohydrates have little chromium content and people eating processed foods will have low intakes.

Interestingly, chromium levels are highest just after birth, then rapidly decrease especially after the age of ten. Levels then become increasingly low with age[1]. Some experts believe that this finding reflects a widespread nutritional deficiency and may be related to premature ageing[2].

Chromium deficiency is thought to be common. One estimate suggests that 90 per cent of adults are deficient as most people get less than 50 mcg from their diet, and only around 2 per cent of this is in an absorbable (trivalent) form. Intestinal absorption is low (0.5–2 per cent) except where chromium is present in the form of GTF. Symptoms that may be due to chromium deficiency include glucose intolerance, alcohol intolerance, abnormal blood fat levels, muscle weakness, hunger pangs, weight gain, nervousness,

1. Davis S et al. Metabolism 1997; 46:469–73
2. Preuss HG. J Am Coll Nutr. 1997; 16;5:397–403

irritability, confusion, depression, thirst, decreased sperm count and impaired fertility.

Trivalent chromium is an essential trace element that is needed in minute amounts to form an organic complex known as the Glucose Tolerance Factor (GTF). This complex also contains vitamin B3 (niacin) plus amino acids, and is also known as chromium dinicotinic acid glutathione. GTF interacts with the pancreatic hormone, insulin, to regulate the uptake of glucose by cells. It increases insulin binding to cells, insulin receptor number and activates insulin receptors leading to increased insulin sensitivity[1]. It also encourages the production of energy from glucose, especially in muscles, increases protein synthesis and lowers blood fat levels, including harmful LDL-cholesterol. It may also suppress hunger pangs through a direct effect on the satiety centre in the brain.

Benefits

Diabetes: Low levels of chromium have been linked with poor glucose tolerance[2,3,4,5] and a dietary lack of chromium appears to be a risk factor for Type 2 diabetes in some people. Some researchers have even suggested that Type 2 diabetes is an age-related chromium deficiency disease, although this is controversial[6]. Results have been conflicting and it is likely that chromium supplements only have beneficial effects in people with Type 2 diabetes who have a marked chromium deficiency. It may also depend on the genes you have inherited. Even so, 13 out of 15 trials, including 11 randomized controlled trials, involving almost 1,700 people found that those taking chromium supplements showed significant improvements in at least one measure of glycaemic control[7]. A systematic review of 41 studies showed it significantly improved glucose levels in people with diabetes[8].

Coronary heart disease: Chromium levels in people with coronary

1. Anderson RA. Diabetes Metab 2000;26;1:22–7
2. Glinsmann WH, Mertz W. Metabolism 1966;15:510–20
3. Martinez OB et al. Nutr Res 1985;5:609–20
4. Potter JF et al. Metabolism 1985;34:199–204
5. Levine RA et al. Metabolism 1968;17:114–25
6. Davis S et al. Metabolism 1997;46:469–73
7. Broadhurst CL, Domenico P. Diabetes Technol Ther 2006;8(6):677–87
8. Balk EM et al. Diabetes Care 2007;30(8):2154–63

heart disease are lower than in healthy people and it has been suggested that chromium deficiency may be an independent risk factor for cardiovascular disease[1]. Some studies suggest that chromium may help to reduce the risk of coronary heart disease by lowering blood levels of harmful low-density lipoprotein (LDL) cholesterol and raising levels of beneficial high-density (HDL) cholesterol. A systematic review of 41 studies however found no significant effects on lipid metabolism in people without diabetes[2].

Weight loss: Because chromium has an effect on appetite, hunger pangs and fat metabolism, it is widely used as a slimming aid and, when combined with a sensible diet and regular exercise, chromium supplements may help some people to lose weight (especially if they are deficient in chromium). While some studies have shown it to be beneficial in weight loss, others have shown little benefit and a meta-analysis of ten trials found that those taking chromium picolinate lost, on average, 1.1 kg more than those not taking placebo[3]. More research is needed.

Cataracts: Chromium has an antioxidant action which, in addition to improving glucose control, may protect against cataracts. Researchers have recently found that people with diabetes who have cataracts have lower levels of chromium than those without cataracts.

Dose

The newly set EU RDA for chromium is 40 mcg. In general, the more carbohydrate you eat, the more chromium you need. Intakes are generally low, however. One study of 22 people following a 'well-balanced' diet found that the average intake was 13.4 mcg per day[4]. The upper safe level for long-term use from supplements is suggested as 10 mg (10,000 mcg) per day.

Supplements are best absorbed when taken with vitamin C, while calcium-containing supplements will reduce absorption.

Brewer's yeast is a particularly good source of chromium present

1. Simonoff M. 1984. Chromium deficiency and cardiovascular risk. Cardiovasc Res. 18;10:591–6
2. Balk EM et al. Diabetes Care 2007; 30(8):2154–63
3. Pittler MH et al. In J Obes Relat Metab Disord 2003; 27(4):522–9
4. Anderson RA et al. Biol Trace Elem Res 1992; 32:117–21

as it is already in the form of GTF, making it at least ten times more effective than that obtained from other food sources.

Do not exceed the stated dose as this may affect zinc and iron absorption.

Cinnamon
(Cinnamomum verum)

Cinnamon is an evergreen tree whose bark contains unique aromatic substances such as cinnamaldehyde and ethylcinamate. The bark is harvested after coppicing two-year-old trees to promote the formation of shoots from the root. The bark is stripped from these shoots and the inner bark is separated from the outer wood. Strips of inner bark are packed together and curl on drying to form the familiar quills.

Benefits

Type 2 diabetes: Several studies suggest that cinnamon extracts can improve glucose tolerance and insulin resistance. Doses of 3 g produce a significant reduction in insulin secretion, while 1 g has no significant effect[1]. According to one review of three trials, cinnamon appears to lower fasting glucose levels by 10.3–29 per cent[2]. The most promising study, involving 60 people with diabetes, found that taking cinnamon reduced mean fasting glucose by 18–29 per cent, triglycerides by 23–30 per cent, LDL-cholesterol by 7–27 per cent and total cholesterol by 12–26 per cent with no significant changes in those on placebo[3]. However, a 2007 analysis of five clinical trials in humans concluded that there was not enough currently available evidence on which to base a recommendation to use cinnamon for improvement of glycaemic control[4].

Polycystic ovary syndrome: PCOS is associated with insulin resistance. A trial involving 15 women with PCOS compared the effects of cinnamon with placebo over eight weeks. Significant improvements in insulin resistance were seen in those taking cinnamon, but

1. Hlebowicz J et al. Am J Clin Nutr 2009;89(3):815–21
2. Dugoua JJ et al. Can J Physiol Pharmacol 2007;85(9):837–47
3. Khan A et al. Diabetes Care 2003;26(12):3215–8
4. Kleefstra N et al. Ned Tijdschr Geneeskd 2007 151(51):2833–7

not in the placebo group[1]. More studies are needed to evaluate the effect of cinnamon on menstruation in this condition.

Dose
1–6 g daily.

If you have diabetes, monitor blood glucose levels carefully when taking supplements and ensure you know how to adjust your medication if improvements occur.

Cinnamon has been reported to worsen rosacea in some people.

CMO (cis-9-cetyl myristoleate)

CMO is a waxy oil (also known as cetylated fatty acids or CFS) which has a natural anti-inflammatory action. It helps to lubricate joints and is mainly taken to improve joint pain in osteoarthritis and rheumatoid arthritis. It is often taken together with fish or flaxseed oil, vitamin E and glucosamine sulphate and sometimes with an enzyme, lipase, to aid its digestion.

Benefits
Osteoarthritis: In a trial involving 64 people with knee osteoarthritis, taking cetylated fatty acids significantly improved knee flexion (by 10 degrees) and overall joint function compared with those taking placebo (1 degree) after 68 days[2].

Few other trials have been published in reputable journals, unfortunately, though there are plenty of anecdotal reports of benefit.

Dose
Doses of up to 600 mg daily are used. CMO is expensive and I suspect that other supplements such as omega-3 fish oils and glucosamine sulphate may be more cost-effective.

From personal experience I can say that applying CMO cream to painful joints is surprisingly effective!

1. Wang JG et al. Fertil Steril 2007:88(1);240–3
2. Hesslink R Jr et al. J Rheumatol 2002;29(8):1708–12

Coccinia indica

Coccinia indica is a creeper that grows wild in India, Ayurvedic physicians have used it as an antidiabetic drug for centuries. It contains substances that have an insulin-like action on enzymes involved in glucose metabolism.

Benefits
Glucose control: In a study involving 60 people with newly diagnosed Type 2 diabetes (aged 35–60 years) some took 1 g Coccinia extract daily for 90 days, while some took placebo. Those in the Coccinia group showed significant improvements in fasting and post-prandial (after meal) glucose levels compared with controls, with reductions of 16 per cent (fasting) and 18 per cent (post-prandial)[1].

Dose
1 g daily.

May interact with other glucose-lowering agents. People taking hypoglycaemic drugs should use Coccinia with caution, under medical supervision, to avoid hypoglycaemia.

Co-enzyme Q10

Co-enzyme Q10 (CoQ10) – also known as ubiquinone – is a vitamin-like substance that is present in all body cells, with the heart, liver cells and sperm cells containing the greatest amounts. CoQ10 is needed to process oxygen in cells, and to generate energy-rich molecules. Without CoQ10, the energy hidden in food molecules could not be converted into a form of energy in muscle cells, including those of the heart. After the age of 20, levels of CoQ10 start to decrease as dietary CoQ10 is absorbed less efficiently from the intestines and its production in body cells starts to fall. Dietary sources include meat, fish, wholegrains, nuts and green vegetables.

Low levels of CoQ10 mean that cells do not receive all the energy they need. As a result, they function at a sub-optimal level and are

1. Kuriyan R et al. Diabetes Care 2008;31(2):216–20

more likely to become diseased, age and even die. Research suggests that falling CoQ10 levels play a significant role in age-related medical conditions such as coronary heart disease. CoQ10 is now also being added to skin-care preparations to reduce skin damage that leads to premature wrinkles, especially following exposure to UVA in sunlight.

Benefits

CoQ10 acts together with vitamin E to form a powerful antioxidant defence against oxidation damage to body fats – including those in the circulation. Like other antioxidants, CoQ10 seems to protect against hardening and furring up of the arteries (atherosclerosis), to reduce heart disease and is also helpful for those with Raynaud's syndrome.

Reducing statin side effects: CoQ10 is especially important for the increasing number of people taking a statin drug to lower their cholesterol levels. Statins (atorvastatin, fluvastatin, pravastatin, rosuvastatin and simvastatin) reduce cholesterol production in the liver by inhibiting an enzyme, HMG-CoA reductase, which is involved in the synthesis of both cholesterol and co-enzyme Q10[1]. Statins are generally considered safe but, like all medicines, they can have side effects. Ten per cent of people treated with statin drugs experience some form of muscle-related side effects in clinical practice[2]. These range from asymptomatic creatine kinase elevation to muscle pain, weakness and, rarely, rhabdomyolysis in which muscle fibres break down. These side effects can involve heart muscle and may increase the risk of heart failure. These myopathies have been linked to the fact that, as well as reducing cholesterol synthesis, HMG-CoA reductase inhibition reduces co-enzyme Q10 production[3,4,5,6,7]. In fact, taking a statin can halve circulating levels of co-enzyme Q10 within just two weeks[8]. If your doctor suggests

1. Passi S et al. BioFactors 2003;18:113–24
2. Venero V, Thompson PD. Endocrinol Metab Clin North Am 2009;38(1):121–36
3. Langsjoen PH, Langsjoen AM. BioFactors 2003;18:101–11
4. Littarru GP, Langsjoen P. Mitochondrion 2007;7S:S168–74
5. Bliznakov EG, Wilkins DJ. Advances in Therapy 1998;15:218–28
6. Passi S et al. BioFactors 2003;18:113–24
7. Ghirlanda G et al. J Clin Pharmacol 1993;33:226–9
8. Rundek T et al. Arch Neurol 2004;61(6):889–92

you would benefit from taking a statin drug, it's equally important to consider taking a co-enzyme Q10 supplement[1].

Taking co-enzyme Q10 supplements helps to maintain blood levels of this important muscle nutrient while taking statin drugs[2,3,4]. This has the potential to decrease muscle pain associated with statin therapy, and offers an alternative to stopping treatment with this important class of drugs[5]. Evidence shows that the use of a supplemental co-enzyme Q10 could reverse any early muscle weakness and fatigue caused by statin drug therapy[6].This is an important strategy given that, in one study, 75 per cent of over 85,000 patients taking statins for primary prevention of CHD were no longer refilling their prescriptions after just two years[7]. Importantly, taking co-enzyme Q10 does not affect the cholesterol-lowering action of statin drugs[8].

Heart disease: Biopsies of heart muscle from patients with various forms of heart disease have shown that up to 75 per cent are deficient in CoQ10. The more severe the heart disease, the lower the levels of CoQ10. It has therefore been used by some doctors in the USA and Japan to treat coronary heart disease and heart failure.

Hypertension: CoQ10 can reduce hypertension by improving the elasticity and reactivity of the blood vessel wall. Adding 225 mg CoQ10 to existing hypertensive drug regimes was found to produce significant, gradual improvements in BP so that 51 per cent of participants were able to stop between one and three antihypertensive drugs within 4.4 months of starting CoQ10. A meta-analysis of data from 12 clinical trials, involving over 360 patients, found that CoQ10 could reduce BP by up to 17/10 mmHg compared with placebo, without significant side effects[9].

1. Langsjoen PH & Langsjoen AM. BioFactors 2003;18:101–11
2. Bargossi AM et al. Molecular Aspects of Medicine 1994;15S:s187–93
3. Mabuchi H et al. Atherosclerosis 2007;195:182–9
4. Chapidze G et al. Georgian Medical News 2005;118:20–5
5. Caso G et al. Am J Cardiol 2007;99(10):1409–12
6. Silver AM et al. Am J Cardiol 2004;94(10):1306–10
7. Jackevicius CA et al. JAMA 2002;288(4):462–7
8. Bargossi AM et al. Molecular Aspects of Medicine 1994;15S:s187–93
9. Rosenfeldt FL et al. J Hum Hypertens 2007;21(4):297–306

Sperm quality: CoQ10 is vital for production of the energy sperm need for motility. Men with reduced sperm motility showed significant improvements in sperm function when taking CoQ10 supplements, and in fertility treatments their sperm were over twice as likely to fertilize an egg compared with those not taking CoQ10.

Immune function: CoQ10 supplements – both given alone and with vitamin B6 – increase the number of antibodies made after vaccination, and also increase the number of certain immune cells to boost immunity. It may also be useful in weight loss by stimulating lipid metabolism in mitochondria.

Gum disease: Diseased gum tissue has significantly lower levels of CoQ10 compared with healthy gum tissue from the same patient. A trial involving 49 patients with periodontal disease found that, compared with placebo, combining periodontal hygeine treatments plus 60 mg CoQ10 daily for 12 weeks produced significant reductions in the depth of periodontal pockets. CoQ10 was able to reverse periodontal gum disease and save teeth scheduled for surgery[1]. Application of a topical gel containing co-enzyme CoQ10 can also improve probing depths and attachment loss in periodontal pockets[2].

Dose
The optimal dietary intake of CoQ10 is unknown. Average adult dietary intakes of CoQ10 are estimated at 3–5 mg daily among meat eaters and 1 mg daily among vegetarians. Commercially available dietary supplements recommend 10–100 mg CoQ10 daily – often taken as two separate doses. If you are on a statin drug, doses of 100–400 mg may be needed to reduce muscle-related side effects. Higher doses of up to 600 mg daily are used under medical supervision to treat illnesses such as heart disease and high blood pressure.

CoQ10 is best taken with food to improve absorption as it is fat-soluble. It usually takes at least three weeks and occasionally up to three months before the full beneficial effect and extra energy levels are noticed.

1. Iwamoto et al. Biomedical and Clinical Aspects of CoQ10 Vol 3 109–119; Elsevier/North Holland Biomedical Press 1981
2. Hanioka T et al. Mol Aspects Med 1994;15(Suppl):S241–8

Side effects
Only occasional and transient mild nausea has been reported at high doses.

Conjugated linoleic acid

Conjugated linoleic acids (CLA) are fatty acids mainly found in meat and dairy products. CLA cannot be synthesized in the human body. It is formed in ruminant animals with more than one stomach, such as the cow, by the action of an enzyme (linoleic acid isomerase) produced by an intestinal bacteria (*Butyrivibrio fibrisolvens*) which acts on dietary linoleic acid before it is absorbed into body tissues. Changes in farming practices, food processing and reduced consumption of milk and high fat foods mean that our CLA intake has fallen by 80 per cent compared with the amounts eaten by our Stone Age ancestors.

Because it is a fatty acid, CLA is laid down in cell membranes, where it is involved in cell growth. It differs from linoleic acid only in the placement of two double bonds within its fatty acid chain, which changes its biological actions. CLA alters the type of chemicals produced by cells when they react to stimulants such as foreign proteins, injury or even exercise. It has an anti-inflammatory effect by reducing synthesis of a substance called prostaglandin PGE-2.

Benefits
Body fat: CLA helps to promote a healthy body fat composition by increasing the breakdown of fatty tissue (lipolysis) and increasing lean body mass (muscle). It is thought to work by regulating the action of enzymes in fat cells so that less fat is laid down in these fat cells, and more is broken down and discharged from the cell, although the exact mechanism is not yet known. Once released, the fatty acids are then transported to muscle cells to act as an energy source – building muscle at the expense of fat. Research has confirmed that CLA reduces the size of fat cells. In animals, CLA consumption reduces body fat, and it has been referred to as the 'missing link' in weight-loss management. Some researchers have even claimed that obesity is a CLA deficiency disease, as it is essential for the mobilization and transport of dietary fats away from

fatty tissues to muscle cells where it is burned for fuel. However, clinical trial results are less conclusive in humans. The effect of CLA appears to be dose related, so that the more you take, the more weight you lose over the first six months. A meta-analysis of 18 studies found that taking 3.2 g CLA per day promoted an additional reduction in fact of 0.09 kg (i.e. 90 g) per week compared with placebo[1].

CLA may preferentially help to reduce waist size in people with central obesity. Twenty-five middle-aged men with abdominal obesity were randomized to receive either 4.2 g CLA per day or placebo. After four weeks those taking CLA had a significant decrease in waist size compared with placebo[2].

Insulin sensitivity: CLA appears to have an effect on the regulation of glucose and fatty acid uptake and metabolism. This may explain how CLA might help to reduce obesity and improve insulin sensitivity[3].

CLA and blood fats: One study looking at the effects of CLA in 51 people with normal blood fat levels found that taking 3 g CLA per day produced significant reductions in fasting triglyceride levels compared with controls. There were no effects on LDL-cholesterol, HDL-cholesterol, body weight, plasma glucose or insulin concentrations[4]. This study suggests that CLA can have an effect on triglyceride levels. The blend of isomers used appeared to affect results.

Dose
The average diet supplies around 100–300 mg CLA daily, but beneficial effects occur at intakes of around 3 g daily.

CLA found in supplements is produced commercially from sunflower, safflower and other oils. Trials tend to use 3–6 g daily, divided into two doses.

Products with a strength of at least 75 per cent CLA are most beneficial. Consider taking antioxidants with them to help protect them from oxidation.

1. Whigham LD et al. Am J Clin Nutr 2007;85(5):1203–11
2. Riserus U et al. Int J Obes Relat Metab Disord 2001;25;8:1129–35
3. Brown JM, McIntosh MK. J Nutr 2003; 133;10:3041–6
4. Noone EJ et al. Br J Nutr 2002;88;3:243–51

Contraindications

CLA should not be taken during pregnancy as its effects are unknown.

Copper

Copper is an essential trace element obtained from a number of dietary sources, including crustaceans and shellfish (prawns, oysters, lobster, crab), nuts, pulses, wholegrain cereals, avocado, artichokes, radishes, garlic, mushrooms and green vegetables grown in copper-rich soil. Brewer's yeast is also a good source.

Bioavailability of dietary copper is low, however, as up to 70 per cent of dietary intake remains bound to other bowel contents such as sugars, sweeteners, refined flour, raw meat, vitamin C, zinc and calcium. Supplementation is therefore important, especially if the diet is deficient.

Copper balance in the body is now known to be controlled by two genes. It plays an important role in oxygen transportation and cellular respiration within cells. It is a component of many anti-oxidant enzymes, including copper-zinc superoxide dismutase, providing important antioxidant protection against free radicals. It is also involved in iron transport, cholesterol and glucose metabolism and contraction of heart muscle. It is also needed to synthesize brain chemicals, and the two pigments melanin and haemoglobin. It is also involved in regulating blood cholesterol levels and may help to protect against hardening and furring up of the arteries (atherosclerosis).

Copper is involved in vitamin C metabolism and the synthesis of collagen – a major structural protein. It is therefore needed to maintain healthy bones, cartilage, hair and skin – especially their elasticity. In fact, if vitamin C intakes are optimal, copper deficiency can quickly occur if dietary intakes are limited.

Research

Coronary heart disease: Copper is an important antioxidant nutrient for both heart and circulatory health. Typical Western diets providing around 1 mg copper per day have been associated with reversible, potentially harmful changes in blood pressure control, cholesterol and glucose metabolism, as well as developing abnormal electrocardiograms which predispose towards coronary heart disease. Animal and human studies suggest that copper deficiency or an imbalance between zinc and copper is a cause of coronary heart disease. Dietary copper intake may be a powerful determinant of raised cholesterol as, when copper levels are low, activity of the cholesterol-making enzyme hydroxymethylglutaryl-coenzyme A reductase (the enzyme blocked by modern statin drugs) is increased.

Bone density: In one trial involving menopausal women, those taking 3 mg copper supplements did not lose significant bone density compared with those taking a placebo, who experienced a significant fall in bone mineral density, suggesting that supplements may help to prevent osteoporosis.

Deficiency

Copper deficiency appears to be relatively common as the dietary sources are not always eaten frequently. Lack of copper can occur in conditions such as Crohn's or coeliac disease or in people with a hereditary inability to process copper properly. This can lead to heart muscle problems (cardiac myopathy). Other problems that may be linked with lack of copper include anaemia, low white cell count, increased susceptibility to infection, fluid retention, loss of taste sensation, raised blood cholesterol levels, abnormal structure and pigmentation of body hair, abnormal pigmentation and loss of elasticity in skin, irritability, impaired fertility and osteoporosis.

Copper-deficient diets have been shown to reduce bone mineralization and strength. Many people with arthritis have low blood levels of copper, and are helped by wearing a copper bracelet so that trace amounts are absorbed through the skin.

Excess copper (e.g. from drinking water supplied through copper pipes) is toxic at levels just twice as high as the norm, and can lead to restlessness, nausea, vomiting, colic, diarrhoea and, in long-term cases, to copper-induced cirrhosis of the liver.

The risk of copper deficiency is greater when zinc intakes are high. The ideal dietary ratio of copper to zinc is 1:10.

Dose

The UK RNI for copper is 1.2 mg for adults aged 19–50 years. The newly set EU RDA for copper is 1 mg. The upper safe level for long-term use from supplements is suggested as 10 mg.

Cranberry
(Vaccinium macrocarpon

Cranberries are sour, red berries native to North America. They are widely used to make sauces and jelly, and are also juiced to make a popular and refreshing fruit drink.

Traditionally, cranberries were used as a poultice to dress wounds, and to prevent or treat scurvy as they have a high content of vitamin C. More recently it was recognized that cranberry juice has a beneficial effect on the urinary tract to reduce the incidence of urinary infections.

Research
Cranberries contain substances known as anti-adhesins, which prevent bacteria sticking to cells lining the urinary tract wall, allowing them to be more easily flushed out. Cranberry is also helpful for reducing the unpleasant odours associated with urinary incontinence.

Urinary tract infections (UTIs): Drinking 300 ml cranberry juice (25 per cent strength) daily can almost halve the risk of developing cystitis. Cranberry fruit solids also have beneficial anti-adhesin properties, and also help to prevent urinary tract infections. A meta-analysis of ten studies, involving 1,049 people, compared cranberry against placebo over a 12 month period. The results showed that cranberry products were significantly better than placebo in reducing the incidence of UTIs in women with recurrent infections.[1] One study, for example, involving 150 sexually active women prone to recurrent urinary infections, found that total use of antibiotics was less in those taking cranberry products, and that cranberry tablets were twice as cost-effective as organic cranberry juice for preven-tion. The review called for a head-to-head trial of cranberry versus low-dose antibiotics to compare their effectiveness. Another study

1. Jepson RG, Craig JC. Cochrane Database Syst Rev 2008;(1):CD001321

was therefore carried out with 137 older women who had experienced two or more recurrent urinary infections in the previous year. This study compared the effects of six months' treatment with cranberry extracts (500 mg) against the usual prophylactic treatment of a low dose antibiotic (trimethoprim). The average time to first recurrence was similar in both groups, although overall more women taking cranberry experienced a UTI (25 versus 14). The authors concluded that the antibiotic had a very limited advantage over cranberry extracts in preventing recurrent UTIs[1]. The antibiotics produced more adverse events, with those taking them being twice as likely to withdraw from the study as those taking cranberry.

Helicobacter pylori: Cranberry anti-adhesins can also help prevent *Helicobacter pylori* sticking to cells in the stomach lining. This may help to flush *Helicobacter* from the stomach so they are expelled more easily to help reduce the risk of gastritis and peptic ulcers. A study involving 189 adults with *H. pylori* infection showed that, after 90 days, more of those taking cranberry juice had cleared the infection compared with placebo (14 per cent versus 5 per cent)[2].

Dose

Cranberry juice: 300 ml (25 per cent strength) daily for treatment; 200 ml for prevention.

Cranberry extracts: 500 mg daily.

Note: If a urinary tract infection is suspected, medical advice should always be sought – especially during pregnancy.

Damiana
(Turnera diffusa aphrodisiaca)

Damiana is a small shrub with aromatic leaves that smell similar to chamomile. It has a long tradition of use as an aphrodisiac and this is reflected in its botanical name, *T. aphrodisiaca*.

The volatile, aromatic oils of damiana are said to have a stimulant

1. McMurdo ME et al. J Antimicrob Chemother 2009; 63(2):389–95
2. Zhang L et al. Helicobacter 2005;10(2):139–45

and gently irritating effect on the genitals to produce localized tingling and throbbing sensations. Its alkaloids may also boost circulation to the genital area and increase sensitivity of nerve endings in the clitoris and penis. Blood flow to the penis is also said to increase so that erections are firmer and more long lasting. These combined effects are said to increase sexual desire, enhance sexual pleasure and stimulate performance.

It is also used as a tonic for the nervous system, mild laxative, anxiolytic, urinary antiseptic and for headaches and bed-wetting.

Benefits

Aphrodisiac: There is evidence to suggest it boosts performance and aids recovery in sexually exhausted rats[1], but as yet there has been little research to look for evidence of a sexual effect in humans.

Mood: When drunk as a tea, damiana produces a mild euphoria and some people use it almost as a recreational drug. It is specifically used in cases of anxiety and depression where there is a sexual problem such as low sex drive, impotence, premature ejaculation and recurrent genital herpes infections.

Dose

Capsules/tablets: 200–800 mg a day, usually taken on an occasional basis when needed rather than regularly, often combined with other prosexual herbs.

Side effects

Some evidence suggests that damiana may reduce iron absorption from the gut and therefore it should not be used long term.

Dandelion

(Taraxacum officinalis)

Dandelion is a well-known perennial weed found throughout most parts of the world. The leaves were traditionally eaten in spring as a cleansing herbal tonic. Dandelion leaf has a diuretic action and is a

1. Estrada-Reyes R et al. J Ethnopharmacol 2009;123(3):423–9

good source of potassium which helps to flush excess sodium through the kidneys. Herbalists use it to treat water retention and bloating – in fact, the medieval name for dandelion was 'piss-a-bed'. Dandelion roots (usually obtained from two-year-old plants) are also used to support liver and kidney detox. It has a gentle laxative action that helps to improve constipation.

Benefits
Liver health: Dandelion has been used to help treat liver problems, including gallstones, jaundice and hepatitis but is best used under medical supervision. It should not be taken during an acute attack of gallstones, or if obstructive jaundice is present, for example.

Hormone balance: Dandelion is traditionally used to relieve symptoms caused by hormone imbalances, especially oestrogen excess, such as endometriosis and cyclical breast pain. However, a pilot study looking at its effects on oestrogen metabolism found no statistically significant changes in oestrogen levels.

Dose
5–10 g fresh root daily, divided between two or three doses, or 500 mg extracts twice a day.

Side effects
Large doses can cause nausea and diarrhoea.

Contraindications
Should not be taken by anyone who has active gallstones or obstructive jaundice.

Devil's claw
(Harpagophytum procumbens)

Devil's claw is named after the sharp hooks that develop on its fruit. It is a South African desert plant whose tap root produces potato-like tubers to store water.

Devil's claw tubers contain compounds known as iridoid glycosides such as harpagoside and harpagide that have a natural anti-inflammatory and painkilling action similar to that of non-steroidal anti-inflammatory drugs (NSAIDs). It appears to regulate the activity of COX-2 enzymes that are involved in the inflammatory process.

Devil's claw is taken to treat low back pain, and painful, inflamed joints due to osteoarthritis, rheumatoid arthritis, gout or sports injuries. It is also traditionally used as a tonic to help digestive problems, headaches and to reduce fevers. Devil's claw has also been found to encourage excretion of uric acid, reducing the risk of recurrent gout.

Research
Osteoarthritis: Devil's claw extracts can significantly improve osteoarthritis and general rheumatic pain and stiffness, with reductions in pain scores for hand, wrist, elbow, shoulder, hip, knee and back pain. It also produces significant benefits in quality of life and general wellbeing, with 6 out of 10 people able to reduce or stop their usual pain medication[1]. A gold-standard Cochrane review of two trials concluded that devil's claw, taken at a dose providing 50 mg or 100 mg harpagoside daily, was more effective than placebo for short-term improvements in pain and the need for rescue medication. It was as effective in reducing low back pain as an NSAID drug[2].

Dose
1–10 g daily, depending on concentration of extract, to provide around 50 mg harpagoside daily.

Contraindications
Devil's claw should not be taken by:
- Sufferers of peptic ulcers or indigestion as it promotes secretion of digestive juices
- Pregnant or breast-feeding women.

Digestive enzymes

An enzyme is a protein that speeds up the rate at which a particular chemical reaction takes place. Within our body, we produce 22

1. Warnock M et al Phytotherapy Res 2007 21(12):1228–33
2. Gagnier JJ et al. Cochrane Database Syst Rev 2006;(2):CD004504

different digestive enzymes. Those known as proteases break down dietary proteins, amylases digest carbohydrates, while lipases break down fats. Many other enzymes with a similar action are found in fruit and vegetables, including cellulases that digest fibre.

We each produce different levels of enzymes depending on our genes, diet, lifestyle, gender and age. As we get older, most people tend to produce less intestinal enzymes so our ability to absorb nutrients decreases. Lack of digestive enzymes has been linked with a number of health problems, from bloating, wind and heartburn to irritable bowel syndrome, candida and rosacea. A number of digestive enzymes are now available to treat a range of conditions in what has become a fashionable therapy.

Enzyme supplements are mainly derived from plants (e.g. pineapple, papaya, kiwi, fungi) or animal sources (e.g. pancreatic enzymes from pigs). Plant enzymes are usually considered superior as they are more stable over a wider range of acidity, and are less likely to be broken down by stomach acids. Products often contain other ingredients that promote enzyme action such as betaine HCL (increases the hydrochloric acid content of the stomach), extract of ox bile (an animal-derived enzyme that stimulates intestinal movements) and fructo-oligosaccharides which promote growth of probiotic bacteria in the bowel.

Benefits

Enzyme products are selected according to symptoms that suggest intolerance to particular food groups (fats, proteins, and carbohydrates), particular foods (e.g. fruit, milk, yeast, gluten-containing cereals). If you feel bloated after eating carbohydrate, for example, select a product that contains carbohydrate-digesting enzymes such as amylase and cellulase. If milk causes a problem, consider a product containing milk-digesting enzymes such as bromelain (from pineapples), papain (from papaya), lipase and lactase. If you are gluten-intolerance, a product supplying gluten protease, cellulase and amylase can help.

If you want to improve general digestion or are not sure which food group is causing the problem, select a mixed digestive enzyme supplement containing lipase (digests fats), amylase (digests carbohydrates), protease (digests protein), lactase (digests milk sugar) and cellulase (digests cellulose).

Enzyme supplements designed to dissolve candida yeasts are also available.

Dose
Normally 1–4 capsules – you may need to experiment to find the best dose to help your symptoms. It is usually best to seek advice from a nutritional therapist to ensure you take the most suitable enzyme mixture for your particular situation.

Check labels for 'activity units' as these show the potency of the enzymes present in a supplement. Those with the highest number of activity units are the most active.

Digestive enzymes are normally taken at the beginning of a meal to help improve digestion-related problems. To treat other problems such as rosacea, you may be advised to take them on an empty stomach. If taking the enzymes for indigestion, don't take an antacid or indigestion remedy within two hours of taking the digestive enzymes as this may reduce the effectiveness of the enzymes.

If your symptoms do not improve within two weeks of taking digestive enzyme supplements, stop taking them and seek medical advice.

Dong quai
(Angelica sinensis)

Dong quai, or Chinese angelica, is native to China and Japan where it is widely used as a female tonic and sometimes referred to as 'female ginseng'. Its aromatic rhizome is harvested after two years' growth. It is traditionally used to ease menstrual cramps, by relieving muscle spasms, and to improve premenstrual syndrome, cyclical breast pain, endometriosis and fibroids. In Asia, dong quai is valued as an adaptogen with hormone and mood-balancing properties. It is second only to Korean ginseng in popularity and is frequently combined with other herbs (e.g. chasteberry, liquorice, Siberian ginseng). However, there appears to be little published research to support its use.

Research
Menopause: Chinese angelica is traditionally combined with other herbs as a natural form of hormone replacement therapy for women

experiencing menopausal symptoms such as hot flushes and night sweats. However, studies have consistently failed to show a significant benefit, compared with placebo, when treating menopausal symptoms with dong quai as a single agent. It does not appear to pave an oestrogen-like action in its effect on the female reproductive tract.

Dose
Capsules standardized to 9000 ppm ligustilide: 200 mg three times daily.

Contraindications
Dong quai should not be taken by:

- Anyone who has peptic ulcers
- Pregnant or breast-feeding women
- Women who experience heavy menstruation, abnormal bleeding or who take anticoagulants such as coumarin or aspirin regularly.

Note: Chinese angelica contains anticoagulants and should not be taken in large quantities. It also contains psoralene, a compound that increases skin sensitivity to sunlight and may cause a skin rash on exposure to sun in some people, especially those with fair skin; they should only, therefore, take small quantities.

Echinacea
(Echinacea purpurea)

Echinacea, or purple coneflower, is a traditional remedy first used by native American Indians such as the Sioux to treat blood poisoning, snake bites, boils, fever, eczema and to relieve allergic reactions.

Echinacea contains several unique polysaccharides known as echinacins that help to stimulate the immune system by increasing the number and activity of white blood cells responsible for attacking viral, fungal and bacterial infections. It stimulates phagocytosis – the process in which white blood cells ingest bacteria and viruses before destroying them – and also boosts production of a natural anti-viral substance called interferon. It also contains flavonoids that have an antioxidant action.

Echinacea boosts immunity, promotes healing and is now mainly used to help prevent and treat recurrent upper respiratory tract infections such as the common cold, laryngitis, tonsillitis, otitis media or sinusitis, viral infections such as herpes cold sores, and skin complaints.

Research

Common cold: Echinacea has been shown to almost double the length of time between infections compared with those who do not take it, and when infections do occur, they tend to be less severe. A meta-analysis of 14 studies found that Echinacea decreased the odds of developing a cold by 58 per cent, and shortened the duration of a cold by 1.4 days[1]. Another analysis of three trials found that taking Echinacea reduces the likelihood of a cold by 55 per cent[2].

Dose

160–300 mg one to three times daily. Select products standardized to contain at least 3.5 per cent echinicosides/cichoric acid.

Opinions on how to take Echinacea vary. Some suggest taking it continually, some suggest taking it cyclically. It works by stimulating the activity of white blood cells that absorb viruses and bacteria before destroying them. This activity is not depleted by taking it continuously. There is little rationale for taking it cyclically. However, as immune function remains elevated above normal for several days after taking a dose, taking it only on weekdays, and not at weekends, for example, should not reduce its effectiveness. Most evidence suggests it may be taken in low dose, long term to reduce infections, or in a higher dose just when you feel an infection coming on.

There is no evidence of any harm from taking it long term. Always follow manufacturer's guidelines on how to use their products, as they do contain different balances of ingredients which means they should be used in a different way.

Echinacea seems to be safe during pregnancy and breast-feeding

1. Shah SA et al. Lancet Infect Dis 2007;7(7):473–80
2. Schoop R et al. Clin Ther 2006; 28(2):174–83

but, as with all supplements, it should only be taken during pregnancy under supervision from a qualified practitioner.

Elderberry
(Sambucus nigra)

Elder trees are native to northern Europe, and elderberries are a familiar autumn fruit widely used in home-made country wines and jams. Elderberry juice contains anti-viral compounds that can reduce the severity and duration of common cold and influenza infections.

Research
Influenza: Studies have found that elderberry extracts are active against influenza types A and B, including the most virulent strains. Several studies involving both children and adults with respiratory viral infections, including influenza, show that taking elderberry extracts produces clinical improvement within two days, whereas it usually takes six days to achieve similar improvement in those receiving placebo.

For example, a trial involving 60 people aged 18–54 years with flu-like symptoms for 48 hours or less found that those taking elderberry syrup were relieved of influenza symptoms on average four days earlier than those taking the placebo[1]. Levels of antibodies were found to be significantly higher in those taking elderberry extracts than in those on placebo.

Elderberry extracts also seem to be active against *Herpes simplex* viruses and HIV.

Dose
Standardized elderberry syrup: 15 ml four times a day starting as soon as possible after symptoms occur.

Essential Fatty Acids

Essential fatty acids (EFAs) belong to a group of oils known as long-chain polyunsaturated fatty acids. They are called essential because

---

1. Zakay-Rones Z et al. J Int Med Res 2004;32(2):132–40

you cannot make enough to supply your needs and they must therefore come from your diet.

The essential fatty acids come in two main types, omega-6s and omega-3s, which are named after their chemical structure. Put simply, if the first double bond in their structure (where hydrogen atoms are missing) is in position 6 on the molecule, they are called omega-6s, and if the first double bond appears in position 3, they are known as omega-3s.

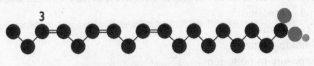

Alpha-Linolenic acid (omega-3)

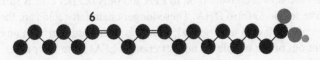

Linoleic acid (omega-6)

There are two main EFAs:

- Linoleic acid – an omega-6 fatty acid
- Linolenic acid – an omega-3 fatty acid

Omega-6s are mainly derived from vegetable oils such as sunflower, safflower and corn oils (which are commonly found in processed foods). The omega-3s are mainly derived from nuts (especially walnuts), flaxseed and fish oils (having originally come from the plankton on which these fish feed).

The essential fatty acids can be converted on to form longer chain fatty acids in the body. Linoleic acid can only be converted into other omega-6 fatty acids, such as gamma-linolenic acid (GLA) and arachidonic acid (AA), however, while linolenic acid can only be converted on to other omega-3 fatty acids such as eicosapentaenoic acid (EPA) and docosahexaenoic acid (DHA). Unfortunately, the metabolic reactions involved are not that efficient, and the enzymes involved (e.g. delta-6-desaturase) are readily blocked by a number of factors associated with an unhealthy diet, lifestyle and toxicity, including:

- Excess intakes of saturated (animal) fat
- Excess intakes of trans-fatty acids (e.g. found in hydrogenated margarines)
- Excess intakes of sugar
- Drinking too much alcohol
- Dietary lack of vitamins and minerals, especially vitamin B6, zinc and magnesium
- Crash dieting
- Smoking cigarettes
- Exposure to pollution.

As a result, it is estimated that only around 5 per cent dietary linolenic acid is converted on to EPA and only 0.5 per cent is further converted on to form DHA. These longer chain fatty acids are therefore often classed as essential, too. It is estimated that as many as eight out of ten people do not get enough EFAs from their diet.

EFAs act as building blocks to make cell membranes, sex hormones, and hormone-like chemicals (prostaglandins) found in all your body tissues. Because of the position of their double bonds, your body handles omega-6 and omega-3 oils in different ways. Most omega-6s are converted into a series of substances (series 2 prostaglandins and series 4 leukotrienes) that promote inflammation in the body, while omega-3s are converted into substances (series 3 prostaglandins and series 5 leukotrienes) that are less inflammatory. The omega-6 fatty acid, gammalinolenic acid (GLA), is one of the few omega-6s that can reduce inflammation if intake is sufficiently high[1].

Because we cannot convert excess omega-6s to omega-3s, we ideally need to balance our intakes of these two types of essential fatty acids to damp down, rather than stimulate, formation of inflammatory chemicals in the body. Consuming fewer omega-6s and more omega-3s has been shown to discourage formation of the

1. Belch JJ, Hill A. Am J Clin Nutr 2000;71(1 Suppl), 352S–6S

inflammatory substances that, as well as increasing pain in arthritic joints, also increase joint damage by breaking down cartilage and bone, for example[1]. And eating more omega-3s derived from fish oils has been shown to reduce the presence of these chemicals within arthritic joints[2].

Unfortunately, in the UK, intakes of inflammation-promoting omega-6s have risen over the last thirty years as vegetable oils and spreads have replaced the traditional butters. In men, for example, intake of one particular omega-6 (linoleic acid) has risen from around 10 g per day to 15 g per day. At the same time, the average adult only eats a third of a portion of oily fish per week, and 70 per cent of adults eat no oily fish at all. Average intakes of the long-chain omega-3s, EPA and DHA, which are especially beneficial for people with arthritis, are therefore well below the 3–6 g per day needed for good anti-inflammatory effects. In fact, the National Diet and Nutrition Survey showed that the average British adult eats just 50 g of oily fish per week, supplying a meagre one gram of the most important long-chain omega-3s, EPA and DHA.

Deficiency

When you do not get enough EFAs from your diet, the metabolism can make do with the next best fatty acids available (e.g. those derived from saturated fats) but these are less flexible and have less optimum effects on cell membranes and hormone function. When essential fatty acids are in short supply, you are more likely to experience dry, itchy skin, flare-ups of chronic inflammatory diseases (e.g. rheumatoid arthritis, psoriasis, eczema, asthma) and women are more likely to experience period pains and cyclical breast pain.

Clinical features associated with EFA deficiency include:

- Thirst
- Urinary frequency
- Dry, scaly, itchy skin
- Keratosis pilaris (pimply, 'goosebump' skin on the upper arms and legs)

1. Calder PC, Zurier RB. Cur Opin Clin Nutr Metab Care 2001;4:115–121
2. James MJ et al. Prostaglandins Leukot Essent Fatty Acids 2003;68(6):399–405

- Lack-lustre, straw-like hair
- Dandruff
- Soft, frayed or brittle fingernails
- Impaired immunity with frequent infections
- Atopic tendencies (eczema, hay fever, asthma)
- Visual difficulties (poor night vision, sensitivity to bright light, visual disturbances when reading)
- Attention problems (distractibility, poor concentration, poor working memory)
- Emotional sensitivity (depression, excessive mood swings, undue anxiety)
- Sleep problems (e.g. difficulty settling at night and waking in the morning).

Lack of EFAs during infancy and childhood has also been linked with an increased risk of allergies such as eczema, asthma and hay fever in later life, and may also be linked with cradle cap – a scaly scalp condition – in newborn infants and dyslexia. Studies suggest that male babies have a higher need for EFAs than females as they metabolize these fatty acids less efficiently.

EFAs are especially important in pregnancy, as they are needed for the development of a baby's eyes and brain. Unfortunately, research in many countries, including the UK, USA and Netherlands, shows that even in normal pregnancy, a mother's EFA status is marginal. As pregnancy requires such high levels of EFAs, and as intakes are generally low, maternal essential fatty acid status declines throughout successive pregnancies: stores are not readily replenished and, with each subsequent pregnancy, essential fatty acid deficiency becomes increasingly marked. EFA deficiency is especially likely with multiple pregnancies when the needs of two or more babies must be met.

Some researchers have observed that first babies are often more intelligent than their younger siblings and have speculated that lack of EFAs – especially DHA – may be involved. Research in the Netherlands involving 244 women who were pregnant for up to the seventh time showed that maternal blood levels of DHA were significantly lower in those women who had previously given birth compared to those pregnant with their first child. Blood samples from the umbilical artery and vein also showed significantly higher

DHA levels in first children compared with those born afterwards. Birth order was found to play a significant role in determining how much DHA was available to the developing baby. Further research is needed to see what effect this has on the intellectual potential for children born second or later in a family. Certainly women planning a second or subsequent pregnancy are well advised to take essential fatty acid supplements to protect themselves and their baby from the potential effects of deficiency.

During pregnancy, women lay down over 5 kg fat. The composition of fats in these stores will depend on their dietary intake. By eating the right sorts of fats – especially essential fatty acids – EFA reserves will be stored to help top up the amount present in their breast milk. In other words, any excess eaten over and above the baby's immediate needs during pregnancy will not be wasted. A significant proportion can be stored and mobilized later, while breast-feeding, to continue the supply needed for eye and brain development during the first four to six months of the baby's life after birth. After this time, a baby's metabolism is mature enough to start making small amounts of DHA from other dietary essential fatty acids, assuming these are available.

Dose

A healthy adult needs around 6–10 g EFAs a day. During pregnancy and while breast-feeding, these needs are increased to an average of 14 g a day (equivalent to about 4000 g per pregnancy). For more information, see Evening primrose oil (page 127) and Fish oils (page 137).

Advice

Improve your essential fatty acid balance by consuming more omega-3s, which are found in:

- Oily fish (2–4 portions per week) such as mackerel, herring, salmon, trout, sardines, pilchards, fresh tuna (not tinned), see the table on page 138
- Wild game meat such as venison and buffalo
- Grass-fed beef
- Omega-3 enriched eggs
- Omega-3 fish oil supplements.

At the same time, cut out excess omega-6s by consuming less:

- Omega-6 vegetable oils such as safflower oil, grape-seed oil, sunflower oil, corn oil, cottonseed oil or soybean oil (replace with healthier oils such as rapeseed, olive, walnut or macadamia oils)
- Margarines based on omega-6 oils such as sunflower or safflower oil
- Convenience foods
- Fast-foods
- Manufactured goods such as cakes, sweets and pastries.

Eucalyptus
(Eucalyptus globulus)

There are over 700 different types of eucalyptus of which over 500 produce essential oils. The blue gum (*Eucalyptus globulus*) is most widely used medicinally.

Benefits

Eucalyptus, sometimes known as the fever tree, is a traditional Aboriginal medicine used as an antiseptic, fumigant, to reduce fever, and as a decongestant to treat catarrh and the common cold. In addition to its antiseptic, antibacterial, anti-inflammatory and expectorant properties, it also stimulates blood flow, is mildly antispasmodic and helps to dilate the small airways (bronchioles) of the lungs.

It is also used to deter mosquitoes.

Eucalyptus leaf medicinal tea is taken for bronchitis and sore throat. It is sometimes included in herbal cough mixtures.

Dose

Infusion: 2–3 g in 150 ml water, twice a day.
Tincture 1:5 (g/ml): 10–15 ml, twice a day.
Extract 5:1 (w/w): 500 mg, twice a day.

Evening primrose oil

The evening primrose plant (*Oenothera biennis*) is native to North America. Its seed oil is a rich source of gamma-linolenic (also known as gamolenic) acid, or GLA – one of the few omega-6 oils with an anti-inflammatory action (similar to that of omega-3s) if intakes are sufficiently high[1]. GLA is metabolized in the body to form hormone-like substances known as prostaglandins which are found in all body tissues and play a major role in mediating inflammation, blood clotting, hormonal balance and are involved in the immune response against infections. Unlike other dietary omega-6 fatty acids, GLA is converted into Series 1 prostaglandins, which relax blood vessels, lower blood pressure, decrease inflammation, improve nerve function and circulation, as well as regulating calcium metabolism. GLA also prevents the release of arachidonic acid from cells, which, in turn, reduces production of Series 2 prostaglandins from unwanted blood clotting and inflammation.

While your body can make small amounts of GLA, this process is easily blocked by factors such as increasing age, smoking, pollution, lack of certain vitamins and minerals or excessive intakes of saturated fat, sugar or alcohol. Evening primrose oil (EPO) is one of the most popular and useful food supplements available as up to 10 per cent of its essential fatty acid content is GLA (other sources include blackcurrant seed oil and starflower oil).

Benefits
EPO is used to help a wide range of problems. When combined with fish oils, the beneficial effects of EPO are increased.

Arthritis: The anti-inflammatory action of GLA can reduce joint pain. In one trial, 60 per cent taking GLA were able to stop NSAID therapy completely, while another 25 per cent were able to cut their NSAID dose in half. Interestingly, taking both evening primrose and fish oils together was only slightly more effective than taking EPO alone[2]. Later studies using higher doses found that GLA was able to

---

1. Belch J, Hill A. Am J Clin Nutr 2000;71(1 Suppl), 352S–6S
2. Belch J et al. Annals Rheum Disease 1988; 47:96–104

reduce the number of joints that were tender or swollen[1,2].

Diabetic neuropathy: Abnormal EFA metabolism occurs in people with diabetes, especially the conversion of dietary linoleic acid to GLA and on to dihomo-GLA and arachidonic acid. These disturbances are associated with a variety of vascular, and clotting abnormalities that can lead to reduced blood flow and lack of oxygen transport to nerve cells which may play a role in diabetic neuropathy[3]. Twenty-two people with diabetic polyneuropathy took either 360 mg GLA or placebo for six months. Compared with the placebo group, those taking GLA showed significant improvement in neuropathy symptom scores, and the speed of conduction of nerve messages. The researchers concluded that GLA may have a useful role in the prevention and treatment of diabetic neuropathy[4]. In a larger trial[5] involving 111 people with diabetic neuropathy one group took 480 mg GLA per day for one year while the other group took placebo. Thirteen out of sixteen different measures of nerve function significantly improved in those taking GLA over the year, but not with placebo. Treatment response was greatest in those whose diabetic control was good rather than poor.

Dry eyes: EPO appears to be helpful for reducing dry eyes, especially in contact lens wearers. A study involving 76 women who took either EPO or placebo (olive oil) for six months, found that those taking EPO showed significant improvement in dryness and overall lens comfort. Viscosity of tears was also increased.

Skin and eczema: If your skin is lacking in essential fatty acids, it becomes scaly, rough, itchy, prematurely wrinkled and dry (xerosis). It also becomes more prone to spots as oil gland ducts become distorted and trap grease. Taking evening primrose oil helps to keep skin feeling soft and some preliminary evidence suggests that it can reduce the appearance of skin wrinkles. A review of nine studies found that evening primrose oil frequently reduced the symptoms of dry itchy skin/eczema after several months of use, with the greatest

1. Leventhal L. et al. Annals Intern Med 1993; 119:867–73
2. Zurier R et al. Arthritis Rheum 1996;39:1808–17
3. Jamal GA Diabet Med 1994; 11;2:145–49
4. Jamal GA, Carmichael H. Diabet Med 1990;7;4:319–23
5. Keen H et al. Diabetes Care 1993;16;1:8–15

improvement seen in reducing the level of itching[1]. A positive correlation was found between improvements in clinical score and a rise in fatty acid levels. In a double blind, cross-over study in which adults with eczema received either 2 g, 4 g or 6 g EPO daily, and children took either 2 g or 4 g EPO daily, there was significant clinical improvement, especially at the higher intakes[2]. Anecdotal evidence suggests that taking EPO during pregnancy may help to reduce the formation of stretch marks by maintaining the suppleness of skin and connective tissue cell membranes.

Heart disease: It has been suggested that combining omega-3 fish oils with evening primrose oil may be more effective in combating heart disease than taking fish oil supplements alone[3]. In one study, two similar groups of people with Type 1 diabetes were compared when one was given 3 g linoleic/GLA mixture per day for two months. No changes were found in the control group but improvements in beneficial HDL-cholesterol and platelet stickiness were seen in those receiving the essential oil mix[4].

Hormone balance: Evening primrose oil provides building blocks for making sex hormones, and some evidence suggests it is helpful in premenstrual syndrome[5]. One study found that supplements relieved bloating and mastalgia in 95 per cent of women, irritability in 80 per cent, low mood in 74 per cent, swollen peripheries in 79 per cent and anxiety in 53 per cent[6]. It is also taken for both cyclical and non-cyclical breast pain (mastalgia). The Cardiff Mastalgia Clinic reported that 92 per cent of 324 patients with cyclical mastalgia and 64 per cent of 90 women with non-cyclical mastalgia obtained a clinically useful response to therapy. Danazol was the most effective drug, with bromocriptine and evening primrose oil having equivalent efficacy. Adverse events were much less common with EPO than danazol or bromocriptine, however[7].

1. Morse PF et al. Br J Dermatol 1989;121:75–90
2. Fiocchi A et al. J Int Med Res 1994;22:24–32
3. Laidlaw M, Holub BJ Am J Clin Nutr 2003;77;1:37–42
4. Uccella R et al. Clin Ter 1989;129;5:381–8
5. Horrobin DF et al. J Nutr Med 1991;2:259–264
6. Larsson B et al. Current Therapeutic Research 1989;46 (1):58–63
7. Gateley, C A et al. J R Soc Med 1992;85(1): 12–5

Prostate: A pilot study involving men with benign prostate enlargement showed improvement in urinary frequency. Before treatment, urinary frequency averaged 14.8 times per day and 4.8 times per night. After taking evening primrose oil for six months, daytime frequency reduced to 9.8 and nocturia to 2.2. It appears to work by suppressing conversion of testosterone to dihydrotestosterone within prostate cells[1].

Dose
500–1000 mg EPO per day (equivalent to 40–80 mg GLA) for preventive health.

Up to 3000 mg (equivalent to 240 mg GLA) per day to help breast pain, pre-menstrual syndrome or menopausal symptoms – may take up to three months to notice a beneficial effect.

As an oil, it is best taken with food to boost absorption. The action of GLA is boosted by vitamin E which also helps to preserve it. Certain vitamins and minerals are also needed during the metabolism of essential fatty acids. These are vitamins C, B6, B3 (niacin), zinc and magnesium. If you are taking evening primrose oil, you should therefore ensure that your intake of these is adequate.

Contraindications
Do not take EPO if you have a rare form of epilepsy, known as temporal lobe epilepsy, or if you are taking medication for schizophrenia as it may make these conditions worse (although EPO has been used diagnostically to differentiate between TLE and schizophrenia[2]).

See also: **Essential Fatty Acids**.

1. Pham H, Ziboh VA. J Steroid Biochem Mol Biol 2002; 82(4–5):393–400
2. Holman CP, Bell AFJ. J Orthomol Psychiatr 1983;12:302–4

Fenugreek
(Trigonella foenum-graecum)

Fenugreek is a strongly aromatic herb from northern Africa and the Mediterranean which is also widely cultivated in India. Its seeds have a wide number of traditional uses in Ayurvedic and Chinese medicine. It has an anti-diabetic action and can lower cholesterol levels. Improvements in glucose control appear to result from activation of insulin-signalling pathways in liver and fat cells.

Benefits

Glucose control: In people with Type 1 diabetes, adding fenugreek seed powder to a controlled diet for ten days significantly reduced fasting blood glucose levels and improved the glucose tolerance test compared with the same diet given without fenugreek seed powder. Urinary analysis also showed a 54 per cent reduction in glucose excretion[1]. These changes did not occur in the diet-only controls. Powdered fenugreek seed has also been shown to reduce blood glucose levels in people with Type 2 diabetes. Insulin levels also tended to be lower[2]. When 25 people with newly diagnosed Type 2 diabetes following dietary and lifestyle advice were randomly given either 1 g fenugreek seed extract or placebo for two months, there was a significant improvement in glucose control and reduced insulin resistance in those taking fenugreek[3]. Triglyceride levels decreased and HDL-cholesterol also increased significantly.

Cholesterol levels: In people with Type 1 and Type 2 diabetes, fenugreek seed powder significantly reduced total cholesterol, LDL-cholesterol and triglycerides levels while HDL-cholesterol increased.

Athletic performance: Adding fenugreek seed extracts to a glucose beverage was found to increase glycogen synthesis in muscles after exercise[4].

1. Sharma RD et al. Eur J Clin Nutr 1990;44(4):301–6
2. Madar Z et al. Eur J Clin Nutr 1988;42(1):51–4
3. Gupta A et al. Assoc Physicians India 2001;49:1057–61
4. Ruby BC et al. Amino Acids 2005;28(1):71–6

Dose

1–25 g powdered whole seed extracts per day.

Mild flatulence and diarrhoea have been reported as a side effect in 10–20 per cent of people using defatted extracts, but powdered whole seed seems to be well tolerated.

Allergic reactions have been reported.

May interact with other glucose-lowering agents. People taking hypoglycaemic drugs should use fenugreek with caution, under medical supervision, to avoid hypoglycaemia.

Feverfew
(Tanacetum parthenium)

Feverfew is a common European plant belonging to the daisy family. Feverfew leaves contain a substance called parthenolide that is believed to either inhibit release of a neurotransmitter, serotonin, in the brain circulation, or to block the serotonin receptor. This prevents sudden changes in blood vessel diameter that are involved in the development of migraine, and helps to reduce the severity and frequency of attacks.

Feverfew also has powerful anti-inflammatory actions that are useful to help treat painful menstrual cramps.

Benefits

Migraine: In clinical trials, 70 per cent of people taking feverfew leaf extract found that it either prevented headaches or lessened their severity, as well as the related symptoms of nausea and vomiting. In a trial involving 170 people with migraine, taking feverfew extracts for 16 weeks reduced the average number of migraine attacks per month by 1.9 (compared with 1.3 in those on placebo)[1]. In three out of four trials, feverfew extracts lessened the severity of headaches as well as related symptoms of nausea and vomiting.

Dose

125–250 mg daily depending on strength of extract. Select a product containing at least 0.2 per cent parthenolide for every 125 mg

1. Diener HC et al. Cephalalgia 2005;25(11):1031–41

feverfew extract. Non-standardized supplements may contain very little parthenolide.

It may take four to six weeks before benefits are noticed, and feverfew usually needs to be taken long term to prevent a recurrence of migraine attacks.

Contraindications
- Feverfew should not be taken during pregnancy or breast-feeding as it may affect contraction of the uterus.
- Feverfew should not be taken by anyone who is on anticoagulant drugs as it may inhibit blood clotting.

Fibre

Dietary fibre – or roughage – consists of the fibrous plant substances that pass through our small intestines undigested. There are two main types of fibre: soluble fibre (e.g. pectins, gums) which forms a gel when mixed with liquid, and insoluble fibre (e.g. cellulose) which does not. We lack the enzymes necessary to break down either type of fibre, but once soluble fibre reaches the large bowel, bacterial enzymes start to ferment it, releasing odoriferous gases. Insoluble fibre is largely excreted unchanged.

Dietary sources of fibre include wholegrain cereals, nuts, seeds, root vegetables and fruits. These all contain both soluble and insoluble fibre, though some sources are richer in one type than another. Oats, figs, barley, apples, prunes and kidney beans, for example, are rich in soluble fibre, while wheat, brown rice, rhubarb, leafy vegetables, peas and chickpeas are sources of insoluble fibre.

Foods containing 3 g of fibre or more per 100 g are considered high-fibre choices. These include:

- Bran (40 g fibre per 100 g portion)
- Dried apricots (18 g)
- Prunes (13 g)
- Brown bread (6 g)
- Walnuts (6 g)
- Peas (5 g)
- White bread (4 g)

• Cooked wholemeal spaghetti (4 g).

While fibre provides little in the way of energy or nutrients, it aids the digestion and absorption of other foods. Soluble fibre is important for the function of the stomach and upper intestines, where it absorbs fats and sugars to slow the rate at which they pass into the circulation. This helps to reduce the rate at which blood glucose levels rise after a meal. It also encourages the muscular contractions that propel digested food forwards. Insoluble fibre is more important in the large bowel, where it absorbs water, bacteria and toxins, bulks up the faeces and hastens stool excretion.

Dietary fibre provides nutrients for bacterial growth, and much of the increased bowel motion bulk due to a high-fibre diet is due to increased bacterial multiplication in the gut. For every gram of fibre eaten, bowel motions increase by around 5 g in weight.

If the diet is lacking in fibre, very little bulk will reach the lower bowel. Instead of the small muscular contractions needed to move bulky stools downwards, the intestinal walls have to squeeze tightly to propel the smaller pellets on their way. This may trigger prolonged muscle spasm and pain in some people with irritable bowel syndrome (IBS). There is no consistent link between symptoms of IBS and fibre intake, however, and it is unlikely that lack of fibre is the sole cause.

Benefits
Irritable Bowel Syndrome: Increasing fibre intake can relieve both diarrhoea (by absorbing excess fluid) and constipation (by bulking bowel contents and stimulating movement). Overall, following a high-fibre diet helps around one third of people with IBS, but in up to a quarter of sufferers, changing to a high-fibre diet initially makes bloating and distension worse. This effect does disappear after two or three weeks so it's worth persevering gradually so that the bowel has time to get used to the higher intake. If you cannot tolerate bran – as at least half of IBS sufferers can't – taking supplements containing other forms of fibre such as psyllium (Plantago ovatum, also known as ispaghula) or sterculia is often effective. Psyllium seed/powder is an excellent and popular fibre source as it quickly swells in the bowel to produce a gentle scouring action. A meta-analysis exploring the effectiveness of

fibre supplements found that if six people took psyllium supplements, one would be prevented from having persistent symptoms[1]. Wheat bran was ineffective.

Constipation: Inulin (20 g per day) has been shown to reduce functional constipation in elderly people and to increase bowel movements from 1–2 per week to 8–9 per week in 70 per cent of patients (impressive!). Stools were soft with no diarrhoea, only mild-to-moderate flatulence and no discomfort[2].

Cholesterol: Fibre binds to cholesterol and other fats in the bowel to reduce their absorption. Just 10 g psyllium seed taken daily for at least six weeks can reduce LDL-cholesterol levels by between 5 and 20 per cent. Oatbran also helps to lower cholesterol levels[3]. Eating pulses can significantly reduce total cholesterol by at least 7 per cent, with reductions in 'bad' LDL-cholesterol and increases in 'good' HDL-cholesterol. These benefits are largely attributable to their soluble fibre content[4].

Ulcerative colitis: A study involving 102 people with ulcerative colitis found that taking 10 g of these seeds per day may be as effective in maintaining remission in ulcerative colitis as a standard drug treatment (mesalamine)[5].

Cancer: A low-fibre (which is also usually high-fat) diet is associated with relatively high levels of circulating oestrogen. As a result, people following this type of eating pattern are more likely to develop hormone-dependent cancers such as those of the breast or prostate gland. This is because sex hormones pass from the bile into the gut from which they are absorbed back into the circulation. This so-called 'enterohepatic circulation' helps to maintain relatively high sex hormone levels. If the gut contains dietary fibre residues, however, these mop up a significant amount of sex hormones so that

1. Ford AS et al. BMJ 2008;337:a2313
2. Kleessen et al. Am J Clin Nutr 1997;65:1397–1402
3. Lepre F, Crane S. Med J Aust 1992; 157(5):305–8
4. Anderson JW, Major AW. Br J Nutr 2002;88 Suppl 3:S263–71
5. Fernandez-Banares F et al. Am J Gastroenterol 1999; 94(2):427–33

more are excreted and less reabsorbed. As a result, oestrogen levels tend to be lower and a high-fibre diet helps to protect against both breast and prostate cancer. For example, one study involving almost 1,300 men found that those with the highest intake of soluble fibre were 11 per cent less likely to develop prostate cancer than those with the lowest intakes[1]. Whether or not a high-fibre diet protects against colon and rectal cancer is controversial. According to the World Health Organization, a weak association has been observed between the risk of colorectal cancer and high consumption of fruits and vegetables and/or dietary fibre, but the results of large, prospective studies are inconsistent. On balance, current evidence suggests that intake of fruits and vegetables probably reduces the risk for colorectal cancer.

Menopause: Women who have followed a lifelong low-fibre diet are more likely to have menopausal symptoms of oestrogen withdrawal – their tissues are used to a relatively high level of circulating hormones, and they seem to tolerate the menopausal drop less well. However, switching to a healthier, low-fat, high-fibre diet around the time of the menopause can also make symptoms of oestrogen withdrawal worse (by lowering oestrogen levels further), unless the amount of plant hormones (e.g. isoflavones obtained from soy) eaten is also increased.

Dose

Our ancestors followed a diet that provided 100 g or more of fibre per day[2]. According to the World Health Organization, the recommended intake of fruits, vegetables and wholegrains is likely to provide more than 25 g per day of total dietary fibre. The recommended intake for UK adults is currently 18 g but our average intake is around 12 g.

Sources of fibre found in supplements include bran, inulin (from chicory), psyllium seed and husks (also known as ispaghula), wheat dextrin, linseed and prune juice.

When switching to a high-fibre diet, go slowly. Start with a small increase in fibre intake, e.g. 2 g with each meal, and slowly increase to obtain the desired effect. An intake of between 18–30 g a day

1. Pelucchi C et al. Int J Cancer 2004; 109(2):278–80
2. Leach JD. Eur J Clin Nutr. 2007;61(1):140–2

(*including* that obtained from your diet) is considered optimum for health.

When increasing fibre intake it is also important to drink at least two to three litres of fluids per day to help bulk up the fibre for optimum effect. Some people experience feelings of bloating and distension on increasing their fibre intake; this effect normally disappears after two or three weeks and can be avoided altogether if fibre intake is increased very gradually.

Bowel bacteria quickly adapt to the types of roughage in your diet, so it is important to eat as many different sources of fibre as possible. If you mainly eat fibre of one type (e.g. bran) bowel bacteria will respond within a week or two by increasing their output of enzymes to ferment this. The fibre reaching your colon will then be broken down more quickly so that you lose some of the benefit.

Safety
- Fibre in the bowel absorbs large quantities of water and can dry the gut out. Fluid intake must also be increased to avoid problems.
- It is possible that a high-fibre diet may reduce absorption of calcium and iron in the bowel.
- Fibre supplements – especially psyllium – should not be taken within two hours of any prescribed medication as they may interfere with its absorption.

Fish oils

Fish oils are a rich source of two long-chain, omega-3 polyunsaturated fatty acids: eicosapentaenoic acid (EPA) and docosahexaenoic acid (DHA).

Omega-3 fish oil is extracted from the flesh of oily fish such as salmon, herrings, sardines, pilchards and mackerel. These beneficial oils are derived from the micro-algae on which the fish feed.

Typical Omega-3 Fatty Acid Content Of Fish

Food	Portion size (Grams)	Total long-chain omega-3s per portion (Grams)
Kippers	150 g	3.89 g
Salmon	150 g	3.25 g
Mackerel	150 g	2.89 g
Pilchards in tomato sauce	110 g	2.86 g
Herring	150 g	1.97 g
Tuna (fresh)	150 g	1.95 g
Trout	150 g	1.73 g
Sardines in tomato sauce	100 g	1.67 g
Salmon (canned in brine)	100 g	1.55 g
Plaice	150 g	0.45 g
Cod	150 g	0.38 g
Haddock	150 g	0.24 g
Tuna (in oil, drained)	45 g	0.17 g
Tuna (in brine, drained)	45 g	0.08 g

The flesh of white fish, such as cod, and tinned tuna, which has been processed, contain very little omega-3 oil. As its name implies, cod liver oil is derived only from the liver of cod. It naturally contains around three times less omega-3 essential fatty acids than is found in oily fish products, but these can be concentrated during processing to increase their percentage. Cod liver oil also contains high amounts of vitamin A and vitamin D.

Healthy staple foods such as margarines, bread and even milk containing omega-3 oils are available in a number of countries to help boost intakes in those who do not each much fish. However, few of these contain the long-chain omega-3s (EPA and DHA) which provide the proven health benefits. Many of these products contain only tiny amounts of omega-3s, usually of the short-chain variety (ALA) derived from vegetable oils. Less than 5 per cent of these are converted on to EPA in the body, and less than 0.5 per cent are transformed into DHA.

Benefits

Omega-3 fatty acids, especially DHA and EPA, are converted in the body into substances (series 3 prostaglandins and series 5 leukotrienes) that reduce inflammation.

This helps to balance the action of omega-6 fatty acids (mostly derived from vegetable oils) which are converted into substances that promote inflammation (see page 122). Omega-3s therefore offer some benefit against long-term inflammatory diseases such as asthma, rheumatoid arthritis, psoriasis and coronary heart disease which is linked with low-grade inflammation in artery walls.

Omega-3 oils reduce blood pressure, blood stickiness, inflammation and are prescribed to lower abnormally high blood fat levels. They may also protect against certain abnormal heart rhythms, especially in heart muscle receiving a poor blood supply[1].

Coronary heart disease: Even a modest increase in dietary intakes of oily fish can help to prevent death due to coronary thrombosis (heart attack). In those who have already had a heart attack, eating more fish significantly reduces the chance of a second heart attack. If one does occur, the chance of dying from this second heart attack is significantly decreased. An intake of at least 1 g omega-3 fish oils per day (from eating oily fish twice a week, or from pharmaceutical grade supplements) has consistently been shown to reduce the risk of sudden cardiac death by 40 per cent to 45 per cent[2,3,4]. As a result, the American Heart Association and the European Society of Cardiology both recommend a daily intake of 1 g omega-3 fish oils to prevent a first heart attack, and to prevent further problems if you have already experienced one. Researchers have analysed the data from 25 studies and found that levels of DHA are 'consistently and significantly' lower in people experiencing a heart attack than in those not experiencing a cardiac event[5]. EPA levels do not show the same association, which suggests that DHA may be more important than EPA for heart health. Fish oil supplements are often prescribed to lower blood triglyceride levels and, at a typical dose of 4 g per

1. Raitt MH. Cardiovasc Drugs Ther 2009;23:1–3
2. Von Schacky C, Harris WE. Cardiovascular Research, 2007; 73(2):310–5
3. Weber HS et al. Herz 2006;31 Suppl 3:24–30
4. Verboom CN et al. Herz 2006; 31 Suppl 3:49–59
5. Harris WS et al. Atherosclerosis 2007; 193(1):1–10

day (supplying 465 mg DHA and 375 mg EPA), can lower triglyceride levels by up to 45 per cent.[1]

Stroke: People who eat oily fish regularly are less likely to die from stroke than those who do not. A meta-analysis of data from six studies suggests that eating any fish on a weekly basis reduces the risk of stroke by 12 per cent, with possible additional reductions of 2 per cent per serving per week[2].

Joints: Increasing intake of omega-3 fish oils reduces the level of inflammatory chemicals within arthritic joints that are responsible for increased blood flow, heat and pain, and which stimulate the breakdown of cartilage and bone[3,4]. EPA and DHA have an action similar to that of non-steroidal anti-inflammatory drugs in that they can inhibit COX-1 enzymes by 92 per cent and 65 per cent respectively, and COX-2 enzymes by 91 per cent and 95 per cent respectively[5]. By reducing inflammation, they reduce the migration of white blood cells into joints to damp down pain and swelling. As a result, consuming more omega-3s may even slow the progression of osteoarthritis. A number of studies have also shown that taking fish oils supplements can reduce the need for taking NSAID painkillers. High intakes of 3–6g EPA and DHA are needed per day for good anti-inflammatory effects in joints[6,7].

Brain health: DHA plays an important structural role within brain cell membranes, improving their fluidity so that messages are passed on more rapidly from one cell to another. EPA is involved in cell signalling and also improves communication between brain cells. Adding fish oils (2 g per day) to usual drug treatment for depression has been shown to significantly improve symptoms within two weeks, compared with placebo[8].

1. Sadovsky R, Kris-Etherton P. Postgrad Med 2009;121(4):145–53
2. Bouzan C et al. Am J Prev Med 2005; 29(4):347–52
3. Calder PC, Zurier RB. Curr Opin Clin Nutr Metab Care 2001;4:115–121
4. James MG et al. Prostaglandins, Leukot Essent Fatty Acids 2003;68(6):399–405
5. McPhee S et al. Comp Biochem Physiol 2007;146:346–56
6. Cleland LG, James MJ. J Rheumatol 2000; 27, 2305–7
7. Kremer JM.Am J Clin Nutr, 2000;71(1Suppl):349S–51S
8. Nemets B et al. Am J Psychiatry 2002:159(3):477–9

Attention deficit hyperactivity disorder: Some trials have shown no apparent benefit from DHA alone in children with ADHD, although inclusion criteria were strict, and those showing problems such as clinical symptoms of essential fatty acid deficiency were excluded – the very children who might have benefited. Benefits were seen in a trial involving 50 children with ADHD (on medication) who received either a fish oil formula (480 mg DHA, 80 mg EPA, 40 mg AA, 96 mg GLA plus 24 mg antioxidant vit E) or placebo for four months. Those receiving fish oils showed significant improvements in conduct (parent ratings) and attention (teacher ratings) with 75 per cent no longer showing oppositional defiant behaviour (clinical ratings). Ability to listen to, and follow, instructions also significantly improved[1]. Clear improvements were also shown in a trial involving children with specific learning difficulties (mainly dyslexia) and above-average ADHD ratings. Those receiving fish oils showed significant improvements in cognitive scores and general behaviour problems, and significantly reduced ADHD-related symptoms such as anxiety, inattention and disruptive behaviour problems[2]. Taking fish oil supplements may help some children with learning and behavioural difficulties – but possibly only those with clinical features of essential fatty acid deficiency (see page 382).

Diabetes: Recent research shows that taking 3 g omega-3 fish oils daily can lower levels of homocysteine by 22 per cent in people with diabetes (compared with 1 per cent with placebo)[3]. Glucose tolerance was also improved.

AMD: Omega-3 fish oils, especially DHA, may protect against progression of age-related macular degeneration. A meta-analysis of nine studies, involving almost 89,999 people, found that a high dietary intake of omega-3 fatty acids reduces the risk of developing late AMD by 38 per cent. Eating fish at least twice a week reduced the risk by 24 per cent[4].

1. Stevens LJ et al. Lipids 2003;38:1007–1021
2. Richardson AJ, Puri BK. Prog Neuropsychopharmacol Biol Psychiatry 2002;26(2):233–9
3. Pooya S et al. Nutr Metab Cardiovasc Dis 2009; Epub doi:10.1016/j.numecd. 2009.04.002
4. Chong EW et al. Arch Ophthalmol 2008;126(6):826–33

Psoriasis: Taking omega-3 fish oils can significantly reduce psoriasis patches within four to eight weeks.

Menstrual pain: Painful periods seem to be worse in women who do not eat much fish, and taking omega-3 fish oil supplements has been shown to significantly improve painful periods in teenage girls. This is because omega-3 essential fatty acids have a beneficial effect on the types of prostaglandins produced in the womb lining (endometrium) to reduce muscle spasm.

Cancer: Fish oils may have a role in reducing the risk of cancer, by interfering with the growth of tumour cells and reversing the weight loss that can occur in people with cancer. In one study, pre-cancerous polyps of the colon also responded dramatically to treatment with fish oils and reduced in frequency by 50 per cent. A meta-analysis of the data from a number of trials suggests that each additional 100 g of fish consumed per week lowers the risk of colorectal cancer by around 3 per cent[1].

Pregnancy: DHA is vital for development of normal brain and eye function, especially during the last three months of pregnancy. The placenta extracts them from the maternal circulation and concentrates them in your baby's circulation, so that foetal levels of DHA are twice as high as in the mother. DHA is transported to the baby's central nervous system and incorporated into brain cell membranes to make up 10–15 per cent of the weight of the baby's cerebral cortex. It is found mainly in the areas of membrane occurring in synaptic connections between brain cells. DHA is also concentrated in the light-sensitive cells at the back of a developing baby's eyes where it makes up 50 per cent of the weight of each retina.

It is now believed that a low-fat diet providing too few essential fatty acids during pregnancy may be linked with an increased risk of the offspring developing dyslexia, attention deficit hyperactivity disorder, autism spectrum and possibly schizophrenia. If a pregnant woman is lacking in DHA, the baby's needs will be met from the mother's richest store – her own brain. This may account for the

1. Geelen A et al. Am J Epidemiol 2007;166(10):1116–25

slight shrinkage (2–3 per cent) in maternal brain size seen in some pregnant women, causing the poor concentration, poor memory, forgetfulness and vagueness that many women experience during the last few months of pregnancy.

Boosting dietary intake of essential fatty acids throughout pregnancy can help to:

* Improve the development of the baby's eyes and brain
* Improve the baby's visual acuity
* Reduce the risk of pregnancy-associated high blood pressure (pre-eclampsia)
* Reduce the risk of a preterm delivery
* Reduce the risk of a low-birthweight baby
* Reduce fluid retention during pregnancy (oedema)
* Reduce the risk of maternal poor concentration towards the end of pregnancy
* Reduce the risk of dry, itchy skin problems
* Possibly reduce the risk of stretch marks
* Possibly increase the baby's intelligence through improved brain development.

It is important to only take a DHA supplement designed for use in pregnancy however. Do not take cod liver oil (too much vitamin A) and do not take a supplement containing high amounts of EPA (may increase bleeding time). Check with a pharmacist if you are unsure whether you are taking an appropriate omega-3 supplement for pregnancy.

Dose

Omega-3 fish oils: 1–4 g a day.

For severe inflammatory diseases such as inflammatory bowel disease and rheumatoid arthritis, doses of 6 g daily may be recommended.

Cod liver oil: 1–1.5 g per day (because of its high vitamin A content).

The UK Food Standards Agency (FSA) currently recommends

that we obtain the equivalent of 450 mg long-chain omega-3 fish oils (DHA and EPA) per day[1]. However, the American Heart Association and the European Society of Cardiology both recommend a daily intake of 1 g omega-3 fish oils to prevent a first heart attack (primary prevention), and to prevent further problems if you have already experienced one (secondary prevention).

Obtaining these higher levels from your diet is difficult unless you eat oily fish on a daily basis. For example, the FSA also recommends that boys, men and women past reproductive age can eat one to four portions (140 g each) oily fish per week, girls and women of child-bearing age should only eat up to two portions of oily fish a week – this lower amount is to reduce foetal exposure to marine pollutants. Few of us achieve these levels of consumption. The average adult only eats a third of a portion of oily fish, supplying a meagre 1 g fish oils per week[2]. And 70 per cent of adults eat no oily fish at all[3].

For their heart health benefits, omega-3 fish oil supplements should almost be mandatory!

Select a pharmaceutical grade omega-3 fish oil supplement to ensure it is virtually free from marine pollutants. Those offered in the triglyceride (TG) form are most easily absorbed and used in the body.

Typically a 1 g capsule of high-strength fish oil contains around 500 mg of the important long-chain omega-3 fatty acids, EPA and DHA (check label claims).

NB: If choosing to take cod liver oil, those described as high or extra high strength provide the highest amount of omega-3 fatty acids. If taking a multivitamin as well, check the total amounts of vitamin A and D you are taking do not exceed recommended doses. Vitamin A is best limited to less than 5,000 IU (1,500 mcg) per day although intakes of up to 10,000 IU (3,000 mcg) are considered safe. The EU RDA for vitamin D is 5 mcg (200 IU) but those over the age of 50 need double this amount (10 mcg = 400 IU) as blood levels fall with increasing age.

1. Food Standards Agency advised by SACN/COT 2004
2. Henderson L et al (2002) National Diet and Nutrition Survey: adults aged 19–64 years 2003
3. SACN 2004

Shaking fish oil together with milk or juice will emulsify it – break it down into tiny suspended globules that will aid absorption. This is the process that naturally occurs in the stomach and helps to avoid 'fishy burps'. Emulsified fish oil supplements are also widely available.

Safety
- Cod liver oil products should not be taken during pregnancy as they contain vitamin A, an excess of which can be harmful to a developing baby.
- Some research suggests that fish oils increase blood sugar levels in diabetics. However, omega-3 fish oils protect against the increased risk of coronary heart disease that occurs in diabetes. Several large scale analyses have now concluded that taking a fish oil supplement has no significant effect on glucose control in people with Type 2 diabetes.
- Because of their blood thinning effect, people with clotting disorders or on blood-thinning medication such as warfarin should only take an omega-3 fish oil supplement under supervision by a doctor. However, no significant increase in blood clotting time is expected at total daily intakes of EPA and DHA of 3 g per day, or less[1].
- Fish oils may worsen asthma in people who are sensitive to aspirin. However, some evidence suggests that omega-3 fish oils can improve bronchial reactivity and protect against exercise-induced asthma.

See also: **Essential Fatty Acids**.

Flaxseed
(Linum usitatissimum)

Also known as linseed, the seed of the flax plant is a rich source of alpha-linolenic acid (ALA), an omega-3 essential fatty acid. It also contains the omega-6 essential fatty acid, linoleic acid (ratio omega-3: omega-6 is around 3:1).

---

1. Blonk MC et al. AM J Clin Nutr 1990;52(1):120–7

Flaxseed oil is a rich source of oestrogen-like plant hormones known as lignans. Flax seeds are a good fibre source and are useful for improving constipation, diverticular disease and irritable bowel syndrome. Flaxseed is a gentle yet effective laxative.

Flaxseed oil is often suggested as an alternative source of omega-3 fatty acids for those unable or unwilling to take fish oils. Although it is a source of short-chain omega-3 essential fatty acids, only 5 per cent of ALA is converted on to eicosapentaenoic acid (EPA) and even less – just 0.5 per cent – is converted on to docosahexaenoic acid (DHA) which are the beneficial long-chain omega-3s found in oily fish. When 86 adults took either 2 g flaxseed oil, fish oil, hempseed oil or placebo per day, for 12 weeks, blood levels of the long-chain omega-3 fatty acids DHA and EPA did not alter significantly with flaxseed oil, but levels of ALA increased transiently[1].

Benefits
Skin: The essential fatty acids in flaxseed oil are incorporated into cell membranes to make them more fluid and supple. Taking flaxseed oil has beneficial effects on skin quality, improving hydration and reducing skin roughness and scaling[2].

Menopause: Flaxseed may reduce hot flushes. A study involving 28 women who took 40 g crushed flaxseed per day found that it halved the frequency of hot flushes from 7.3 to 3.6 per week[3]. However, there was no placebo group with which to compare these results. Half those involved experienced abdominal distension, 30 per cent experienced diarrhoea and 21 per cent withdrew because of side effects.

Cardiovascular disease: Most evidence suggests that increased consumption of omega-3s from alpha-linolenic acid does not reduce the rates of all-cause mortality, heart attack, and possibly stroke in the same way that fish oils do[4]. Flaxseed may have a modest and short-lived effect in lowering 'bad' LDL-cholesterol, but studies involving people with Type 2 diabetes show that taking up to 30 g

1. Kaul N et al. J Am Coll Nutr 2008; 27(1):51–8
2. De Spirt S et al. Br J Nutr 2009; 101(3):440–5
3. Pruthi S et al. J Soc Integr Oncol 2007; 5(3):106–12
4. Wang C et al. Am J Clin Nutr 2006; 84(1):5–17

flaxseed oil per day produces no significant changes in glucose levels, blood pressure, cholesterol or triglyceride levels[1,2,3].

In 2007, the Natural Standard Research Collaboration stated that, although flaxseed and flaxseed oil may have several promising uses for future study, current evidence does not support its recommendation for any conditions at this time[4].

Note:
Flaxseed oil degrades on exposure to light and if not processed and stored properly quickly turns rancid.

Liquid flaxseed oil must be stored carefully (e.g. in the fridge in opaque bottles).

Avoid oil that is past its use by date, or which has a strong odour.

Dose
Oil: 1 teaspoon–1 tablespoon once or twice a day.

Flax seeds: 1–2 tablespoons with water twice a day.

Best taken with food to enhance absorption.

Taking it in the form of seeds or as capsules is most convenient. Do not exceed stated doses.

Fluoride

Fluoride is a mineral that is important for healthy bones and teeth. It binds to tooth enamel and strengthens it to help prevent decay. In the same way, small amounts of fluoride can bind to bone to produce calcium fluoroapatite which is more resistant to reabsorption.

Dietary sources of fluoride include tea leaves (which provide 70 per cent of average intakes), fluorinated water supplies, seafood (especially oysters), milk, eggs, lettuce, cabbage, lentils and wholegrains.

People who drink large amounts of tea may gain some benefit in the long-term prevention of osteoporosis.

1. Alekseeva RI et al. Vopr Pitan. 2000; 69(6):32–5
2. Kaminskas A et al. Vopr Pitan. 1992;5–6:13–4
3. McManus RM et al. Diabetes Care 1996; 19(5):463–7
4. Basch E et al. J Soc Integr Oncol 2007;5(3):92–105

Dose

There is currently no EU RDA for fluoride. Intakes of 1.5–4 mg have been suggested as desirable. Fluorination of drinking water supplies 1–3 mg fluoride a day.

Excess

Excess fluoride can cause formation of abnormal, weakened bone and discoloured teeth (fluorosis). Fluorosis seems to triple the risk of osteoporotic fractures and may also increase the risk of bone cancer.

Folic acid

Folic acid is a water-soluble vitamin. It is the synthetic (monogluta-mate) form of the naturally occurring folate vitamin (polyglutamate form) found mainly in green leafy vegetables and wholegrains. Folic acid is more readily absorbed and used more efficiently in the body and is therefore preferable in supplement form.

It is difficult to obtain optimum amounts of folate from dietary sources alone, as foods originally rich in folate typically retain less than a third of their folate content after processing and cooking.

Folic acid is involved in the synthesis and metabolism of proteins, sugar and nucleic acids during cell division. Like vitamin B12, it is especially needed by cells that are dividing rapidly. When folic acid is in short supply, newly replicated chromosomes are more likely to be abnormal and cells – especially red blood cells – become larger than normal which can lead to a form of anaemia. Folic acid is particularly essential during the first few weeks of a baby's develop-ment in the womb to help prevent a type of developmental abnor-mality known as a neural tube defect (e.g. spina bifida) which arises between the 24th and 28th day after conception. It is also possible that taking folic acid supplements increases the chance of twin conceptions surviving, although this is by no means certain.

Folate is needed to process an amino acid, homocysteine, to ensure levels are optimally low. If allowed to rise, homocysteine damages artery walls and is as important a risk factor as cholesterol for developing coronary heart disease, stroke, peripheral vascular disease and other conditions associated with abnormal blood clotting. Homocysteine is formed in the body from the breakdown of the dietary amino acid, methionine. Homocysteine becomes highly reactive and toxic as it accumulates in the circulation, causing oxidation damage to the lining of artery walls so they become narrow and inelastic. Normally, its level is tightly controlled by three different enzymes that convert homocysteine to cysteine – a safe end product used by cells for growth.

Two of the three enzymes that control homocysteine levels depend on folate for their activity. Those who do not obtain enough folate/folic acid for optimal enzyme function will have a raised homocysteine level and consequently an increased risk of atherosclerosis. Low blood levels of folic acid have also been linked with an increased risk of depression and dementia. The risks associated with an elevated homocysteine level are comparable to those of an abnormally raised cholesterol level, but is more easily corrected through dietary intervention.

Because of its effects on cell division, folic acid may also help to protect against certain cancers.

The body stores very little folic acid and dietary lack rapidly causes deficiency – it is probably the most widespread vitamin deficiency in developed countries. Lack of folic acid causes a variety of symptoms, including a red, sore tongue, tiredness, exhaustion, cracking at the corners of the mouth, diarrhoea, insomnia, weakness and muscular cramps. Emotional symptoms of irritability, forgetfulness, confusion and depression can also occur.

Benefits

Birth defects: A meta-analysis of data from four trials found that taking 4 mg folic acid per day could prevent 87 per cent of recurrent neural tube defects in women who consistently take folic acid supplements before and during a subsequent pregnancy[1].

Homocysteine: Data from 25 trials show that daily doses of 200 mcg lower homocysteine levels by 60 per cent and a dose of 400 mcg lowers them by 90 per cent. A dose of 800 mcg folic acid or more is needed for maximum reduction of blood homocysteine concentrations[2]. Adding in 400 mcg per day vitamin B-12 produced a further

---

1. Grosse SD, Collins JS. Birth Defects Res A Clin Mol Teratol 2007;79(11):737–42
2. Homocysteine lowering trialists' collaboration: Am J Clin Nutr 2005; 82(4):806–12

7 per cent reduction in homocysteine concentrations, but vitamin B6 had little effect.

Coronary heart disease: The Nurses' Health Study[1], involving over 80,000 women, found that women with the highest intakes of folate were 45 per cent less likely to have a heart attack than those with the lowest intakes. Results from trials have been conflicting, and even after analysis of data from 12 clinical trials, it is still unclear whether or not folic acid supplements can reduce the risk of heart disease in those with a previous history of cardiovascular disease[2].

Stroke: A meta-analysis of data from eight trials suggests that taking folic acid supplements can significantly reduce the risk of stroke by 18 per cent. Greater benefit is seen in those taking it for more than three years, and when homocysteine levels were reduced by more than 20 per cent[3].

Peripheral vascular disease: A study involving 392 men over the age of 50 years, of whom 86 (22 per cent) had peripheral arterial disease, found that folate intakes were significantly lower in those with peripheral arterial disease (288 mcg daily compared with 324 mcg daily in those without peripheral arterial disease). The researchers concluded that daily folate (and vitamin B6) were independent risk factors for peripheral arterial disease after taking other risk factors such as age, blood pressure, cholesterol levels, diabetes, and smoking status into account[4].

Depression: There is growing evidence that low folate intake increases the risk of depression. A meta-analysis of 11 studies, involving over 15,000 people, found that lack of folate increased the risk of depression by 55 per cent[5].

Breast cancer: Some studies, but not others, suggest that an increase of 200 mcg dietary folate per day can lower the risk of breast cancer

1. Rimm EB et al. JAMA 1998; 279(5):359–64
2. Bazzano LA et al. JAMA 2006;296(22):2720–6
3. Wang X et al. Lancet 2007;369(9576):1876–82
4. Wilmink AB et al. J Vasc Surg. 2004;39(3):513–6
5. Gilbody S et al. J Epidemiol Community Health 2007;61(7):631–71.

by 20 per cent. This effect may be related to alcohol intake (which increases the risk of breast cancer and also lowers folate levels). Analysis of results from four studies suggests that, among women with a moderate or high alcohol consumption (14 or more grams per day) those with the highest folate intake were half as likely to develop breast cancer as those with low or no alcohol consumption[1].

Other cancers: Analysis of results from over 20 trials suggests that folate may play a role in protecting against cancers of the stomach, oesophagus and pancreas[2].

Cataracts: People with the highest intake of folic acid appear to be 60 per cent less likely to develop cataracts severe enough to need extraction compared to those with the lowest intakes[3].

Cognitive function: A study assessed over 200 people of whom 55 did not have dementia, 81 had mild cognitive impairment, 74 had Alzheimer's disease and 18 had vascular dementia[4]. Those with the lowest folate concentration were 3.1 times more likely to have mild cognitive impairment and 3.8 times more likely to have dementia than those with higher folate levels. Having raised homocysteine levels also significantly increased the risk of dementia around four-fold. The researchers concluded that folate deficiency may precede the onset of Alzheimer's and vascular dementia. This raises the possibility that folate supplementation may slow or even prevent the onset altogether. However, systematic reviews of the evidence have not yet shown consistently that folic acid has a beneficial effect on cognitive function in older people – mostly because trials were relatively short. Long-term use of folic acid may improve cognitive function in healthy older people with high homocysteine levels[5].

Diabetes: Taking metformin to improve insulin resistance in Type 2 diabetes increases homocysteine levels. This effect can be counter-acted with folic acid supplements. Taking 250 mcg folic acid per day

1. Larsson SC et al. J Natl Cancer Inst 2007;99(1):64–76
2. Larsson SC et al. Gastroenterology 2006;131(4):1271–83
3. Tavani A et al. Ann Epidemiol.1996; 6(1):41–6
4. Quadri P et al. Am J Clin Nutr. 2004;80(1):114–22
5. Malouf R, Grimley-Evans J. Cochrane Database Syst Rev 2008;(4):CD004514

was shown to reduce homocysteine by 13.9 per cent after four weeks' treatment and of 21.7 per cent after 12 weeks' treatment[1].

Allergies: Recent research involving over 8,000 people (aged 2–85) suggests that those with the highest levels of folate have lower levels of IgE (antibodies associated with allergy) and are over 40 per cent less likely to experience wheezing, 16 per cent less likely to have asthma and 31 per cent less likely to have atopic allergies than those with low levels[2].

Vitiligo: A raised level of homocysteine has been linked with skin depigmentation in vitiligo. Treatment with folic acid, vitamin B12 and safe, sensible exposure to the sun, can result in repigmentation without side effects. In one study involving 100 people, repigmentation occurred in 52 per cent and was most evident on sun-exposed areas[3].

Dose

The EU RDA and the UK RNI for folic acid is 200 mcg for adults. Women of fertile age who could become pregnant are advised to take supplements providing 400 mcg.

Doses of 800 mcg per day are needed for maximum lowering of homocysteine levels (see above).

Folic acid is generally considered safe, even at high doses, but long-term use of high doses can mask vitamin B12 deficiency as it prevents the occurrence of red blood cell changes that usually allow lack of vitamin B12 to be detected. Lack of vitamin B12 damages the nervous system, especially the spinal cord, and is masked by taking folic acid supplements. Therefore, the upper safe level for long-term use from supplements is suggested as 1000 mcg (1 mg) daily. Supplements providing higher doses of 4 mg per day or more may be advised under medical supervision (e.g. for women who have previously conceived a child with certain developmental abnormalities).

Safety

Some anti-epilepsy drugs result in low levels of folic acid. People taking drugs to treat epilepsy should tell their doctor if they take

1. Aarsand AK, Carlsen SM. J Intern Med. 1998;244(2):169–74
2. Matsui EC, Matsui W. J Allergy Clin Immunol 2009; 123(6):1253–9
3. Juhlin L, Olsson MJ. Acta Derm Venerol 1997: 77(6):460–2

folic acid supplements so blood levels of their medication can be monitored where appropriate. For women on anti-epileptic drugs, it is vitally important to obtain advice about taking extra folic acid supplements before trying to conceive a baby.

Fo-ti
(Polygonum multiflorum)

Fo-ti – also known as *he shou wu* – is one of the oldest Chinese tonic herbs whose dried roots are harvested when they are three to four years old. Raw fo-ti roots are laxative and also toxic but curing the root – for example, by boiling for hours in black soybean broth – converts it into a highly valued tonic that has mostly lost its laxative and toxic effects.

Benefits
Fo-ti is famous for its rejuvenating and revitalizing properties. It is widely used in the East as a general restorative, to promote fertility, sexual function and boost a low sex drive. Research shows that it can reduce abnormally raised cholesterol and may have some antibiotic effects against tuberculosis and malaria. It is also used to reduce premature greying of hair. It is often taken together with *Panax ginseng (see Ginseng)*.

Dose
Tablets: 5 g daily.

Garlic
(Allium sativum)

Garlic is an important component of the Mediterranean diet, and is such a popular culinary herb that, worldwide, average consumption is equivalent to one clove per person per day.

Garlic is a source of the powerful antioxidant, allicin. Allicin is not present in whole garlic cloves, but is formed from an odourless precursor called alliin, which is an amino acid unique to the garlic family. Alliin is stored within garlic cells, separated from the enzyme (alliinase) that breaks it down. It is only when alliin and alliinase come together that beneficial allicin (diallyl thiosulphinate) is made. This natural reaction occurs as soon as a clove of garlic is cut or crushed, to release the characteristic odour. If garlic is cooked immediately after peeling, however, allinase is inactivated and some of the beneficial effects are lost.

Allicin prevents cells from taking up cholesterol, reduces cholesterol production in the liver and hastens excretion of fatty acids, thereby discouraging atherosclerosis.

Sulphur compounds formed from the degradation of allicin also have beneficial effects, and are incorporated into long-chain fatty acid molecules, to act as antioxidants. Researchers recently discovered that these sulphur compounds react with red blood cells to produce a substance (hydrogen sulphide) which relaxes blood vessels and helps keep blood flowing easily. An interesting study found that garlic powder tablets can increase the elasticity of the aorta so that the heart has to work less hard to pump blood out into the body.

Another benefit of garlic is that it helps to improve the circulation, especially through small arteries (arterioles) and small veins (venules). Garlic dilates the arterioles by an average of 4.2 per cent and the venules by 5.9 per cent. As a result, it can improve blood flow to the skin by almost 50 per cent (helpful for sufferers of Raynaud's syndrome and chilblains) and to the nail folds by as much as 55 per cent. Platelet clumping is significantly decreased after a dose equivalent to half a clove of garlic and lasts for three hours. Some of the ingredients in garlic (ajoene, methylallyl trisulphide and dimethyl trisulphide) seem to be as potent as aspirin in this respect.

Garlic has a number of medicinal uses and is antioxidant, antiseptic, antibacterial and anti-viral. It is used to treat viral warts, stomach and respiratory infections but its most important effect is its ability to maintain a healthy circulation and reduce the risk of coronary heart disease and stroke.

Benefits

As an antioxidant, garlic extracts protect blood LDL-cholesterol molecules against oxidation and reduce their uptake by scavenger cells to protect against atherosclerosis. Research suggests that garlic supplements also have beneficial effects on blood vessel dilation, blood stickiness, blood pressure, and may improve cholesterol balance.

Blood pressure: Studies looking at the effects of garlic extracts on blood pressure have produced conflicting results. However, a meta-analysis of the results from ten trials suggests that, compared with placebo, garlic extracts can reduce blood pressure by an average of 16.3/9.3 mm Hg in people with hypertension[1]. It does not seem to have effects on blood pressure in people without an elevated systolic blood pressure.

Cholesterol: Some, but not all, studies have suggested that garlic can lower cholesterol levels. This discrepancy may be related to the different garlic preparations used, the dose, and the duration of the trial. One review found that, in six out of ten studies, there was a 9.9 per cent average drop in total cholesterol, 11.4 per cent drop in LDL-cholesterol and 9.9 per cent fall in triglycerides[2]. One meta-analysis of 13 trials involving almost 800 people found a significantly greater effect with garlic than with placebo, equivalent to a 5.8 per cent reduction in total cholesterol levels[3]. However, a recent analysis of data from 13 trials, involving over 1,000 people, suggests that garlic has a neutral effect on cholesterol and triglyceride levels[4]. The evidence is therefore not conclusive.

Coronary heart disease: Taking a garlic preparation for 12 months has been predicted to reduce the risk of heart attack and sudden death by 50 per cent in men and 30 per cent in women, based on changes in blood cholesterol levels[5]. When effects on blood pressure and blood vessel dilation are also taken into account, the protective effects are likely to be even higher.

Cancer: Garlic constituents can suppress formation of carcinogenic substances in the body called nitrosamines. Laboratory evidence suggests that garlic can arrest the growth of human colon cancer cells. A meta-analysis of results from 18 studies suggests that those consuming more than 28.8 g garlic per week were 31 per cent less likely to develop colorectal cancer, and 47 per cent less likely to develop

1. Reinhart KM et al. Ann Pharmacother 2008;42(12):1766–71
2. Alder R et al. J Am Acad Nurse Pract 2003; 15(3):120–9
3. Stevinson C et al. Ann Intern Med 2000 133(6):420–9
4. Khoo YS, Aziz Z. J Clin Pharm Ther 2009;34(2):133–45
5. Sobenin IA et al. Klin Med (Mosk) 2007;85(3):25–8

stomach cancer than those consuming less than 3.5 g garlic per week[1].

Colds: A recent review of the evidence looked at results from 146 people who either took garlic supplements or inactive placebo for 12 weeks[2]. Only 24 of those taking garlic developed a cold, compared with 65 of those taking dummy tablets. On average those taking garlic had colds lasting 1.5 days while those taking a placebo had colds lasting 5 days. Quite how it protects against colds is unclear and more research is needed to confirm these findings.

Dose
600–900 mg standardized garlic powder tablets a day.

Enteric coating of garlic powder tablets reduces garlic odour on breath and protects the active ingredients from degradation in the stomach.

Note: If applying raw garlic juice or oil to warts, protect surrounding skin with petroleum jelly. Some people are allergic to topical application of garlic.

Ginger
(Zingiber officinale)

Ginger is obtained from the rhizome of a perennial, tropical plant native to the jungles of south-east Asia. It contains a variety of unique chemicals such as gingerol, zingerone and essential oils.

Benefits
Ginger has analgesic, antihistamine, stimulating, anti-inflammatory and anti-nauseant properties. It also has a warming action that promotes sweating, and is popular for treating chilblains, Raynaud's syndrome, colds and fevers.

Ginger is frequently used to quell motion sickness, morning sickness during pregnancy, and to relieve postoperative nausea. It appears to work both by stimulating contraction of the stomach and

---

1. Fleischauer AT et al. Am J Clin Nutr 2000;72(4):1047–52
2. Lissiman E et al. Cochrane Database Syst Rev 2009;(3):CD006206

accelerating gastric emptying, and by reducing release of the hormone, vasopressin, during circular vection.

It can also help to relieve indigestion, flatulence, diarrhoea, suppressed menstruation, poor circulation, dizziness and migrainous headaches. Gingerol has a similar structure to aspirin, and may help to reduce blood clotting, boosting the circulation and lowering blood pressure.

Its anti-inflammatory action is helpful in relieving muscle and joint aches and pains, including those of rheumatoid and osteoarthritis.

Benefits

Arthritis: Ginger has an anti-inflammatory action, helping to block the release of inflammatory chemicals within synovial, cartilage and white blood cells[1]. A study involving 247 people with moderate osteoarthritis of the knee found that a standardized ginger extract produced a moderately significantly reduction in pain on standing, compared with inactive placebo[2].

Nausea: Analysis of five trials involving over 360 people found that a dose of at least 1 g ginger was more effective than placebo for preventing postoperative nausea and vomiting[3]. Ginger has also been shown to help prevent nausea in pregnancy (1 g per day)[4] and motion sickness[5].

Cholesterol: Recent evidence suggests that ginger can lower cholesterol and triglyceride levels significantly more than placebo.

Dose

Powdered ginger root standardized for 0.4 per cent volatile oils: 250 mg, two to four times a day.

Fresh powdered ginger: 1–2 g every four hours as necessary, up to 6 g per day.

Note: Do not exceed more than 1 g daily during pregnancy.

1. Phan PV et al. J Altern Compl Med 2005; 11(1):149–54
2. Altman RD, Marcussen KC Arthritis Rheum 2001;44(11):2531–8
3. Chaiyakunapruk N et al. Am J Obstet Gynecol 2006;194(1):95–9
4. Ozgoli G et al. J Altern Complement Med 2009;15(3):243–6
5. Lien HC et al. Am J Physiol Gastrointest Liver Physiol 2003;284(3):G481–9

Ginkgo
(Ginkgo biloba)

The ginkgo, or Maidenhair tree, is among the oldest living tree species, dating back over 270 million years. It is often referred to as a living fossil, as it was thought to have been wiped out during the last Ice Age. Specimens survived in remote parts of China, however, where they can live for several thousand years when carefully tended by monks.

Ginkgo's fan-shaped leaves contain a variety of unique anti-oxidants – flavonoid glycosides and terpenoids – known as ginkgolides and bilobalides. These compounds have been shown to stabilize cell membranes, relax blood vessel walls and increase the flexibility of red blood cells, so that oxygen-rich blood flows more freely through the tiny capillaries that supply the outer reaches of the body. Ginkgolides also reduce the effects of platelet activating factor (PAF) – a blood clotting substance that has been linked to allergies, asthma and blood clotting disorders such as heart attack and stroke.

Benefits

Circulation: By improving blood flow to the hands and feet, ginkgo helps to overcome poor circulation linked with hardening and furring up of the arteries, chilblains, Raynaud's disease and erectile dysfunction. Researchers have found that blood flow to the digits is significantly increased (by 57 per cent) within just one hour. Some trials, but not others, have shown benefits in intermittent claudication. A meta-analysis of 14 trials, involving over 700 people, found that people taking ginkgo supplements could walk, on average, a further 64.5 metres on a flat treadmill (with an average speed of 3.2 km per hour) before developing leg pains, compared with those on placebo[1]. While small, this effect would be welcome by most sufferers. However, the researchers concluded that there was no evidence of a clinically significant benefit in people with peripheral arterial disease.

Dementia: By improving blood flow to the brain, ginkgo extracts may help to improve memory, concentration and thought processes,

---

1. Nicolai SP et al. Cochrane Database Syst Rev 2009;(2):CD006888

especially in older people. Some trials involving people with dementia show that ginkgo extracts can improve apathy/indifference, anxiety, irritability, depression, sleep and night-time behaviour compared with placebo. In a meta-analysis of 34 clinical trials, 21 trials showed significant results in favour of the ginkgo in more than half of tested outcomes, eight were significant for less than half of measurements, four showed a trend in favour of ginkgo, and two found no advantage for ginkgo, compared with placebo[1]. A Cochrane review, however, of 36 trials concluded that many early trials used unsatisfactory methods and that, overall, the evidence that ginkgo is beneficial for people with dementia or cognitive impairment is inconsistent and unreliable.

Glucose control: The effect of ginkgo biloba on insulin secretion by pancreatic beta-cells was investigated in people with Type 2 diabetes[2]. Ginkgo biloba reduced circulating insulin levels during an oral glucose tolerance test in those taking oral hypoglycaemic drugs, but not those using dietary control only. The researchers suggest that ginkgo biloba may improve insulin production in those with pancreatic exhaustion. Whether this is due to 'resuscitation' of previously exhausted islets or due to increased activity of the few remaining functional islet cells remains unclear.

Blood clotting: Taking 120 mg of standardized ginkgo biloba extract for three months was found to have a beneficial effect on platelet clumping in people with Type 2 diabetes[3].

A previous study involving 20 people with raised blood clotting factors from a variety of underlying conditions showed significant improvement in blood stickiness – a coronary heart disease risk factor[4].

Eye problems: Ginkgo biloba improves peripheral blood flow, making it of likely benefit in a number of eye conditions, including glaucoma, cataracts, retinopathy and macular degeneration. A double-blind trial involving ten people compared ginkgo biloba extracts with placebo and, even though numbers were small, found

1. Bornhoft G et al. Z Gerontol Geriatr 2008; 41(4):298–312
2. Kudolo GB. J Clin Pharmacol.2001;41(6):600–11
3. Kudolo GB et al. Thromb Res 2002;108(2–3):151–60
4. Witte S et al. Fortschr Med 1992;110(13):247–50

a significant improvement in long distance visual acuity in those taking ginkgo biloba extracts[1].

In a larger trial involving 99 people with macular degeneration, visual acuity was assessed after six months' treatment with either 240 mg per day or 60 mg per day of a ginkgo biloba extract. Marked improvement in vision occurred in both treatment groups after just four weeks, with a more pronounced improvement in those taking the higher dose[2]. No serious side effects occurred.

Hardening and furring up of the carotid arteries can lead to lack of blood flow to the back of the eye – a condition known as chronic cerebral retinal insufficiency. In a study involving 24 people the effects of ginkgo biloba were assessed at two doses. In those taking 160 mg per day a significant increase in retinal sensitivity was observed within four weeks. In those on the lower dose (80 mg per day) this beneficial change did not occur, but was seen after increasing the dose to 160 mg a day. Both doctors and patients noticed a significant improvement after the treatment. The results suggest that damage to the visual field in this condition is reversible[3].

Tinnitus: By improving blood flow to the inner ear, ginkgo extracts can help some people with vertigo and tinnitus, where symptoms are linked with abnormal circulation. The effects appear to be small however. An analysis of six trials found that 21.6 per cent of those taking ginkgo experienced benefit, versus 18.4 per cent on placebo.

Sexual dysfunction: In the laboratory, ginkgo biloba extract has been shown to have a relaxant effect on the smooth muscle cells of human corpus cavernosal (penile) tissue which would be expected to allow more blood to flow into the area during erection[4].

Some, but not all, studies have found that ginkgo extracts improve sexual dysfunction in both men and women experiencing problems as a side effect of antidepressant medication. In one study, success rates were achieved of 91 per cent in men and 76 per cent in women, with positive effects on desire, excitement,

1. Lebuisson DA et al. Presse Med 1986;15(31):1556–8
2. Fies P, Dienel A. Wien Med Wochenschr 2002;152(15–16):423–6
3. Raabe A et al. Klin Monatsbl Augenheilkd. 1991;199(6):432–8
4. Paick JS, Lee JH. J Urol 1996;156(5):1876–80

orgasm and resolution[1]. However, there was no placebo group with which to compare results. A study using a placebo group did not find statistically significant results after 12 weeks' treatment, as some spectacular individual responses were recorded in both groups[2]. In one study, 60 men with erectile difficulties who had not responded to penile injections with papaverine took ginkgo extracts. After six months, half of men taking it had regained full potency with another 20 per cent responding to papaverine after the ginkgo treatment[3]. A similar study involving 50 males found that all those who had previously relied on injectable drugs (papaverine) to achieve an erection regained potency after taking ginkgo for nine months. Of the 30 men who were not helped by medical drugs, 19 regained their erections with ginkgo[4]. In another trial, taking 240 mg ginkgo extracts per day for nine months failed to produce significant improvement compared with placebo[5].

Dose
120–240 mg.

Select extracts standardized to provide a known amount of ginkgolides: e.g. at least 24 per cent.

Effects may not be noticed until after ten days' treatment and it may take up to 12 weeks for ginkgo to have a noticeable beneficial effect.

Side effects
A Cochrane review of the effects of ginkgo biloba analysed all the published randomized controlled trials available. The meta-analysis found no significant differences in side effects between ginkgo and placebo. The conclusion was that ginkgo biloba appears to be safe[6].

If taking ginkgo and using hypoglycaemic drugs, it is important to monitor blood glucose levels closely.

Seek medical advice before taking ginkgo if you are taking blood thinning treatment such as warfarin or aspirin, although at usual

1. Cohen AJ, Bartlik B. J Sex Marital Ther 1998; 24(2):139–43
2. Wheatley D. Hum Psychopharmacol 2004; 19(8):545–8
3. Sikora R et al. J Urol 1989;141:188A
4. Sohn M, Sikora R. J Sex Ed Ther 1991;17(1):53–61
5. Sikora R et al. J Urol 1998;159(suppl 5):240
6. Birks J et al. Cochrane Database Syst Rev 2002;4:CD003120

therapeutic doses of ginkgo biloba, no effects on blood clotting have been found.

Do not combine with MAOI antidepressants.

Do not use unprocessed *ginkgo* leaves from the garden, as these contain powerful chemicals that can cause allergic reactions.

Ginseng
(Panax ginseng; P. quinquefolium)

Ginseng is one of the oldest known herbal medicines, used as a revitalizing and life-enhancing tonic for over 3,000 years. The botanical name of Chinese, Korean or Asian ginseng (*Panax ginseng*) is derived from the Greek word *panacea*, meaning 'cures everything' and the Chinese word *ginseng* meaning 'man-like'. The roots, which contain the active ingredients, are often distinctly human-shaped. The closely related American ginseng (*P. quinquefolium* from the woodlands of east and central US and Canada) has a similar action and is, in fact, generally preferred in Asia as it is sweeter tasting.

High quality ginseng roots are collected in the autumn from plants that are five to six years old. White ginseng is produced from air-drying the root, while red ginseng (which is more potent and stimulating) is produced by steaming and then drying the root. The strain with the highest medicinal value is Panax ginseng C A Meyer, named after the sixteenth century German botanist who first described it in the West.

Ginseng roots contain substances known as ginsenosides (triterpenoid saponin glycosides) of which 29 different constituents have been identified. These make up 3–6 per cent of the dry weight of the root and belong to two main groups:

- Those with a relaxing, sedative action (e.g. Rb1, Rb2, Rc, Rd) that are mostly derived from small lateral roots
- Those with a more stimulating action (e.g. Rg1, Re, Rf, Rg2) which are mostly derived from the large (main) root.

Korean ginseng contains more of the stimulating ginsenosides, while American ginseng contains more of the relaxing ginsenosides.

Ginseng is classed as an adaptogen, which means it helps the body adapt to physical or emotional stress and fatigue. It has a normalizing action on many body systems, improving oxygen-usage in cells to boost the production of energy. In particular, ginseng improves adrenal gland function during times of stress. Researchers believe it has a direct action on the pituitary gland, to increase secretion of adrenocorticotrophic hormone (ACTH) which kick-starts the adrenal glands[1]. Some of the ginsenosides in ginseng also have an antioxidant action.

American ginseng is said to be best for fatigue caused by nervous conditions, anxiety and insomnia, while Korean ginseng is better for fatigue with general weakness and loss of energy.

Benefits

Traditionally, ginseng is described as stimulant, restorative and energizing, helping to improve strength, stamina, alertness and concentration.

Alertness: Research suggests ginseng may help to improve alertness and awareness.

A group of hospital nurses who took ginseng extracts were better able to stay awake and perform their night duties than those not taking it[2]. A study involving 112 adults aged 40 to 60 years found that those taking 400 mg ginseng for eight weeks showed significantly improved ability to analyse and solve problems at an abstract level, and to be mentally flexible under changing conditions, than those taking placebo. Those taking ginseng made 17.6 per cent fewer mistakes than those in the control group, and also showed significantly improved reaction times in a simple auditive test suggesting increased alertness and awareness[3].

Immunity: Ginseng helps to stimulate the activity of white blood cells against viral and bacterial infections. Research involving over 300 adults suggests that ginseng may boost immunity against the common cold. Those taking American ginseng extracts were half

1. Sandberg F, Dencker L. Zeitschrift fur Phytotherapie 1994;15(1):38–42
2. Hallstrom C et al. AJCM 1978;6(4):277–282
3. Sorensen H, Sonne J. Curr Ther Res 1996;57(12): 959–68

as likely to develop a cold during the four month study period, than those taking inactive placebo[1]. And when a cold did develop, the severity of symptoms was reduced in those taking ginseng extracts.

Diabetes: Ginseng is thought to lower blood glucose levels by stimulating the release of insulin[2] from the pancreas and by increasing the number of insulin receptors on cells to reduce insulin resistance. In people with newly diagnosed Type 2 diabetes, taking 100 mg or 200 mg ginseng was found to improve mood, vigour, well-being and psychomotor performance compared with placebo and, with 200 mg, also improved physical activity. Those receiving ginseng experienced a reduced fasting blood glucose, with eight of those given ginseng achieving a normal fasting blood glucose. Blood glucose levels returned to the normal range in a third of those taking ginseng without any changes in blood insulin levels. This suggests that ginseng improves the way cells respond to insulin. No adverse events were reported[3]. The main glucose lowering activity appears to be due to five glycans (named panaxans A to E) rather than the ginsenosides. It is therefore important not to select a highly concentrated extract (above 7 per cent ginsenosides) as this may not contain as many of the active panaxans.

Erectile dysfunction: Several studies suggest ginseng increases levels of nitric oxide (NO) in the spongy tissue of the penis. NO is a nerve communication chemical (neurotransmitter) that is essential for a number of physiological processes, including increasing blood flow to the penis for normal erectile function and sexual arousal. This action is similar in effect to that of anti-impotence drugs such as sildenafil. In a study involving 45 males with erectile dysfunction, taking Korean red ginseng (900 mg three times a day) improved penile tip rigidity, penetration and maintenance of erection significantly more than when taking placebo. Overall, 60 per cent of participants found that Korean red ginseng improved their

1. Predy GN et al. CMAJ 2005; 173(9):1043–8
2. Vuksan V et al. J Am Coll Nutr. 2001;20(5) Suppl:370S–380S; discussion 381S–383S
3. Sotaniemi EA et al. Diabetes Care 1995; 18(10):1373–1375

erections[1]. A systematic review of seven trials confirms evidence for effectiveness of red ginseng in the treatment of erectile dysfunction although the reviewers state that more rigorous studies are necessary[2]. Since then, a study involving 143 males found that taking 1 g Panax ginseng CA Meyer produced significantly greater improvements than placebo[3].

Aphrodisiac: Ginseng is prized as an aphrodisiac, sexual balancer and fertility enhancer. These effects are believed to relate to its steroidal compounds that are similar in structure to human sex hormones. Studies in laboratory animals show that ginseng increases libido and copulatory frequency. As well as its effect on nitric oxide in the penis (and, probably, the clitoris) ginseng also increases nerve ending sensitivity, lowers prolactin secretion (nature's anti-sex hormone) and facilitates the secretion of hypothalamic catecholamines involved in driving sexual behaviour[4].

Muscle metabolism: Ginseng appears to improve oxygen utilization in working muscles. In a study involving 50 healthy male volunteers (aged 40 to 58 years), taking ginseng extracts for eight weeks significantly reduced the concentration of lactic acid in working muscles compared to the start of the trial and compared with placebo[5].

Dose
Start with a low dose and work up from 200–1000 mg standardized extracts.

Select products standardized to contain at least 4–7 per cent ginsenosides. These will generally be more expensive, but cheap versions may contain very little active ingredient.

Doses are usually divided in two and taken twice daily. Optimum dose usually around 600 mg daily.

Traditionally, ginseng is not usually taken for more than six weeks without a break. In the East, ginseng is taken in a two weeks on, two weeks off cycle. Some practitioners recommend taking it in a six weeks on, eight weeks off cycle.

1. Hong B. J Urol 2002;168(5):2070–3
2. Jang DJ et al. Br J Clin Pharmacol 2008; 66(4):444–50
3. Kim TH et al. Asian J Androl 2009;11(3):356–61
4. Murphy LL, Lee TJ. Ann N Y Acad Sci 2002;962:372–7
5. Branth S. Biomed 1992; 3:1–4

For those who find Chinese ginseng too stimulating, try American ginseng which seems to have a more gentle action.

Safety

A review of all the studies shows that single ginseng extracts have a low incidence of side effects at usual therapeutic doses, and those that do occur are usually mild and transient[1].

It is best to avoid taking other stimulants (e.g. caffeine) while taking ginseng.

Ginseng is not advised if you have high blood pressure (may make hypertension worse), a heart rhythm abnormality, or if you have an oestrogen dependent condition (e.g. pregnancy, cancer of the breast, ovaries or uterus) as it contains oestrogenic compounds.

Like all ginseng products, it should not be used by women who are pregnant or breast-feeding, or by children under the age of 12, except under medical advice.

Always seek medical advice if taking prescribed medicines.

Glucosamine

Glucosamine sulphate is a substance that is naturally made in the body from a sugar (glucose) and an amino acid (glutamine). It is needed to produce molecules (glycosaminoglycans) for laying down new framework tissues in damaged joints. Glucosamine is essential for the production of new cartilage and synthesis of the joints' oil (synovial fluid). Larger quantities are needed when damaged joints are healing and, as production of glucosamine is normally a slow process, it is often in short supply.

Glucosamine sulphate has been shown to stimulate formation of cartilage and the connective tissues that bind joints together. It is also important for the production of synovial fluid, making it thicker, more cushioning and protective. Researchers now also believe that glucosamine suppresses the activity of immune cells involved in joint inflammatory reactions, to reduce the inflammatory breakdown of cartilage.

Glucosamine supplements are widely taken as a source of the

---

1. Coon JT, Ernst E. Drug Safety 2002;25(5):323–44

materials needed to boost repair of cartilage and joint tissues. The two main forms available are glucosamine sulphate and glucosamine hydrochloride. Two other versions, N-acetyl glucosamine and glucosamine chlorohydrate are also available. Glucosamine supplements can be synthesized in the laboratory, but most are produced commercially from the shells of crustaceans (lobster, crab and prawns).

Benefits

There is a polarization between experts in favour of glucosamine sulphate and those that prefer glucosamine hydrochloride. When either supplement is digested by stomach hydrochloric acid, however, around half dissociates into neutral glucosamine and half into ionized glucosamine. If recovered, most would be in the form of glucosamine hydrochloride because of its interaction with stomach acid. The question therefore remains whether or not the sulphate component of glucosamine sulphate has an additional anti-inflammatory action of its own, similar to that of MSM (see page 229), which might provide additional benefits.

Possible reasons for the conflicting results seen in trials using glucosamine sulphate and glucosamine hydrochloride include differences in study design, length of trial, and different strengths and quality of the supplements used. While most trials used pharmaceutical grade glucosamine salts, this was not always the case, leading to some uncertainty about the dose used. Independent laboratory analyses have shown that many products do not contain the amounts stated on the label[1]. It is also possible that glucosamine can only work when cartilage is still present within an osteoarthritis joint, which is not the case in more severe disease.

At present, most studies have used the glucosamine sulphate form, and therefore most evidence supports the use of glucosamine sulphate rather than glucosamine hydrochloride. This could change as new studies are published, however. Interestingly, the two supplements have not yet been directly compared in a head-to-head trial.

Osteoarthritis and glucosamine sulphate: Many studies indicate that glucosamine sulphate has a beneficial structural effect in

---

1. Das A, Hammad TA. Osteoarthritis Cartilage 2000; 8(5), 343–50

osteoarthritis. A landmark trial published in *The Lancet* looked at the effects of taking 1500 mg glucosamine sulphate per day, versus inactive placebo, for three years, on the long-term progression of knee osteoarthritis in 212 patients[1]. Those randomized to receive inactive placebo showed progressive narrowing of their knee joint space over the three-year trial period, while those taking glucosamine sulphate showed no significant loss of joint space. Those receiving glucosamine sulphate enjoyed significant improvements in pain and disability which was sustained for the three year duration of the trial; in contrast, those taking placebo experienced a significant worsening of symptoms. The authors concluded that, 'The long-term structure-modifying and symptom-modifying effects of glucosamine sulphate suggest that it could be a disease modifying agent in osteoarthritis'. A later analysis of the results suggests that glucosamine sulphate may be most effective in modifying joint structure where joints are less severely affected with osteoarthritis when significant amounts of cartilage are still present[2]. People who had taken 1500 mg glucosamine sulphate for up to three years in these studies were then followed for a further five years, on average, after stopping the supplements. Those who had formerly taken glucosamine sulphate underwent fewer surgical knee replacements than those taking placebo, and used fewer painkillers and anti-inflammatory drugs[3].

A meta-analysis of 15 trials looked at the effects of combining glucosamine sulphate with chondroitin sulphate in 1,775 people with osteoarthritis of the knee[4]. This analysis confirmed the results of previous studies that glucosamine appears to reduce joint pain and preserve joint space in people with OA of the knee.

Two years later, another meta-analysis of 20 randomized controlled trials looked at the effects of taking glucosamine in 2,596 adults with knee and hip osteoarthritis with an average age of 61 years[5]. Most used an oral dose of 1500 mg glucosamine sulphate daily. Overall results found that glucosamine was more effective than inactive placebo, with a significant reduction in pain of 28 per

1. Reginster JY et al. Lancet 2001; 357: 251–56
2. Bruyere O et al. Osteoarthritis Cartilage 2003;11(1), 1–5
3. Bruyere O et al. Osteoarthritis and Cartilage 2008; 16(2), 254–60
4. Richy F et al. Archives of Internal Medicine 2003; 163(13), 1514–22
5. Towheed TE et al. Cochrane Database Syst Rev 2005; CD002946

cent and a 21 per cent improvement in joint mobility, compared with the start of the study, when measured using a scoring system known as the Lequesne Index. Less impressive effects were found when another scoring system (WOMAC) was used however. In four studies comparing glucosamine sulphate with non-steroidal anti-inflammatory drugs (NSAIDs, mostly ibuprofen), glucosamine was superior in two and equivalent in two. Adverse events and drop-out rates were much higher in the NSAID treatment groups than in the glucosamine sulphate groups however, showing the superior tolerance to glucosamine treatment.

NB: Some trials allowed participants to take paracetamol which neutralizes the sulphur component of glucosamine sulphate and may reduce its effectiveness[1].

Osteoarthritis and glucosamine hydrochloride: Trials using glucosamine hydrochloride (usually together with chondroitin sulphate) have produced less favourable results. The Glucosamine/chondroitin Arthritis Intervention Trial (GAIT) was set up to assess short-term effectiveness (24 weeks) on pain and joint function and long-term (a further 18 months) effects on progression of knee OA, compared with an NSAID drug. Over 1,500 adults, aged 40 and over, with knee pain of at least six-months' duration (and X-ray evidence of knee OA) were randomly assigned to receive either glucosamine hydrochloride or chondroitin, both supplements, an NSAID (Celecoxib) or inactive placebo. No overall benefit was seen from either supplement alone, or in combination, after the first six month period. Benefit for the combination of glucosamine hydrochloride and chondroitin sulphate was found in a subgroup of patients with moderate-to-severe knee pain, however[2]. About 79 per cent had a 20 per cent or greater reduction in pain versus about 54 per cent taking placebo. At the end of the longer, two year period, which was designed to assess X-ray outcomes in 572 of the participants with knee osteoarthritis, no statistically significant difference in loss of joint space width on knee X-ray was seen in any treatment group[3]. The authors concluded that the effect of the combination of glucosamine hydrochloride plus chondroitin sulphate may be less

1. Hoffer LJ et al. Metabolism 2001;50(7), 767–70 2001
2. Clegg DO et al, N Eng J Med 2006; 354(8), 795–808
3. Sawitzke AD et al. Arthritis Rheum 2008; 58(10):3183–91

active than the effect of each treatment singly. However, glucosamine hydrochloride plus chondroitin sulphate has shown benefits in some studies[1,2].

Sports injuries: When just over 100 athletes were given 1500 mg glucosamine or placebo to treat an acute knee injury, there was significant improvement in knee flexion and extension after 28 days with glucosamine compared with placebo.

Inflammatory bowel disease: Inflammatory bowel disease has been linked with reduced activity of an enzyme, glucosamine synthetase, that is involved in bowel wall repair[3]. A pilot study in which children with chronic inflammatory bowel disease took N-acetyl glucosamine supplements showed promise as a safe, inexpensive treatment, with 8 out of 12 children showing clear benefit in symptoms and in the appearance of their bowel wall[4]. This is by no means proven, however, as large trials are needed to confirm this finding in both children and adults. It is important to take N-acetyl glucosamine supplements, not glucosamine sulphate (the more common form available) as there is some evidence that sulphur sources may worsen IBD.

Dose
1500 mg a day.

Safety
Glucosamine salts are well tolerated, and the incidence of side effects is similar to that of inactive placebo. Benefits may be seen within one month, although some studies show effects within two weeks. If, after two months, there is insufficient pain relief, you may wish to add in, or switch to, a chondroitin sulphate supplement to see if that suits you better.

1. Das A & Hammad TA. Osteoarthritis Cartilage 2000; 8(5), 343–50
2. Leffler CT et al. Military Medicine 1999; 164(2), 85–91
3. Russell AL. Med Hypotheses 1999;52(4):297–301
4. Salvatore S et al. Aliment Pharmacol Ther 2000; 14(12):1567–79

L-glutamine

Glutamine is an amino acid that can be synthesized in the body but may become essential during times of stress, and when recovering from injury, infection or surgery. It is the most abundant free amino acid in muscle, cerebrospinal fluid and in the circulation. Food sources include meat, chicken and eggs but only in the raw form – once heated, glutamine becomes inactive. Its precursor, glutamic acid, is present in grains, grapes, nuts and chocolate.

Glutamine has several important roles in metabolism. Its synthesis (from glutamate) is the main pathway for removing toxic ammonia from the body. Glutamine plays a role in maintaining normal blood glucose and acid levels, and if glucose is in short supply, brain cells can burn glutamine for energy instead. Glutamine is also used by the brain to make chemical messengers (neurotransmitters) and helps to overcome mental fatigue, anxiety and improve mood.

Glutamine is used as a source of energy and for synthesis of genetic material in rapidly dividing cells, such as those lining the gut. If glutamine is in short supply, the intestinal lining becomes 'leaky' and when it was first discovered, glutamine was initially referred to as 'intestinal permeability factor'. Other rapidly dividing cells that need good supplies of glutamine include red blood cells, immune cells, and those in hair follicles.

Glutamine is an important muscle-building amino acid and helps replenish muscle glycogen stores after exercise. Some researchers consider glutamine may have an anti-ageing effect by preserving muscle, encouraging fat metabolism and boosting growth hormone levels by up to four-fold.

Benefits

Cancer: Glutamine has been used to reduce side effects of chemotherapy and to support people undergoing bone marrow transplantation.

Inflammatory bowel disease: Gutamine has been used to improve permeability of the gut in people with ulcerative colitis or Crohn's disease. The evidence of benefit is conflicting, however, and most studies show little benefit.

Dose

0.5–2 g daily.

People with diabetes may have abnormal glutamine metabolism, with more glutamine being broken down for the production of glucose. People with diabetes should not take glutamine supplements except under medical advice.

People with chronic renal failure should avoid glutamine supplementation.

Goji berries
(Lycium barbarum; L. chinense)

Goji berries (also known as Wolf berries and red medlars) are the fruit of a plant belonging to the nightshade family, making them related to tomatoes and the potato family. They grow naturally in China, Tibet and the Himalayas, and are found in many UK gardens (sometimes referred to as the Duke of Argyll's Tea Tree, as the leaves are used to make a tea). They have been used as a nutritious food in Asia for more than 2,500 years, and as a Chinese medicine are said to have anti-ageing benefits on the eyes, kidneys and liver.

Goji berries contain a number of vitamins, minerals, carotenoids (including lutein, lycopene and zeaxanthin), essential fatty acids and antioxidants, including vitamin C. They also contain polysaccharides that have been shown in the laboratory to protect nerve cells from degenerative changes, and stimulate the activity of a variety of immune cells.

Benefits

Antioxidant: The antioxidant capacity of dried Goji berries is 25,300 ORAC units (microTE/100g)[1].

Weight loss: Although often marketed as a weight loss supplement, there is no clinical evidence that it is effective. A study involving 34 people which looked at effects on body measurements found that taking Goji berry extracts for 15 days produced no significant

---

1. www.oracvalues.com

changes in body weight, body mass index, blood pressure, pulse rate or visual acuity compared with placebo[1].

Well-being: The same trial quoted above also looked at measures of well-being, including energy levels, athletic performance, quality of sleep, ease of awakening, ability to focus, mental acuity and calmness plus feelings of health, contentment and happiness. They found significant improvements over the 15 days in all of these parameters, together with reduced fatigue and feelings of stress. In contrast, those on placebo only showed two significant changes over the 15 days (heartburn and happiness). This suggests that consuming Goji berry extracts can increase subjective feelings of general well-being and improve mental performance.

Dose
1–2 g concentrated extracts daily.
  Juice: 30 ml twice daily.
  Dried berries: 10–30 g daily.

Goldenseal
(Hydrastis canadensis)

Goldenseal is a plant native to North America, but which has been collected so extensively it is now cultivated commercially. The dried root contains many unique substances, including alkaloids such as hydrastine and canadine, as well as berberine.

Benefits
Goldenseal has a natural antibacterial and anti-viral action, and boosts immunity by activating scavenger cells known as macrophages. It also increases blood circulation to the spleen, where bacteria and other foreign substances are rapidly filtered from the blood. Goldenseal is widely used to overcome infections such as sinusitis, cold sores, common cold, influenza, urinary tract and eye

1. Amagase H, Nance DM. J Altern Complement Med 2008;14(4):403–412

infections. As an immune booster, it is often helpful against chronic fatigue syndrome, recurrent herpes attacks and shingles. It is also helpful against nausea and vomiting.

Freshly prepared goldenseal infusion (i.e. tea) may be strained and used as an eyewash to relieve infections such as conjunctivitis or styes, while goldenseal tincture (prepared using alcohol) may be applied topically to treat mouth ulcers and warts.

Dose

125 mg extract, twice to four times daily (standardized to at least 8 per cent alkaloids or 5 per cent hydrastine).

Goldenseal is only usually taken for up to two weeks at a time. It is often taken with Echinacea (*see also* **Echinacea**). Goldenseal is usually only taken when symptoms are present, and stopped as soon as they have improved, except when it is being alternated with Echinacea (e.g. two weeks on, two weeks off) to maintain immune vigour.

Side effects

Very high doses may cause mouth dryness.

Contraindications

Goldenseal should not be used during pregnancy, breast-feeding, or by sufferers of high blood pressure or glaucoma.

Gotu kola
(Centella asiatica)

Gotu kola is an important Ayurvedic herb that is referred to as the Fountain of Youth, as it is reputed to increase longevity. In Asia, many people regularly eat one leaf of gotu kola a day in the hope of prolonging their life though, unfortunately, there is little evidence that it is effective in this respect.

The dried leaves, stems and flowers contain glycosides and triterpenoids which are present in concentrations of 1–8 per cent. Gotu kola is not related to the kola nut (*Cola nitida* or *Cola acuminata*) and does not contain caffeine.

Benefits

Wound healing: When used externally, gotu kola promotes healing of wounds, chronic ulcers, burns, psoriasis plaques and keloid scars. It also improves cellulite by acting directly on fibroblasts (fibre-producing cells) to improve connective tissue structure and reduce connective tissue hardening (sclerosis) which makes it especially helpful for symptoms associated with varicose veins. Several studies have shown that at least eight out of ten people with varicose veins show significant improvement.

Anxiety: Gotu kola is taken to relieve anxiety and depression, improve memory and concentration and to promote calm and relaxation. A study involving 40 people found that those taking gotu kola showed a reduced startle response to a loud noise compared with those on placebo, suggesting that it has anxiolytic activity.

Dose

60–200 mg a day of standardized extracts.

Side effects

High doses may cause headache.

Grapefruit seed

The seeds of the common grapefruit (*Citrus paradisi*) were first investigated when it was noted that they did not rot when thrown on a compost heap.

Benefits

Antimicrobial: Grapefruit seed extracts have a natural broad-spectrum antibacterial, anti-fungal, anti-viral and anti-parasitic action that may be used internally or externally. They have been proven effective against candida yeasts, herpes viral infections, the parasite *Giardia lamblia*, and the following bacteria: *E. coli*, *Staphylococci*, *Streptococci*, *Salmonella*, *Pseudomonas*, *Klebsiella*, *Shigella*, *Chlamydia*, *Helicobacter*. They are non-toxic and may be helpful for people with recurrent infections such as candida or cystitis. A small trial involving just four patients with bacterial urinary tract infections found that taking grapefruit seeds for two weeks cleared the infection in three of the four patients.

Dose

3–15 drops liquid extract, diluted into water or juice, daily.

Grapefruit seed extracts may be applied undiluted to warts and corns (one drop, twice daily).

Safety

Grapefruit seed extracts should not be taken by people who are on warfarin.

Grapeseed Extracts

Extracts from the seeds of red grapes (*Vitis vinifera*) contain antioxidant flavonoids (proanthocyanidins) which are more concentrated than those that give red wine its widely appreciated health properties. Although grapeseeds constitute less than 5 per cent of the weight of a grape, they contain two-thirds of their flavonoid content.

Benefits

Cardiovascular health: Antioxidant flavonoids found in grapeseed are similar to those found in grape juice and wine. They have a beneficial effect on the circulation, by inhibiting oxidation of 'bad' LDL-cholesterol, inhibiting formation of unwanted blood clots and relaxing blood vessel linings through an effect on nitric oxide (NO). They also appear to strengthen fragile capillaries and protect cell structures from damaging oxidation reactions[1].

They may be helpful in conditions associated with poor circulation, such as diabetes, impotence, varicose veins, thread veins, rosacea, macular degeneration, peripheral vascular disease, intermittent claudication and leg cramps.

Dose

100–300 mg daily (standardized extracts containing at least 92 per cent proanthocyanidins).

1. Kar P et al. Int J Clin Pract 2006;60(11):1484–1492

Grapeseed oil also has beneficial properties and taking 30 ml daily can both increase levels of beneficial HDL-cholesterol (which protects against coronary heart disease), and reduce triglyceride levels by around 15 per cent within one month.

Green-lipped mussel
(Perna canaliculus)

Interest in green-lipped mussels arose when it was noticed that Maori living in coastal regions, who regularly consumed these mussels, suffered fewer arthritic symptoms than those living inland. Freeze-dried extracts of raw New Zealand green-lipped mussels contain glycoproteins that damp down inflammation in arthritic joints. Extracts contain a series of omega-3 fatty acids with anti-inflammatory activity, including EPA (eicosapentaenoic acid), DHA (docosahexaenoic acid) and some additional recently-identified unique omega-3 variants of ODA (octadecatetraenoic acid), NDA (nondecatetraenoic acid), ETA (eicosatetraenoic acid) and HPA (heneicsapentaenoic acid)[1] which inhibit the production of inflammatory cell substances (cytokines such as leukotrienes). These lipids have an action similar to that of non-steroidal anti-inflammatory drugs in that they can inhibit COX-1 and COX-2 enzymes. By reducing inflammation, they reduce the migration of white blood cells into joints to damp down pain and swelling.

Benefits
Osteoarthritis: Several studies suggest that green-lipped mussel extracts produce significant reductions in pain and stiffness in people with osteoarthritis. A systematic review of the data suggests that, as an adjuvant to conventional treatment, green-lipped mussel extracts produce clinical benefits in mild to moderate osteoarthritis[2]. However, a recent review suggests that placebo-controlled trials show about a 20 per cent reduction in osteoarthritis symptoms after three months' use, and suggests there is little to choose between these extracts and cheaper omega-3 fish oils[3].

1. Treschow AP et al. Comp Biochem Physiol 2007;147:645–56
2. Brien S et al. QJM 2008;101(3):167–79
3. Doggrell SA. Evid Based Complement Alternat Med 2009 doi:10.1093/ecam/nep030

Asthma: By reducing formation of leukotrienes, green-lipped mussel extracts would be expected to improve asthma symptoms. A trial involving 46 people with atopic asthma found that taking green-lipped mussel extracts significantly decreased daytime wheeze compared with placebo[1].

Dose

200–1250 mg a day.

Green-lipped mussel extracts do not produce gastric side effects and may even protect against NSAID induced ulceration.

Green tea

Green, white and black tea are similar in that they are made from the young leaves and leaf buds of the same shrub, *Camellia sinensis*. Two main varieties are used, the small-leaved China tea plant (*C. sinensis sinensis*) and the large-leaved Assam tea plant (*C. sinensis assamica*).

Green tea is made by steaming and drying fresh tea leaves immediately after harvesting, while black tea is made by crushing and fermenting freshly cut tea leaves so they oxidize before drying. This allows natural enzymes in the tea leaves to produce the characteristic red-brown colour and reduced astringency.

White tea is similar to green tea, in that it is not fermented, but is only made from new tea buds, picked before they open. These have a white appearance due to the presence of fine, silvery hairs. The buds are gently dried and make a tea that is pale, straw coloured and delicately fragrant – described as light and sweet. White tea does not develop the characteristic 'grassy' flavour of green tea.

Over 30 per cent of the dry weight of green tea leaves consists of powerful flavonoid antioxidants such as catechins. These are converted into less active antioxidants (such as theaflavins and thearubigins) during fermentation but even so, drinking four to five cups of black tea per day provides over 50 per cent of the total dietary intake of flavonoid antioxidants (other sources include fruit and vegetables, especially apples and onions).

1. Emelyanov A et al. Eur Respir J 2002;29(3):596–600

The antioxidants in green tea extracts appear to be at least 100 times more powerful than vitamin C, and 25 times more powerful than vitamin E.

Tea is also a source of the trace element, manganese, and one of the few dietary sources of fluoride.

Benefits

Coronary heart disease: Research suggests that drinking either type of tea has beneficial effects on blood lipids, blood pressure, blood stickiness and can decrease the risk of coronary heart disease and stroke. Researchers have suggested that people who drink at least four cups of tea a day are 50 per cent less likely to have a heart attack than non-tea drinkers (its antioxidants reduce oxidation of LDL-cholesterol so less is deposited in artery walls) and are also less likely to suffer from high blood pressure. A meta-analysis of data showed that drinking three or more cups of tea per day can reduce the risk of coronary heart disease and for improved antioxiant status with intakes of from one to six cups of tea per day[1].

Cancer: High intakes (around eight to ten cups a day) of green tea were thought to protect against cancer, but despite positive evidence from laboratory and non-human studies, recent large analyses of data have failed to confirm significant protective effects against stomach or colon cancer. Analysis of results from four studies suggests that women with the highest intake of green tea are 22 per cent less likely to develop breast cancer[2].

Weight loss: Extracts from green tea leaves (*Camellia sinensis*) can boost the rate at which the body burns calories by as much as 40 per cent over a 24 hour period. This is due to its ability to inhibit a metabolic enzyme (catechol-0-methyl transferase) so that levels of noradrenaline increase to stimulate the amount of energy burned in body cells (thermogenesis). It may also block the activity of intestinal enzymes (gastric and pancreatic lipases) needed to digest dietary fat, so that less fat is absorbed. Several trials have suggested

1. Gardner EJ et al. Eur J Clin Nutr 2007;61(1):3–18
2. Sun CL et al. Carcinogenesis 2006;27(7):1310–5

that adding green tea extracts to a weight loss regime helps to improve fat loss. For example, a study involving 60 obese adults following a prepared diet of three meals a day found that, compared with placebo, those taking green tea extracts lost an additional 2.7 kg during the first month, 5.1 kg during the second month and 3.3 kg during the third month[1].

Dose

Drink four cups of green tea daily, or take supplements of 500 mg daily (standardized to contain at least 50 per cent polyphenols).

White tea contains around 15 mg caffeine per cup, compared to 20 mg for green tea and 40 mg for black tea.

Guarana
(Paullinia cupana)

Guarana is derived from a Brazilian bush and known locally as the 'food of the gods'. The dried seeds contain a complex of natural stimulants, including caffeine (trimethyl xanthene), guaranine (tetramethyl xanthene), theobromine, theophylline and saponins similar to those found in Korean and American ginseng. It also contains unique flavone glycosides not found in other plants.

Guarana increases physical, mental and sexual energy levels and relieves fatigue.

Benefits

Alertness: Taking guarana extracts can increase energy levels and improve stress responses. In a study involving 26 adults, doses of 37.5 mg and 75 mg guarana extracts produced greater improvements in mood, memory and cognition (ability to think straight) than placebo. The researchers also suggest that these effects cannot be attributed to caffeine alone[2].

Guarana is useful for preventing jet lag, when taken before, during and after a long-distance flight. Some research suggests it has a blood thinning action which may make it helpful for reducing the

---

1. Auvichayapat P et al. Physiol Behav 2008;93(3):486–91
2. Haskell CF et al. J Psychopharmacol 2007 21(1):65–70

incidence of abnormal blood clotting associated with so-called economy-class syndrome.

Dose
1 g a day.

Note: Guarana is a restricted substance for some sports.

Gymnema sylvestre

Gymnema is a woody vine used in Ayurvedic medicine. When applied to the tongue, it reduces the ability to detect sweet sensations for up to 90 minutes, blocking both the taste of sugars and artificial sweeteners. These taste-blocking effects are believed to result from the presence of several unique, oily saponins[1]. It has also been suggested that it may help regeneration of insulin-producing beta-cells in the pancreas, and to increase natural production of insulin.

When given to healthy volunteers it does not seem to have an effect on blood glucose levels, but when given to people with Type 1 or Type 2 diabetes, it improves glucose control and reduces the amount of hypoglycaemic medication needed.

Benefits
Glucose control: Extracts of Gymnema sylvestre can reduce fasting blood glucose levels in people with diabetes, so that insulin requirements reduce[2]. Cholesterol and triglyceride levels also improved in those taking extracts. When added to the usual hypoglycaemic drug regimes of people with Type 2 diabetes, all showed improved glucose control compared with a similar group using drugs alone. Natural insulin production increased and most had to reduce the dose of the oral hypoglycaemic drugs they were taking[3].

Dose
200–400 mg a day.

1. Ye W, Liu X et al. J Nat Prod 2001; 64;2:232–5
2. Shanmugasundaram ER et al. J Ethnopharmacol 1990;30(3):281–94
3. Baskaran K et al. J Ethnopharmacol 1990;30(3):295–300

Side effects/Safety

Long-term use may reduce iron absorption leading to iron deficiency anaemia.

Most research has therefore occurred with an extract known as GS4 which has had components removed that are believed to interfere with iron absorption.

No adverse effects reported in trials where it was taken by some for 30 months.

Monitor blood glucose levels closely and adjust medication dose as necessary, under medical supervision.

Hawthorn

(Crategus oxycantha; C. laevigata; C. monogyna)

The flowering tops and berries of the hawthorn provide one of the most beneficial herbal remedies available for treating the heart and circulation. Hawthorn extracts contain flavonoids, such as vitexin, which are used to treat cardiovascular problems such as high blood pressure and heart failure. It does not contain cardiac glycosides such as those found in the foxglove, and therefore has low toxicity. Hawthorn is also used to treat insomnia and anxiety.

Benefits

Heart failure: Hawthorn extracts increase the strength and efficiency of the heart's pumping action. A meta-analysis of the results from ten trials, involving 855 people, show that taking hawthorn extracts reduced heart work load, improved shortness of breath and fatigue, and increased exercise tolerance more than placebo[1].

Blood pressure: Hawthorn helps to reduce high blood pressure by relaxing peripheral blood vessels and dilating coronary arteries through its ability to block the action of an enzyme (ACE or angiotensin-converting enzyme), which improves blood circulation to heart muscle and the peripheries. It has a mild diuretic action that discourages fluid retention, and can also slow or possibly even reverse the build-up of atheromatous plaques to reduce hardening

1. Pittler MH et al. Cochrane Database Syst Rev 2008; (1):CD005312

and furring up of the arteries (atherosclerosis). In a group of 80 people with Type 2 diabetes, who were taking an average of 4.4 hypoglycaemia and/or hypotensive drugs, half were randomized to receive 1200 mg hawthorn extract, and half placebo. Those taking hawthorn showed greater reduction in blood pressure (3.6/2.6 mmHg) versus the placebo group (in whom systolic BP reduced by 0.8 mmHg and diastolic blood pressure increased by 0.5 mmHg).

Dose

500–1200 mg a day (standardized to at least 1.8 per cent vitexin).

Larger amounts are usually divided between three doses. It may take up to two months for hawthorn extracts to show an appreciable effect.

Safety

Should only be used under medical supervision. Side effects are uncommon, and include nausea, dizziness, sweating and skin rashes.

Hempseed oil
(*Cannabis sativa*)

Oil from the seed of the non-drug strain of cannabis, known as the hemp plant, contains both omega-6 and omega-3 essential fatty acids. The ratio of omega-6: omega-3 is around 3:1 – the opposite to that found in flaxseed oil. However, a significant amount of the omega-6 oil is in the form of anti-inflammatory gammalinolenic acid (GLA).

Hempseed oil is often suggested as an alternative source of omega-3 fatty acids for those unable or unwilling to take fish oils. Although it is a source of short-chain omega-3 essential fatty acids, only 5 per cent of ALA is converted on to eicosapentaenoic acid (EPA) and even less – just 0.5 per cent – is converted on to docosahexaenoic acid (DHA) which are the beneficial long-chain omega-3s found in oily fish.

Benefits

Hempseed oil has similar uses to evening primrose and flaxseed oils. It is used to correct hormone imbalances and to improve skin condition. Individuals who use hempseed oil long term have reported improved fingernail strength and thicker hair as well as improved skin condition.

Cardiovascular: When 86 adults took either 2 g hempseed oil, flaxseed oil, fish oil or placebo per day, for 12 weeks, blood levels of the long-chain omega-3 fatty acids DHA and EPA did not alter significantly with hempseed oil[1]. Hempseed oil does appear to have a beneficial effect on the ratio of total-to-HDL cholesterol[2].

Eczema: In a small group of 20 people, taking hempseed oil (30 ml daily) for eight weeks was shown to significantly improve levels of anti-inflammatory lipids (GLA, ALA) in the circulation, and improved symptoms of atopic dermatitis (itching, dryness) and a reduced need for emollient creams, compared with a similar period in which they took placebo (olive oil)[3].

Dose
10–30 ml a day, best taken with food.

Safety
Hempseed oil supplements contain small amounts of the psychoactive chemical (tetrahydrocannabinol, or THC) found in marijuana strains of the cannabis plant. Independent testing of commercially available hempseed oil products in the US found THC in all eight oils (some bottled oils, some capsules) in concentrations ranging from 11.5–48.6 mg/g[4]. Some THC was also found in the urine of volunteers taking 15 ml doses of these oils, with urinary concentrations ranging from 1–49 ng/ml. Drug test screening for THC typically uses a cut off of 50 ng/ml for a positive result, and consumption of large amounts of hempseed oil could raise urine levels above this range. Positive tests have been reported with the use of hempseed oil products.

Some oils are labelled as having undetectable amounts of THC (below 3 parts per million).

1. Kaul N et al. J Am Coll Nutr 2008; 27(1):51–8
2. Schwab US et al. Eur J Nutr 2006; 45(8):470–7
3. Callaway J et al. J Dermatolog Treat 2005;16(2):87–94
4. Bosy TZ, Cole KA. J Anal Toxicol 2000;24(7):562–6

Holy basil
(Ocimum sanctum and Ocimum album)

Holy basil (also known as tulsi) is a sweet culinary herb from India that is related to the European garden basil. It is used in Ayurvedic medicine to lower blood glucose levels, reduce high blood pressure and to relieve fevers, bronchitis, asthma, stress and mouth ulcers. It has anti-inflammatory effects.

Benefits

Glucose control: Holy basil is believed to increase uptake of glucose by cells and to improve pancreatic beta cell function and insulin secretion. In one trial 40 people with Type 2 diabetes were given either holy basil leaves or placebo (spinach) for eight weeks – all other diabetic medication was stopped. Holy basil was shown to reduce average fasting blood glucose levels by 17.6 per cent during the trial, while post-meal glucose levels fell by 7.3 per cent[1]. In another trial involving 27 people with Type 2 diabetes, holy basil was said to lower blood glucose levels by 20 per cent, LDL-cholesterol by 14 per cent and triglycerides by 16 per cent after 30 days[2]. The researchers suggest that holy basil leaves may be used together with dietary or drug treatment in mild to moderate Type 2 diabetes.

Anxiety: When 35 people with generalized anxiety disorder took 500 mg holy basil extracts twice a day after meals, for 60 days, significant improvements in stress, anxiety and depression were recorded[3]. There was no placebo group with which to compare, however.

Dose

500 mg extracts twice a day.

1. Agrawal P et al. Int J Clin Pharmacol Ther 1996;34(9):406–9
2. Rai V et al. J Nutr Environ Med 1997;7:113–8
3. Bhattacharyya D et al. Nepal Med Coll J 2008;10(3):176–9

Hoodia gordonii

Hoodia is a spiny, succulent cactus-like plant from South Africa that is used as a natural appetite suppressant. It was traditionally chewed by the Khomani San bushmen of the Kalahari desert as a food to stave off hunger pangs on long hunting trips. It contains several unique substances (known as hoodigosides and hoodistanalosides) that have been shown to suppress appetite and produce significant weight loss in animal studies.

Benefits

An active extract, known as P57, is in development to produce an anti-obesity drug which is particularly attractive because, unlike many other appetite-suppressant drugs in the past, it is non-stimulating.

Initial clinical studies in 60 human volunteers found that it could produce a 30 per cent reduction in calorie intake and a significant reduction in body fat of 1 kg over a 15 day period[1].

Dose

2000–8000 mg per day.

Horsechestnut
(Aesculus hippocastanum)

Horsechestnut seed extracts are derived from the common deciduous tree. The main active ingredients are triterpene saponins together known as escin (aescin). These are used to tighten small blood vessels and reduce excessive permeability, to help stop fluid leakage from the circulation into the peripheral tissues. They may also reduce the activity of enzymes that lead to excessive breakdown of supporting tissues (proteoglycans) around capillary walls to produce a strengthening effect on tissues supporting peripheral blood vessels.

---

1. Harbeck M. Drug Discov Today 2002;7(5):280–281

Benefits

Extracts are used to treat varicose veins, venous insufficiency, venous ulcers, haemorrhoids and may help to reduce nosebleeds. They have also been used to reduce swelling following sprains and strains.

Venous insufficiency: A review of five clinical studies shows that horsechestnut extracts significantly reduce fluid exudation across capillaries compared with placebo, and that extracts can reduce sensations of tiredness, heaviness, tension, itching, cramping, pain and swelling in the legs in those with varicose veins and chronic venous insufficiency[1]. A meta-analysis of data from seven trials showed significant improvements in leg pain[2]. One trial suggests that horsechestnut extracts may be as effective as treatment with compression stockings.

Dose

20–50 mg, daily, corresponding to 100 mg escin daily.

Select extracts standardized to contain 16–21 per cent escin where possible.

Side effects

Occasional side effects of itching, nausea, and indigestion may occur.

5-hydroxy-tryptophan

5-hydroxy-tryptophan (5-HTP) is derived from an amino acid, l-tryptophan, which is found in small amounts in foods such as turkey, chicken, meat and dairy products such as cheese. Preformed 5-HTP is only found in two places in nature, however – in the human body, and in the seeds of a West African medicinal plant, *Griffonia simplicifolia*. The 5-HTP found in supplements is extracted from the latter source.

Once absorbed into the circulation, some 5-HTP travels to the

1. Suter A et al. Adv Ther 2006; 23(1):179–90
2. Pittler MH, Ernst E. Cochrane Database Syst Rev 2006; (1):CD003230

brain, where it is converted into the 'happy' chemical messenger, serotonin (5-hydroxytryptamine or 5-HT), which helps to regulate mood, behaviour, appetite, sleep and impulse control. Low levels of serotonin are associated with depression, insomnia, anxiety, premenstrual syndrome, binge eating disorders, fibromyalgia, and migraine. Serotonin levels in the brain are dependent on levels of 5-HTP which readily crosses the blood-brain barrier. Supplements supplying 5-HTP may help to overcome these conditions by increasing serotonin synthesis.

The most commonly prescribed antidepressant drugs, SSRIs (selective serotonin re-uptake inhibitors) work by raising levels of serotonin in the brain, but rather than increasing serotonin synthesis, they block its re-uptake so that levels within the communication gaps (synapses) between brain cells increase. If you are making very little serotonin, however, SSRIs may not produce a significant response, or may do so only slowly. As 5-HTP helps to boost production of serotonin in the brain, it tends to have a faster onset of action than prescription-only SSRI anti-depressant drugs. Because of its mode of action, it often produces good results in people who have not previously responded to standard SSRI antidepressant drugs.

Levels of other important brain chemicals also increase after taking 5-HTP, including melatonin, dopamine, norepinephrine and beta-endorphin.

Benefits

Depression: Several trials have shown that 5-HTP supplements have a positive effect on low mood, and are better than placebo at alleviating depression. These trials, involving over 500 people with depression, showed significant improvement in 56 per cent of participants[1]. In a study involving 74 people with unipolar or bipolar depression, 69 per cent improved, with most responding within two weeks[2]. A meta-analysis of data suggests that 5-HT is better than placebo but that more well-designed trials are urgently needed to assess its effectiveness[3].

1. Birdsall TC. Altern Med Rev 1998;3(4):271–280
2. Sano I. Folia Psychiatr Neurol Japan 1972;26:7–17
3. Shaw K et al. Aust N Z J Psychiatry 2002;36(4):488–91

Headache: 5-HTP has been used to help prevent chronic daily headache, tension headache and migraine. By boosting serotonin production it promotes vaso-constriction in the brain to relieve pounding migraine headaches linked with vasodilation. 5-HTP is also thought to increase pain thresholds by increasing levels of endorphins – the brain's own morphine-like painkillers. In a study involving 78 people with tension headaches, when taking 5-HTP for two weeks there was a significant reduction in the need for analgesics than when taking placebo[1]. In a study involving 124 people treated with either 5-HTP or the antimigraine drug, methysergide, 71 per cent taking 5-HTP and 74 per cent of those taking methysergide experienced significant improvement with either prevention or substantially decreased numbers of attacks. Side effects were less frequent with 5-HTP, and it was effective in reducing the intensity and duration of attacks[2]. It has been used successfully to treat headache in pubertal children[3].

Sleep: 5-HTP is used to help treat insomnia. It is involved in the production of melatonin, the sleep hormone, and improves the architecture of sleep. In particular, it extends the period of time spent in REM (rapid eye movement, or dreaming) sleep so you wake up feeling more refreshed. 5-HTP has also been used successfully to treat 'sleep terrors' in young children, and sleep disorders and headaches in children[4]. However, an estimated 2.5 per cent of people taking 5-HTP experience insomnia and in some people it may trigger vivid dreams.

Fibromyalgia: People with fibromyalgia have low serotonin levels and sleep disturbances which can respond to 5-HTP, with three trials showing improvement in pain, number of tender points, morning stiffness, sleep patterns, anxiety and fatigue[5,6,7].

Appetite: Raised levels of serotonin help to trigger feelings of satiety, so you feel more full, less hungry and with decreased interest

1. Ribeiro CA. Headache 2000; 40(6):451–6
2. Titus F et al. Eur Neurol 1986;25(5):327–9
3. Longo G et al. Pediatr Med Chir 1984;6(2):241–5
4. De Giorgis G et al. Drugs Exp Clin Res 1987;13(7):425–33
5. Nicolodi M et al. Adg Exp Med Biol 1996;398:373–379
6. Puttini PS et al. J Int Med Res 1992;20:182–189
7. Caruso I et al. J Int Med Res 1990;18:201–208

in food. This may make 5-HTP helpful for people with binge eating disorder. It has been shown to decrease carbohydrate cravings and binge eating even in the absence of a structured diet[1].

Dose

It is usually taken for up to three months, followed by a break. 50 mg three times a day, initially, increasing to 100 mg three times a day after two weeks, if necessary.

For insomnia: 100–200 mg before bedtime.

Safety

5-HTP should not be taken at the same time as prescription anti-depressant drugs, except under medical advice and supervision.

Since 5-HTP may cause drowsiness, it should not be used while driving a car or operating heavy machinery.

In the late 1980s, researchers found an unknown contaminant in some 5-HTP supplements that was referred to as 'Peak X'. This was associated with a serious illness known as eosinophilia myalgia syndrome (EMS) which caused muscle and joint pain, fever, weakness, swelling and shortness of breath. The contaminant was traced to a single Japanese manufacturer and appeared to arise during their filtration process. All 5-HTP sources are now screened to ensure they are 'Peak X free'.

Iodine

Iodine is an essential trace element that has only one known function in the body: it is vital for the production of the two thyroid hormones, thyroxine (T4) and tri-iodothyronine (T3). These hormones control the metabolic rate, the conversion of food and fat stores into energy and how much body heat is produced.

Dietary sources of iodine include marine fish, seaweed products, iodized salt and crops or cattle reared on soils exposed to sea spray. Lack of iodine is common in many parts of the world, however.

---

1. Cangiano C et al. Am J Clin Nutr 1992;56:863–867

Benefits
Iodine plays a major role in preventing lethargy, tiredness, and excessive weight gain. The normal range for thyroxine hormone is wide, and sub-optimal intakes of iodine may account for feelings of lethargy and difficulty in losing weight in many whose T4 level is in the low normal range.

Deficiency
Symptoms that may be linked with iodine deficiency include under-active thyroid gland, swollen thyroid gland (goitre), tiredness, lack of energy, weight gain, muscle weakness, susceptibility to the cold, coarse skin, brittle hair and nails, breast tenderness and increased production of mucus.

Lack of iodine in pregnancy leads to an underactive thyroid which shows up after birth as a condition known as cretinism. As well as an underactive thyroid, the child's brain cannot develop properly, leading to severe mental retardation. This is a serious problem in some parts of the world, including parts of Europe, New Zealand, Brazil and the Himalayas. In some areas, iodine deficiency affects nine out of ten of the population. In Indonesia, for example, there are currently an estimated 1.5 million severely mentally retarded children and 800,000 with cretinism. This is a devastating condition that is entirely preventable if expectant mothers are given injections of iodized oil – preferably during the preconceptual period. Treatment must be given before the sixth month of pregnancy to protect the brain against the effects of iodine deficiency. When treatment is not given until the last three months of pregnancy, it does not seem to improve brain function. In the Western world, newborn babies are screened for cretinism as part of the heel-prick test carried out soon after delivery.

Gross iodine deficiency leading to swelling of the thyroid gland (goitre) may occur in people who restrict their salt intake and who do not eat iodine-rich foods (e.g. seafood).

Supplements providing iodine act as a mild thyroid stimulant and may encourage a more efficient metabolism if your iodine intake has been sub-optimal. It is therefore included in many products designed to aid weight loss. It may also improve energy levels and quality of skin, hair and nails.

Selenium plays a role in the metabolism of thyroid hormones, and the effects of iodine deficiency are made worse by low selenium intakes.

Dose

The UK RNI for iodine is 140 mcg per day for adults. The EU RDA for iodine is 150 mcg a day. Those who are physically active may need more iodine than people who are inactive as iodine is lost in sweat – an athlete in heavy training can lose 150 mcg iodine in sweat alone. The upper safe level for long-term use from supplements is suggested as 500 mcg per day.

Iodine is best obtained from natural extracts of kelp, bladder-wrack (*Fucus*) or from an A to Z-style vitamin and mineral supplement.

Up to 3 per cent of people are allergic to iodine, and taking supplements long term (especially those derived from kelp) can cause sensitivity reactions.

Excess

Excess iodine may lead to a metallic taste in the mouth, oral sores, headache, diarrhoea, vomiting, rash and – as with a deficiency – can also lead to thyroid swelling (goitre).

Iron

Iron is an essential mineral needed for the production of haemoglobin (the red blood pigment which transports oxygen and the waste gas, carbon dioxide, around the body), myoglobin (a muscle pigment), cytochrome enzymes, and plays an important role in energy production in cells. Two-thirds of the body's iron stores are present in haemoglobin.

Dietary sources of iron include shellfish, red meats, sardines, wheatgerm, wholemeal bread, egg yolk, green vegetables and dried fruit. Currently, iron fortification of white and brown flour is mandatory in the UK (not less than 16.5 mg iron/kg flour). Some manufacturers also fortify breakfast cereals on a voluntary basis (typically 70–120 mg/kg). Infant formulas and follow-on milks are fortified by EU law. Fortification accounts for around 10 per cent iron intake in adults and more than 20 per cent in preschool children. .

There are two main forms of dietary iron:

- Haem – from animal sources
- Inorganic – from plant sources and enriched cereals.

Haem is absorbed via a specific haem receptor 2–3 times more efficiently than non-haem iron. However, most dietary iron is obtained in inorganic form, 48 per cent from cereal products, 16 per cent from vegetables.

Inorganic iron exists in two oxidation states: ferrous (Fe^{2+}) and ferric (Fe^{3+}) which have separate uptake mechanisms. Ferric iron – the form in which most plant-derived iron is obtained – is less well absorbed due to low solubility at higher pH. Iron uptake from a varied diet is therefore low, estimated at 15 per cent. Vitamin C increases absorption by converting ferric iron to ferrous iron. Over boiling vegetables decreases their iron availability by up to 20 per cent.

Deficiency
Vegetarians and those who eat little red meat are at increased risk of iron deficiency. Their intakes are dependent on absorbing inorganic non-haem iron, and food supplements play an important role.

In the UK, dietary iron intakes have fallen over the last 30 years due to decreased meat consumption and reduced energy intake. As a result, iron deficiency anaemia (IDA) is increasingly common. Vulnerable groups include:

- Infants if exclusively breast-fed (formulas/follow-on milks are fortified by EC law)
- Toddlers – studies suggest 28 per cent have no iron stores; 12–30 per cent have IDA
- Adolescents – 64 per cent have low iron stores, 28 per cent have no stores, 20 per cent have IDA
- Menstruating women – 32 per cent have low iron stores, 11 per cent have no stores, 36 per cent have IDA
- Pregnant women
- Vegetarians
- Those with high intakes of iron absorption inhibitors (e.g. phytates)

- Those with excessive, pathological blood losses (e.g. gastro-intestinal disease)
- Elderly – up to 10 per cent living at home have IDA and prevalence is higher in institutions.

IDA is an important public health problem in the UK with potentially serious consequences. In adults, it is associated with fatigue, reduced work performance, impaired immunity, reduced fertility and deranged thermogenesis – a particular problem for the elderly. In childhood, IDA is associated with behavioural problems, poor concentration and learning difficulties. Although psychomotor delay appears to be reversible with iron therapy, later cognitive deficits may be apparent.

Lack of iron quickly leads to the production of red blood cells that are much smaller and paler (due to lack of haemoglobin) than normal. This results in iron-deficiency anaemia with symptoms of paleness, fast pulse, tiredness, exhaustion, dizziness, headache and even shortness of breath and angina if anaemia is severe.

Other symptoms that can occur in iron deficiency include generalized skin itching, concave brittle nails, hair loss, sore tongue, cracking at the corners of the mouth, reduced appetite and difficulty in swallowing.

Worldwide, iron deficiency is the most common nutritional disease, with most cases going unrecognized. Women are more at risk of iron deficiency than men, because of blood loss during menstruation. This can result in a low-grade iron deficiency that is enough to impair immunity, without causing frank iron-deficiency anaemia. If anaemia is suspected, it is important to seek medical advice before taking iron supplements, as the cause needs to be determined and iron supplements may mask iron deficiency.

Lack of iron can trigger pica – a condition characterized by cravings for eating strange things such as soil, coal, paper. This is especially common during pregnancy, and iron deficiency should always be checked for.

Excess
There is no specific mechanism for excreting excess iron. High intakes accumulate in liver storage proteins (haemosiderin, ferritin). Generalized iron overload (excess total body iron greater than 5 g in

adults) and severe iron overload (excess total body iron greater than 10 g) leads to oxidative tissue damage. However, this effect is minimized as most body iron is bound to carrier molecules with antioxidant properties. Also, iron absorption is inversely related to the level of iron stores except in people with haemochromatosis.

Haemochromatosis is an autosomal recessive condition linked with the *HFE* gene. In those inheriting two copies of this gene, absorption of dietary iron is unregulated and excess accumulation of iron can lead to liver cirrhosis, liver carcinoma, diabetes and heart failure.

In Caucasian populations, haemochromatosis affects 1 in 140 people. Another 1 in 100 carry another gene mutation that also increases their risk of iron accumulation, although to a lesser extent. In addition, 1 in 7 people carry one copy of the defective gene and have mildly increased iron stores, although significant iron loading is rare.

Coronary heart disease: Excess iron may cause oxidation changes in 'bad' LDL-cholesterol to promote atherosclerosis. A 2.2-fold increased risk of myocardial infarction was found in Finnish males with elevated serum ferritin levels, after adjusting for confounding factors such as age, exercise level, smoking, blood pressure, glucose and lipid levels. And Finnish males who regularly donated blood (and therefore lost approximately 250 mg haem iron per 500 mg donated) were found to have an 88 per cent reduced risk of CHD compared with non-blood donors. However, individuals with haemochromatosis do not seem to have an increased risk of heart attack (though they are at risk of heart failure) and these findings have not been corroborated by other studies in other populations[1]. A meta-analysis of 12 studies involving 7,800 people with coronary heart disease found no significant differences in risk between those with the highest iron status and those with the lowest iron status[2].

Immunity: Iron plays an important role in immunity as white blood cells use powerful iron-containing chemicals to destroy invading micro-organisms (bacteria, yeasts, viruses) and one of the signs of

1. Sun Q et al. J Nutr 2008;138(12):2436–41
2. Danesh J, Appleby P. Circulation 1999;99(7):852–4

iron deficiency is often increased susceptibility to infection, especially recurrent thrush and *Herpes simplex* virus attacks. As this can occur when levels of iron are not low enough to cause anaemia, it will not be picked up with a simple test to measure haemoglobin levels. Instead, it is necessary to measure the amount of iron binding protein (ferritin) present in the circulation to detect low iron stores.

Pregnancy: Iron requirements are thought to double during pregnancy as a woman's red blood cell and haemoglobin count goes up by 30 per cent although a lot of this will be obtained through the absence of normal losses associated with menstrual bleeding. Pregnancy is also associated with significantly increased iron absorption of up to nine-fold. Although iron is important during pregnancy, many doctors no longer routinely recommend iron supplements to pregnant women, as excess intakes have been associated with an increased risk of developing pre-eclampsia.

Dose

The UK RNI for iron is 8.7 mg for men and 14.8 mg for women. The EU RDA is 14 mg for adults. The upper safe level for long-term use from supplements is suggested as 17 mg per day.

Take a supplement supplying iron in the ferrous (not the ferric) form. Ferrous fumarate and ferrous gluconate are usually better tolerated than ferrous sulphate.

Iron-rich spa water is available as a liquid iron tonic, as are iron-rich solutions/tablets obtained from plant sources (herbal tonics) which are also well tolerated and may act more quickly.

Vitamin C increases the absorption of inorganic (non-haem) iron when taken at the same time, so it is a good idea to wash down supplements with fresh fruit juice.

Phytate fibre, calcium and tannin-containing drinks decrease iron absorption. Coffee, for example, can reduce iron absorption by up to 39 per cent if drunk within an hour of eating. Iron is therefore best taken on an empty stomach unless it causes irritation.

Taking iron supplements alone can decrease absorption of zinc and other essential minerals (such as manganese, chromium and selenium) so it is usually advisable to only take iron in combination with these, e.g. in an A to Z-style vitamin and mineral supplement (unless prescribed individually by a doctor).

Excess

Avoid taking too much iron as this can cause constipation or indigestion and excess is toxic (especially for children).

Keep iron supplements well away from small children – eating just a few has been known to be fatal.

Most men and post-menopausal women do not need to take iron-containing supplements.

Isoflavones

Isoflavones are a class of plant hormones that have a similar structure to human oestradiol. Around a thousand different plant isoflavones have been identified, but we only obtain five dietary isoflavones with oestrogenic activity in significant amounts: genistein, daidzein and glycitein are mainly derived from soy and Japanese Arrowroot (*Pueraria lobata* also known as kudzu), while formononetin and biochanin A (which are metabolized to form daidzein and genistein) are mostly obtained from chickpeas, lentils and mung beans.

In Japan, where soy is a dietary staple, intakes of isoflavones are 50–100 mg per day for both men and women, compared with typical Western intakes of just 2–5 mg isoflavones per day. Blood levels of isoflavones in Japan are therefore as much as 110 times higher than those typically found in the West.

Dietary plant isoflavones are mostly present in an inactive form in which they are attached to sugars to form glycosides. The principal isoflavone glycosides in soy are genistin and daidzin. Once ingested, bacteria in the large intestines break down the sugar-isoflavones, releasing the active forms (isoflavone aglycones) called genistein and daidzein.

Isoflavone metabolism varies greatly among individuals, and absorption is greatest in those with the slowest gut transit time. Some people also possess intestinal bacteria (e.g. Lactobacillus, Bacteroides and Bifidobacterium species) able to metabolize daidzein to a more powerful oestrogen, called equol. People can therefore be divided into two distinct groups: equol producers and nonequol producers. Equol has a higher antioxidant activity than any other isoflavone, and equol producers gain greater health benefits from isoflavones than nonequol producers[1]. This difference may explain some of the contradictory findings obtained from some research studies into the health benefits of isoflavones.

Isoflavones are less active than oestradiol at oestrogen receptor sites. Compared with oestrodiol, the affinity of genistein for oestrogen receptors is 0.82 per cent (around 100 times weaker than oestradiol), while that of daidzein is 0.015 per cent (around 6,666 times weaker than oestradiol)[2]. They have a normalizing effect on oestrogen status as they act as both oestrogen agonists (stimulating the receptors) and antagonists (blocking the receptors from interacting with stronger human oestrogens). They therefore provide a useful oestrogen boost when oestrogen levels are low and, conversely, reduce oestrogen stimulation during high oestrogen states. They also stimulate production of sex hormone binding globulin (SHBG), which reduces the level of active, circulating free oestrogen.

Benefits

Pre-menstrual syndrome: A cross-over study involving 23 women found that isoflavone supplements significantly reduced symptoms of headache, breast tenderness, cramps and swelling compared with placebo[3]. Interestingly, equol production did not enhance symptom reduction suggesting that the mode of action was non-hormonal.

Menopause: A number of studies show that isoflavones can reduce menopausal hot flushes and night sweats. A study involving 50 postmenopausal women found that isoflavones were significantly superior to placebo, reducing hot flushes by 44 per cent versus 10 per cent. After six months, the isoflavone group showed increased oestradiol levels with unchanged FSH, LH, and vaginal cytology. The researchers concluded that isoflavones are an interesting alternative for postmenopausal women in whom conventional HRT is contraindicated[4]. However, perhaps surprisingly, a meta-analysis of data from five trials found no significant differences in frequency of hot flushes compared with placebo[5].

1. Setchell KD et al. J Nutr 2002;132(12):3577–84
2. Hopert A-C et al. Environmental Health Perspectives 1998;106(9):581–6
3. Bryant M et al. Br J Nutr 2005; 93(5):731–9
4. Petri NE et al. Maturitas 2004;48(4):372–80
5. Lethaby AE et al. Cochrane Database Syst Rev 2007;17(4):CD001395

Coronary heart disease: A large body of evidence suggests that isoflavones can reduce the risk of coronary heart disease (CHD) through a variety of independent mechanisms, including their anti-oxidant and anti-inflammatory actions. Isoflavones interact with oestrogen receptors within the circulation, helping to dilate coronary arteries, reduce arterial stiffness, lower blood pressure, reduce homo-cysteine levels, blood stickiness and platelet clumping. A meta-analysis of 23 trials found beneficial reductions in serum total choles-terol, LDL-cholesterol and triglycerides, with increased beneficial HDL-cholesterol[1]. Individual studies which have shown no effect on individual coronary heart disease risk factors may have inadvertently contained a high population of non-equol producers. Although a lot of the research involved postmenopausal women, one study involved 61 Scottish males (aged 45–59), who had relatively high BP and/or total cholesterol levels. Increasing isoflavone intake for just five weeks produced significant reductions in both systolic and diastolic blood pressure and reduced low density lipoprotein cholesterol, compared with an olive-oil placebo. Significant increases in high-density lipoprotein cholesterol were also observed. The authors concluded that increasing the dietary content of soy protein and isoflavones can reduce CHD risk among high-risk, middle-aged men[2].

Osteoporosis: Isoflavones mimic the effects of natural oestrogen on bones and, in theory, should increase the activity of bone-building osteoblasts, and reduce activity of bone-dissolving osteoclasts. A study involving 650 women aged 19–86 found that post-menopausal women with the highest intake of dietary isoflavones had signifi-cantly higher bone mineral density at both spine and hip than those with the lowest intakes after adjusting for age, height, weight, years since menopause, smoking, alcohol consumption, HRT usage, and daily calcium intake[3]. A meta-analysis of ten studies involving over 600 subjects found significant increases in spine bone mineral density in those consuming isoflavones compared with those with low intakes. Favourable effects were greatest in those consuming more than 90 mg isoflavones per day for at least six months[4]. The

1. Zhan S, Ho SC. Am J Clin Nutr 2005; 81(2):397–408
2. Sagara M et al. J Am Coll Nutr 2004;23(1):85–91
3. Mei J et al. J Clin Endocrinol Metab 2001;86(11):5217–5221
4. Ma DM et al. Clin Nutr 2008;27(1):57–64

protective effect of soy in maintaining bone mineral density is more marked in women in later menopause, those with lower body weight or lower calcium intake[1]. Continuous dietary intake of isoflavone may therefore inhibit postmenopausal osteoporosis[2].

Memory: Consuming a high-soy diet improves memory and frontal lobe function in young healthy students (both male and female), men awaiting gender reassignment and in postmenopausal women[3]. In a trial involving 33 postmenopausal women (50–65 years) who were not on HRT, those taking isoflavone supplements for 12 weeks showed significantly greater improvements in memory recall, sustained attention tasks, learning rule reversals, and in planning tasks than those on placebo[4]. A study involving 56 postmenopausal women aged 55–74 years also showed that taking isoflavones has a favourable effect on cognitive function, particularly verbal memory[5].

Prostate cancer: Soy isoflavones contain genistein, a phytoestrogen that may protect against prostate cancer. Genistein decreases the growth of both benign prostatic hyperplasia (BPH) and prostate cancer cells in the laboratory and induces apoptosis (programmed cell death). Research involving 137,000 males found that men with high levels of genistein are 26 per cent less likely to develop prostate cancer than men with lower levels[6]. In a pilot study involving 41 males with newly diagnosed prostate cancer, taking soy isoflavones for an average of 5.5 months reduced the rate of rise of serum PSA (prostate specific antigen) levels[7].

A meta-analysis of data from 24 trials found that non-fermented soy products could reduce the relative risk of developing prostate cancer by 30 per cent and taking isoflavone supplements reduced the risk by 12 per cent[8]. Fermented soy products did not appear to lower the risk. Case-controlled studies in Japan and Korea show that men who

1. Chen YM et al. Menopause 2004;11(3):246–54
2. Yamori Y et al. Am Coll Nutr 2002;21(6):560–3
3. File SE et al. Psychopharmacology 2001;157(4):430–6
4. Duffy R et al. Pharmacol Biochem Behav 2003;75(3):721–9
5. Kritz-Silverstein D et al. Menopause 2003;10(3):196–202
6. Travis RC et al. Br J Cancer 2009; 100(11):1817–23
7. Hussain M et al. Nutr Cancer 2003;47(2):111–7
8. Yan L, Spitznagel EL. Am J Clin Nutr 2009;89(4):1155–63

can degrade daidzein to equol have a lower incidence of prostate cancer than nonequol producers, and that a diet based on soybean isoflavones is useful in preventing prostate cancer[1].

Breast cancer: Blood levels of phytoestrogens in Japan are significantly higher than those typically found in the West and the incidence of breast cancer in Japan is also particularly low. In the UK, the incidence is 87 per 100,000 women per year. In Japan it is 32 per 100,000 women per year. Mortality from breast cancer is also three times lower. Isoflavones may protect against breast cancer by reducing exposure to human oestradiol and protecting DNA from genetic mutations. If breast cancer does develop, isoflavones have a moderating effect on tumour growth factors, so that new blood vessels do not form in developing tumours and tumour cells fail to thrive. They also appear to suppress invasiveness of breast cancer cells.

In a study of 406 women aged 45–74 years, those with the highest soy intake were least likely to show changes on mammography that are associated with high breast cancer risk[2]. Those eating most soy were 60 per cent less likely to have a high risk of breast cancer than those eating the least. Increased isoflavone intake may also reduce the risk of breast cancer in premenopausal women by altering steroid hormone concentrations and menstrual cycle length[3]. In a population based study of 21,852 Japanese women (aged 40–59 years), those with the highest consumption of miso soup and isoflavones were 54 per cent less likely to develop breast cancer than those with the lowest intake, even after adjusting for reproductive history, family history, smoking, and other dietary factors. The protection was highest in post-menopausal women[4].

There has been concern over a possible detrimental effect of isoflavone supplements in women with pre-existing breast cancer due to their oestrogen-like action. However, a recent study, just published, suggests that isoflavones protect against all tumour subtypes of breast

1. Akaza H et al. Jpn J Clin Oncol 2004; 34(2):86–9
2. Jakes RW et al. Cancer Epidemiol Biomarkers Prev 2002;11(7):608–613
3. Kumar NB et al. Cancer 2002;94(4):1166–741
4. Yamamoto S et al. J Natl Cancer Inst. 2003;95(12):906–13

cancer, whether they are oestrogen receptor positive or negative, or whether progesterone receptor positive or negative[1].

A recent study looked at almost 2,000 women who were breast cancer survivors, diagnosed during 1997–2000. They were followed for six years, and 282 developed a recurrence. The researchers found that 'Soy isoflavones consumed at levels comparable to those in Asian populations may reduce the risk of breast cancer recurrent in women receiving tamoxifen therapy, and that supplements appear not to interfere with tamoxifen efficacy'[2].

Another recent study involved 35,000 Singapore Chinese women, of whom 629 developed breast cancer between 1993 and 1998. Women with a high intake of soy isoflavones were 18 per cent less likely to develop breast cancer than those with a low intake (less than 10 mg daily). The protective effect was strongest in postmenopausal women and in those with a higher weight[3].

A review[4] concluded that, overall, there is no impressive data suggesting that adult consumption of soy/isoflavones affects the risk of developing breast cancer or that soy consumption affects the survival of breast cancer patients. The authors stated that, if women with breast cancer enjoy soy products, it seems reasonable for them to continue using them.

Dose
40–100 mg isoflavones a day.

(60 g of soy protein provides 45 mg isoflavones.)

Safety
If you have a history of breast cancer, always follow your own doctor's advice about whether or not to take isoflavone supplements.

1. Zhang M et al. Breast Cancer Res Treat 2009; Feb 28 (Epub) doi:10.1007/s 10549–009–0354–9
2. Guha N et al. Breast Cancer Res Treat 2009; Feb 17 (Epub) doi:10.1007/s 10549–009–0321–5
3. Wu AH et al. Br J Cancer 2008;99(1):196–200
4. Messina MJ, Loprinzi CL. Nutr 2001 Nov;131(11 Suppl):3095S–108S1

Kelp
(Laminaria sp., Fucus vesiculosus)

Kelp (bladderwrack) supplements are obtained from long-leaved seaweeds and form a nutritious supplement containing 13 vitamins, 20 essential amino acids and 60 minerals and trace elements. It is a particularly rich source of calcium, magnesium, potassium, iron and iodine.

Benefits
Its main use is as a source of iodine to improve production of thyroid hormones, which in turn boosts the metabolic rate and may aid weight loss where obesity is related to reduced thyroid function as a result of low iodine intake. The alginates present in kelp also help to promote feelings of fullness and to reduce appetite.

Other benefits of kelp include reducing hair loss, and improving the quality of hair, skin and nails where iodine intakes are low, and it can help to relieve arthritis. It also acts as a chelating agent, to remove heavy metal toxins from the intestines.

Some studies suggest that a kelp-rich diet lowers blood pressure and cholesterol, boosts immune function and wards off cancer but more research is needed.

Dose
200–600 mg daily. Follow manufacturer's guidelines. Skin patches containing iodine derived from kelp extracts are also available.

Safety
Up to 3 per cent of people are allergic to iodine, and taking kelp supplements can cause sensitivity reactions.

Kelp supplements should not be used by people with thyroid problems. Iodine-induced thyrotoxicosis has been reported (in a woman with pre-existing multinodular goitre) after drinking kelp tea. Thyroid overactivity has also been described in people taking kelp tablets.

A case of arsenic toxicity with alopecia and memory loss has been reported in the US, as a result of using kelp supplements.

Krill oil

Krill oil, extracted from the Antarctic crustacean, *Ephausia superba*, is a rich source of omega-3 fish oils and the antioxidant carotenoids, astaxanthin and canthaxanthin. Krill oil consists of around 21 per cent EPA and 20 per cent DHA. In comparison, omega-3 fish oils typically contain between 18 per cent and 20 per cent EPA and between 12 per cent and 28 per cent DHA depending on the level of concentration that occurs during production. In addition, the only antioxidant usually found in omega-3 fish oils is added vitamin E (cod liver oil typically contains 7.5 per cent EPA, 10 per cent DHA plus vitamins A, D and added vitamin E).

Benefits

Anti-inflammatory: Nine people with cardiovascular disease, rheumatoid arthritis or osteoarthritis were randomized to receive either 300 mg krill oil or placebo for 30 days. Their blood levels of a marker for inflammation (c-reactive protein) decreased by 19 per cent after seven days, by 29 per cent after 14 days and by 31 per cent after 30 days in those taking krill oil, but increased by 25 per cent in those taking placebo over the same time period. Significant improvements in joint pain (29 per cent), stiffness (20 per cent) and joint function (23 per cent) accompanied the improvement in CRP levels[1].

Coronary heart disease: CRP is a strong predictor of future cardio-vascular disease suggesting that, like the oil extracted from oily fish, krill oil has the potential to reduce the occurrence of coronary heart disease and stroke. In addition, its astaxanthin content may have beneficial effects on blood lipids. Preliminary studies suggest that krill oil supplements can lower triglyceride, total cholesterol and LDL-cholesterol with no change in HDL-cholesterol. In a study involving 12 people with raised blood lipid levels, one group took 2–3 g krill oil per day (based on their body mass index), one group took 1–1.5 g per day, one group took omega-3 fish oil (3 g daily) and one group took placebo. In those taking krill oil, significant reductions in glucose levels, total cholesterol, triglycerides, LDL-

1. Deutsche L. J Am Coll Nutr 2007;26(1):39–48

cholesterol and HDL-cholesterol were seen compared to lower or equal doses of fish oil and to placebo[1].

PMS: Krill oil has also shown some benefit in treatment of premenstrual syndrome and painful periods. Seventy women with PMS received either 2 g krill oil or 2 g omega-3 fish oil for one month. Over the next two months, they took 2 g of the same oil for eight days before menstruation was expected, and for the first two days of their period (i.e. ten days' treatment per month). Improvements were seen in both groups, with significantly greater improvement in emotional symptoms of PMS, breast tenderness and joint pain in those taking krill oil. Those taking krill oil also needed significantly fewer painkillers for menstrual pain than those taking omega-3 fish oils[2].

Dose
300 mg–3 g daily.

No significant side effects reported. Krill oil should be avoided by those with a seafood allergy.

The down side is the sustainability of intensive Antarctic krill fishing. Krill are at the bottom of the food chain, and many marine animals such as baleen whales, Antarctic fur seals and Adelie penguins require a plentiful supply of krill on which to feed.

Kudzu
(Pueraria lobata)

Kudzu is a Chinese vine whose starchy root is used in soups and stews as a thickening agent, similar to cornstarch. It contains beneficial plant hormones (betasitosterol and isoflavones such as daidzein and formononetin) similar to those found in soya.

Benefits
Alcohol cravings: The main medicinal use for kudzu involves its ability to decrease alcohol cravings. Extracts are used to help treat

1. Bunea R et al. Altern Med Rev 2004;9(4):420–8
2. Sampalis F et al. Altern Med Rev 2003;8(2):171–179

those under the influence of alcohol – both to sober them up, and to reduce their alcohol intake. This traditional use was initially tested in the golden hamster, a species that would otherwise voluntarily increase intakes of alcohol and reduce intakes of water when given a free choice[1]. Results showed it suppressed ethanol intake by over 50 per cent, making it as effective as some anti-alcoholism drugs. The active ingredients were identified as daidzein and daidzin (see Isoflavones, page 197).

An initial pilot study involving 38 males with chronic alcoholism found no differences in craving or sobriety scores, however, between those taking kudzu for one month and those taking placebo[2]. However, this trial was criticized as it did not report the concentration of active isoflavones in their kudzu extract – typical products contain low amounts of less than 1 per cent. Another trial was therefore carried out using a concentrated extract (500 mg capsules containing 25 per cent isoflavones) in 14 volunteers (male and female), who drank an average 25 alcohol beverages per week. Each took the extracts, or a gelatin placebo, three times a day for seven days. They were then invited to a drinking session to see how much beer they consumed. After a few weeks, they performed the same test using the other capsules, so that each participant was tested both with kudzu and with placebo. The researchers found that kudzu significantly reduced the amount of beer consumed (532 ml versus 906 ml) over a 90 minute period. No side effects were recorded[3].

Cluster headache: A pilot trial designed to explore the use of kudzu for treating cluster headaches (a traditional use) found that, out of 235 patients, 16 had used kudzu. Of these, 11 (69 per cent) said it decreased the intensity of their attacks, 9 (56 per cent) said it decreased the frequency and 5 (31 per cent) said it decreased the duration of their attacks[4]. These findings need to be tested against placebo.

Menopausal symptoms: Also used as a source of isoflavones to reduce hot flushes and night sweats. (See Isoflavones, page 197.)

1. Keung WM, Vallee BL. Phytochemistry 1998; 47(4):499–506
2. Shebrek J, Rindone JP. J Altern Complement Med 2000; 6(1):45–8
3. Lukas SE et al. Alcohol Clin Exp Res 2005;29(5):756–62
4. Sewell RA et al. Headache 2009;49(1):98–105

Dose
50–500 mg, three times a day. Lower doses are used to treat menopause, and higher doses to reduce alcohol cravings.

Lapacho
(Tabebuia avellanedae; T. impetiginosa)

Lapacho, also known as pau d'arco, and the 'divine tree', is native to South America. The tree has unusual, carnivorous flowers that feed on insects, keeping it free from parasites and infections.

Lapacho contains both naphthoquinones and anthraquinones, which are not usually found together in the same plant. It grows at high altitudes where few other plants survive. It has adapted to this environment by developing a unique enzyme system which uses ozone to help synthesize lignin, an important constituent of woody tissues. As the reactions involved generate large quantities of free radicals, it has also developed a powerful antioxidant system based around carnosol.

The inner bark of lapacho is also rich in other unique substances: lapachol and ß-lapachone, which interfere with the oxygen metabolism of tumour cells so that free radicals accumulate inside to trigger cell death. It also has an additional anti-viral action against viruses, including those associated with some forms of cancer such as leukaemia.

Benefits
Lapacho has anti-inflammatory, antibacterial, anti-fungal and anti-parasitic actions and is widely used to help treat candida (thrush), skin infections with Gram positive bacteria, colds, warts, herpes cold sores, polio, influenza, boils, urinary tract infections, prostatitis and malaria.

Lapacho's anti-viral actions appear to be due to its ability to block enzymes involved in synthesis of viral genetic material (DNA and RNA) so that replication cannot occur. With other infections, it interferes with oxygen metabolism so pathogens cannot produce enough energy to reproduce. When taken by mouth, lapacho is secreted onto the skin surface in sweat and can even help to treat fungal skin infections, although it is also applied topically as a tincture or infusion.

Substances isolated from the lapacho tree have completed phase II human clinical trials for the treatment of pancreatic cancer, head and neck cancer, and a form of muscle cancer (leiomyosarcoma). It is also being investigated as a possible anti-psoriasis and anti-malaria drug.

Dose

1–2 g powdered bark a day for general use.

Select products standardized to contain at least 3 per cent naphthoquinones or at least 2 per cent lapachol.

Medical herbalists may prescribe higher doses to support the conventional treatment of cancer.

Safety

Higher doses are often combined with vitamin K to reduce the blood thinning that has been noted when high dose extracted lapachol alone (but not whole lapacho) is taken.

Few side effects occur but lapacho may cause nausea or diarrhoea at very high doses.

Lapacho should not be taken by pregnant or breast-feeding women.

Lemon balm
(Melissa officinalis)

Lemon balm is an aromatic herb native to the Mediterranean whose leaves contain a variety of aromatic essential oils. It has been used since ancient times as a healing, soothing herb with calming properties.

Lemon balm has sedative, anti-spasm and antibacterial actions and was also known as the 'scholar's herb' as it was traditionally taken by students suffering from the stress of impending exams. It is widely used to ease a number of stress-related symptoms including digestive problems, nausea, flatulence, depression, tenseness, restlessness, irritability, anxiety, headache and insomnia. Lemon balm tea is also used to stimulate appetite.

Benefits

Sleep: Laboratory tests suggest that lemon balm works by inhibiting enzymes that break down an inhibitory brain chemical, gamma-aminobutyric acid (GABA). This raises GABA levels, and damps down the over-stimulation that can occur during periods of anxiety. Of several herb tests, lemon balm had the greatest activity in this respect – greater than for gotu kola, valerian, chamomile or hops[1].

Dose

650 mg, three times a day.

When combined with valerian, the two herbs work in synergy to reduce symptoms of tension, stress and mild depression. They also have a gentle lowering effect on the raised blood pressure that often accompanies stress.

Lemon balm should not be taken with prescribed sleeping tablets; this may cause mild drowsiness which will affect the ability to drive or operate machinery.

Liquorice
(*Glycyrrhiza glabra*)

Liquorice is a plant that is native to the Mediterranean. Its roots contain a substance known as glycyrrhizin (also known as glycyrrhizic or glycyrrhizinic acid) which makes up 5–9 per cent of its weight. Glycyrrhizin is 50 times sweeter than sucrose and is commonly used in herbal teas and confections in place of sugar. Liquorice root also contains phytoestrogens and antioxidant flavonoids. It also has anti-inflammatory actions.

There are two forms of liquorice extracts available: those that contain glycyrrhizin, and deglycerrizhinated liquorice (DGL) which have different uses.

Traditional uses for DGL extracts include speeding the healing of mouth ulcers and sore throat (lozenges), peptic ulcers (by increasing production of thin mucus to line the stomach), improving upper abdominal bloating, intestinal spasms and indigestion, relieving

---

1. Awad R et al. Can J Physiol Pharmacol 2007;85(9):933–42

flatulence, and as an expectorant to thin phlegm so it is easier to cough up.

Benefits

Stress: Glycyrrhizin-intact liquorice is mainly used to stimulate the adrenal glands, making it especially helpful in times of stress, convalescence and for those with chronic fatigue syndrome or fibromyalgia. A breakdown product of glycyrrhizin, known as glycyrrhetenic acid, is responsible for its action in blocking the inactivation of hydrocortisone hormone. This also results in the most well known side effect of liquorice, which is sodium retention and an increase in blood pressure (pseudoaldosteronism) with prolonged use and at high doses.

Infections: Glycyrrhizin-intact liquorice stimulates immunity by increasing production of the anti-viral substance interferon. This makes liquorice useful in treating respiratory tract infections such as viral bronchitis and the common cold. It is used topically to help reduce recurrence of oral herpes infections as it suppresses production of viral latency proteins and induces more rapid destruction of infected cells.

Hormone balance: As glycyrrhizin has a weak oestrogenic and anti-androgenic action, it is used to help treat premenstrual syndrome, endometriosis and menopausal symptoms. It is used to treat excessive body hair (hirsutism) and to lower testosterone levels in women with polycystic ovary syndrome[1]. It has also been used to reduce the side effects of the drug, spironolactone (a powerful diuretic effect leading to low blood pressure) in the treatment of polycystic ovary syndrome[2].

Dose

5–15 g per day of whole root for short-term use (up to one week). For long-term use, 0.3 g daily.

Extracts: 200–400 mg a day (standardized to 22 per cent glycyrrhizin).

DGL: 760–1520 mg, three times a day.

1. Armanini D et al. Steroids 2004;69(11–12):763–6
2. Armanini D et al. Eur J Obstet Gynecol Reprod Biol 2007;131(1):61–7

Glycyrrhizin-intact liquorice needs to be stopped slowly rather than suddenly to prevent a rebound effect on adrenal function if used in high doses.

Safety

A daily consumption of 95 mg or more glycyrrhetinic acid can increase blood pressure. It has been suggested that, per day, you should consume no more than 10–30 g liquorice, and no more than half a cup of liquorice tea[1].

Glycyrrhizin-intact liquorice should not be used by people with liver disease, low potassium levels, kidney failure or high blood pressure, by those taking diuretics or digoxin, or during pregnancy. This form of liquorice should not be taken long term (e.g. more than a month) except under supervision from a medical herbalist.

Lutein

Lutein is one of 600 naturally occurring carotenoid pigments which have antioxidant properties. It cannot be made in the body and must therefore come from your diet.

Lutein is found in sweetcorn, carrots and other yellow-orange fruit and vegetables, as well as spinach and other dark-green leafy vegetables. One of the richest dietary sources is spinach.

Benefits

Lutein is important for healthy vision. It becomes concentrated in a part of the retina called the macula, where it is partly converted into another carotenoid called zeaxanthin. The macula is responsible for the fine vision needed for reading and recognizing faces. When light stimulates macular cells it triggers a series of chemical reactions which, as well as sending visual images to the brain, also releases a cascade of harmful free radicals. If not neutralized immediately, these free radicals damage and destroy these light-sensitive cells. Lutein and zeaxanthin protect the macula from damage through their antioxidant activity, which mops up free radicals, and because their yellow colour filters out light in the harmful blue region of the

1. Boganen H et al. Ned Tijdschr Geneeskd 2007;151(51):2825–8

visible spectrum which is associated with photo-damage to the eye. That's why lutein is sometimes referred to as 'nature's sunglasses'.

Poor dietary intake of lutein is associated with an increased risk of age-related macular degeneration, and of cataracts.

Macular degeneration: If your intake of lutein is poor, you are at increased risk of developing age-related macular degeneration (AMD) – the leading cause of registered blindness in people over the age of 50 years. There are two types of AMD: 'wet' in which new, fragile blood vessels leak fluid into surrounding tissues, and 'dry' where new blood vessel formation has not occurred. Wet AMD is treated with laser therapy to seal leaking blood vessels. For dry AMD, the mainstay of treatment – and prevention – is to obtain a good dietary intake of lutein-rich foods.

Lutein concentrations in the macula are greater than those found in the circulation and other body tissues. A number of studies examining the association of dietary lutein/zeaxanthin intake with advanced AMD have yielded inverse relationships that are statistically significant. People with macular degeneration have, on average, 70 per cent less macular pigment in their eyes than those with healthy vision.

Good intakes of lutein and zeaxanthin from foods such as spinach, broccoli and eggs, for example, are associated with a significantly reduced risk of age-related macular degeneration of up to 40 per cent[1]. In one study, in which lutein levels in the retina were measured, those with the highest levels were 82 per cent less likely to develop AMD than those with the lowest levels[2].

Lutein supplements are protective, too, and can significantly increase blood levels of lutein, and the amount of macular pigment present in the retina[3]. People taking 10 mg lutein supplements per day have been shown to achieve a 50 per cent increase in macular pigment optical density after one year. Taking the equivalent of 10 mg per day free lutein in supplement form can also increase macular pigment optical density in patients with early AMD, showing that a diseased macula can still accumulate and stabilize lutein and/or zeaxanthin[4]. Follow-up research published in *Optometry* – the Journal of the

1. Moeller SM et al. J Am Coll Nutr 2000;19(5 Suppl):522S–527S
2. Bone RA et al. Invest Ophthalmol Vis Sci 2001; 42(1):235–40
3. Berendschot TT et al. Invest Ophthalmol Vis Sci 2000;41(11):3322–6
4. Koh HH et al. Exp Eye Res 2004; 79(1):21–7

American Optometric Association – showed that taking 10 mg lutein supplements per day can improve visual acuity in those with 'dry' AMD by the equivalent of 5.4 letters on a Snellen chart, compared with no improvement in those taking inactive placebo[1].

Cataracts: A study involving almost 77,500 female nurses aged 45–71 years found that, after age, smoking, and other potential cataract risk factors were controlled for, those with the highest intake of lutein and zeaxanthin were 22 per cent less likely to develop cataracts severe enough to require extraction[2].

Dose
10 mg lutein per day.

According to a recent review, a dietary intake of about 3 mg lutein per day should provide sufficient reserves to provide health benefits if begun early in life[3].

Lycopene

Lycopene is an important dietary carotenoid, that makes up at least 50 per cent of all carotenoids found in the body. It is best known as the red pigment in tomatoes, and is also found in pink guava, papaya, red/pink grapefruit and watermelon.

Cooking tomatoes releases five times more lycopene than is available from raw tomatoes. Tomato ketchup and tomato purée (which are concentrated) are therefore the richest dietary sources of lycopene. Pizza is also an excellent source as lycopene is fat-soluble and olive oil increases dietary absorption of lycopene as much as three-fold.

Benefits
It has been suggested that some of the benefits previously attributed to betacarotene may actually have been due to the presence of lycopene.

1. Richer S et al. 2004. Optometry 75(4):216–30
2. Chasan-Taber L et al. Am J Clin Nutr 1999;70 (4):509–16
3. Chung-jung C, Taylor A. Exp Eye Res 2007; 84(2):229–245

Cancer: A number of studies suggest that an increased dietary intake of lycopene may lower the risk of certain cancers. There are significant correlations between tomato intake and blood lycopene levels and the reduced risk of cancers of the mouth, oesophagus, stomach, lung, colon, rectum, cervix and prostate gland. For example, carotenoid intakes and blood levels were assessed in almost 48,000 male health professionals between 1986 and 1992[1]. Consuming more than ten servings tomato products per week was associated with a significant 35 per cent reduction in the risk of developing prostate cancer compared with men consuming less than 1.5 servings per week. Those with the highest intakes of lycopene (more than 6.5 mg a day) were 21 per cent less likely to develop prostate cancer than those with the lowest intakes (less than 2.3 mg a day). No such associations were found for other carotenoids such as betacarotene, alphacarotene, lutein or beta-cryptoxanthin. When the men were reassessed in 1998, those with the highest lycopene intake were 16 per cent less likely to have developed prostate cancer than those with the lowest intake[2].

Several studies have shown that men with prostate cancer who consumed 30 mg lycopene a day (as a pure tomato extract), for three weeks before surgical removal of the gland, appear to have smaller tumours, which were more likely to be confined to the prostate, and to show signs of regression and decreased malignancy, than in those not taking tomato extracts. Their levels of serum PSA (prostate specific antigen), a common marker used to detect prostate cancer) were also reduced. Results suggest that lycopene is concentrated within prostate cells to reduce DNA damage.

Women with the highest lycopene levels also appear to have five times less chance of developing pre-cancerous changes on their cervical smear than women with the lowest lycopene levels. This finding is associated with more rapid clearance of the human papilloma virus (HPV) associated with cervical cancer.

Similarly, after accounting for smoking, people with the lowest levels of lycopene are three times more likely to develop lung cancer than those with the highest intakes.

While these studies suggest that a tomato-based antioxidant might

1. Giovannucci E et al. J Natl Cancer Inst 1995; 87:1767–1776
2. Giovannucci E et al. J Natl Cancer Inst 2002;94:391–398

play a role in treating as well as preventing prostate cancer, it is not certain that lycopene itself is protective. It may just act as a biomarker for tomato consumption. Tomatoes also provide folate, vitamin C and a variety of other phytochemicals (e.g. phytoene, phytofluene, ß-carotene, quercetin, kaempferol, naringenin) which may contribute to lower cancer risk[1]. It is also important to bear in mind that a tomato-rich diet is likely to be a generally healthy diet, associated with other healthy lifestyle choices such as not smoking, exercising regularly and avoiding excess alcohol.

If lycopene does have an anti-cancer action, it is likely to relate to its antioxidant activity. Lycopene is three times more potent as an antioxidant than vitamin E, and consuming a single serving of tomatoes can reduce DNA oxidative damage by as much as 50 per cent within 24 hours.

Benign prostate enlargement: Lycopene is also beneficial for men with benign prostate hyperplasia (BPH). Taking 15 mg lycopene per day for six months was found to significantly decrease levels of prostate specific antigen (PSA) compared with placebo. In those taking lycopene, the prostate gland did not enlarge and symptoms improved, but in those on placebo, progressive enlargement was noted[2].

Coronary heart disease: People who regularly eat tomatoes and tomato products are 30–47 per cent less likely to develop heart disease than those who eat them infrequently[3,4]. Lycopene is the most likely protective factor. Low plasma lycopene levels are associated with increased thickness of the carotid artery wall[5]. Lycopene also reduces oxidation of low-density lipoprotein (LDL) cholesterol that promotes atherosclerosis (hardening and narrowing of the arteries)[6]. When LDL-cholesterol is oxidized, it is taken up by scavenger cells (macrophages) that form bloated 'foam cells'. These become trapped in artery walls as they try to leave the circulation, contributing to the build-up of plaque which contributes to coronary

1. Campbell JK et al. J Nutr 2004;134:3486S–3492S
2. Schwartz S et al. J Nutr 2008;138(1):49–53
3. Sesso HD et al. J Nutr 2003;133(7):2336–41
4. Kohlmeier L et al. Am J Epidemiol 1997;146(8):618–26
5. Rissanen T et al. Arterioscler Throm Vasc Biol 2000;20(12):2677–81
6. Agarwal S, Rao A V. Lipids 1998; 33:981–984

heart disease. Daily consumption of tomato extracts providing at least 40 mg of lycopene is sufficient to alter LDL oxidation, and could potentially reduce the risk of coronary heart disease and stroke. Recent research involving over 4,400 adults also suggests that high intakes of carotenoids are associated with a lower risk of developing hypertension[1].

Macular degeneration: Like lutein and zeaxanthin, lycopene helps to protect against age-related macular degeneration. Those with low lycopene intakes have more than double the risk of developing AMD than those with high intakes.

Lycopene is depleted in skin exposed to ultraviolet light, suggesting that it also plays a role in protecting the skin from sun damage.

Dose
6–30 mg per day. Or, aim to consume at least five servings of lycopene-rich foods per day (tomato sauce, tomato juice, healthy pizza).

Maca
(*Lepidium meyenii*)

Maca is a root vegetable which grows in the Peruvian Andes at heights of more than 4,000 metres above sea level. It has been used as a dietary staple since before the time of the Incas as it is a good source of carbohydrate, amino acids, fatty acids, vitamins B1, B2, B12, C and E plus the minerals calcium, phosphorus, zinc, magnesium, copper and iron.

Maca's tubers contain a number of steroid glycosides with oestrogen-like actions and are used to increase energy and stamina. Maca has also been used by some athletes as an alternative to anabolic steroids, without the side effects. However, its use does not affect levels of circulating oestrogen, testosterone, progesterone, prolactin, FSH or LH hormones and the way it works is not fully understood[2]. It has long been reputed to act as an aphrodisiac for

1. Hozawa A et al. J Hypertens 2009;27(2):237–42
2. Gonzales GF et al. J Endocrinol 2003; 176(1):163–8

men and women, an aid to female fertility and a treatment for male impotence. It helps to relieve menopausal symptoms and other gynaecological problems related to hormonal imbalances. Some researchers believe maca to be superior to red Korean ginseng, and it is sometimes even referred to as Peruvian ginseng.

Benefits

Erectile dysfunction: A study involving 50 men with mild erectile dysfunction found that those taking maca (2.4 g daily) for 12 weeks experienced a significant improvement in symptoms compared with those taking inactive placebo[1].

Low sex drive: A pilot study involving 16 men and women with low sex drive as a result of antidepressant (SSRI) therapy found that those taking 3 g maca per day had significant improvement in sexual function and libido, but that those taking a lower dose (1.5 g per day) did not[2]. A similar study involving 14 postmenopausal women found that those taking 3.5 g maca per day for six weeks showed significant improvements in anxiety, depression and sexual dysfunction compared with those taking inactive placebo[3]. Another study involving men aged 21–56 showed a significant increase in sexual desire compared with placebo after eight weeks[4].

Sperm health: A small trial involving nine males found that taking maca for four months significantly improves semen volume, sperm count, motile sperm count and sperm motility without affecting blood hormone levels[5].

Dose

1 g, twice or three times a day.

A moderate increase in a liver enzyme (AST) and in diastolic blood pressure has been reported in some people using maca. This effect is prevented by combining it with milk thistle extracts (silymarin)[6].

1. Zenico T et al. Andrologia 2009; 41(2):95–9
2. Dording CM et al. CNS Neurosci Ther 2008; 14(3):182–91
3. Brooks NA et al. Menopause 2008; 15(6):1157–62
4. Gonzales GF et al. Andrologia 2002;34(6):367–72
5. Gonzales GF et al. Asian J Androl 2001;3(4):301–3
6. Valentova K et al. Food Chem Toxicol 2008; 46(3):1006–13

Magnesium

Magnesium is the fourth most common metal found in the body, with 70 per cent stored in the bones and teeth. It is needed for the function of over 300 enzymes, and is vital for every major metabolic reaction from the synthesis of protein and genetic material to the production of energy from glucose. Few enzymes can work without it and magnesium is now known to help maintain healthy tissues, especially those in the muscles, lung airways, blood vessels and nerves. Lack of magnesium leads to cell death due to depletion of energy stores.

One of the most important functions for magnesium is to maintain the integrity of ion pumps that control the flow of sodium, potassium, calcium, chloride and other salt components across cell membranes. By moving ions against gradients, these pumps allow cells to hold an electrical charge and, in the case of nerve cells, to pass electrical messages from one neurone to another. Magnesium is essential for maintaining a cell's electrical stability and is especially important in controlling calcium entry into heart cells to trigger a regular heartbeat.

Magnesium is a co-factor in the metabolism of essential fatty acids, and for the interaction of sex hormones with cell receptors to switch on the genes they regulate. It is involved in the production of brain chemicals (such as dopamine) and helps to maintain normal moods.

Dietary sources of magnesium include beans (especially soy), nuts, wholegrains (although if these are processed they lose most of their magnesium content), seafood, and dark green, leafy vegetables. Chocolate, drinking water in hard-water areas, mineral seasoning salt and brewer's yeast are also important sources.

Lack of magnesium is common and may affect as many as one in ten people. Symptoms that may be due to magnesium deficiency include loss of appetite, nausea, fatigue, weakness, muscle trembling or cramps, numbness and tingling, loss of co-ordination, palpitations, hyperactivity and low blood sugar. It can also lead to diarrhoea (in early deficiency) and constipation (in later deficiency).

Benefits
Blood pressure: High blood pressure is less common in hard-water areas where water has a higher calcium and magnesium content. The

use of low sodium, higher magnesium, higher potassium table salt in Finland was associated with a lower incidence of high blood pressure in the population. However, a meta-analysis of data from 12 trials, involving 545 people found that taking magnesium supplements only reduced blood pressure by 1.3/2.2 mmHg[1]. More research is needed to confirm whether or not magnesium can lower BP significantly. It does, however, appear to be helpful for treating high blood pressure in pregnancy (pre-eclampsia) and reducing seizures (eclampsia)[2].

Heart health: Heart attacks are less common in hard-water areas where water has a higher calcium and magnesium content. People with low magnesium levels are at risk of spasm of the coronary arteries (linked with angina or heart attack) and sudden death (due to abnormal heart rhythms). These effects seem to be more pronounced during times of stress. Magnesium treatment has been given immediately after a heart attack to help prevent dangerous abnormal heart rhythms. It also helps to widen coronary blood vessels, and reduces the formation of platelet blood clots. A meta-analysis of data from 12 trials suggests that intravenous magnesium is effective in improving heart beat rate and rhythm in people with rapid atrial fibrillation[3].

Diabetes: A meta-analysis of data from seven studies involving over 286,000 people found that those with a high intake of magnesium (whether from food or supplements) had a significantly lower risk of developing Type 2 diabetes than those with low intakes. An additional intake of 100 mg magnesium reduced the risk by 15 per cent. Taking magnesium supplements may also improve glucose control and raise 'good' HDL-cholesterol levels in people with Type 2 diabetes[4].

Osteoporosis: As magnesium regulates the movement of calcium in and out of cells, it is important for bone health and the prevention of osteoporosis. Women with osteoporosis appear to have significantly lower magnesium levels than similar women without osteoporosis[5].

1. Dickinson HO et al. Cochrane Database Syst Rev 2006;3:CD004640
2. Chien PF et al. Br J Obstet Gynaecol 1996;103(11):1085–91
3. Onalan O et al. Am J Cardiol 2007;99(12):1726–32
4. Song Y et al. Diabet Med 2006; 23(10):1050–6
5. Odabasi E et al. Ann Acad Med Singapore 2008 37(7):564–7

Taking magnesium supplements for two years has been shown to significantly increase bone mineral density, and prevent bone fractures[1].

Asthma: People with low magnesium levels are more likely to experience spasm of the airways leading to asthma attacks. A review of 24 studies involving people with acute asthma found that magnesium therapy (intravenous or nebulized) in addition to bronchodilator drugs was associated with a strong improvement in respiratory function in children but had only a weak effect in adults[2].

Chronic fatigue: Low levels of red blood cell magnesium have been linked with chronic fatigue. While early small studies suggested that magnesium could improve tiredness and lack of energy, other studies have not found significant differences in magnesium levels between people with chronic fatigue and those without[3].

Fibromyalgia: Early studies suggested that white blood cell magnesium levels were significantly decreased in people with muscle pain due to fibromyalgia. Later studies have not found significant differences in magnesium levels between people with fibromyalgia and those without[3]. Significant increases in magnesium content of platelets have been found, however, leading some researchers to suggest that disturbances in calcium-magnesium flow may be involved[4]. Some people find that taking magnesium supplements reduces the number of tender points.

PMS: Several studies have found that red blood cell magnesium levels are significantly lower in women with premenstrual syndrome (PMS) than those without. Magnesium deficiency is common, with 85 per cent of the fertile, adult female population aged 19–24 years obtaining less than the RNI of 270 mg daily[5].

1. Sojka JE, Weaver CM. Nutr Rev 1995;53(3):71–4
2. Mohammed S, Goodacre S. Emerg Med J 2007;24(12):823–30
3. Moorkens G et al. Magnes Res 1997 10(4):329–37
4. Bazzichi L et al. Clin Biochem 2008; 41(13):1084–90
5. Henderson L 2003. The National Diet & Nutrition Survey: Adults Aged 19 to 64 Years

Researchers have found that red blood cell magnesium concentrations in 105 women with PMS were significantly lower than in the normal population[1]. In a cross-over study involving 38 women, the taking of 200 mg magnesium for two months significantly improved premenstrual symptoms associated with fluid retention (weight gain, oedema, mastalgia, bloating). There were no significant effects on depression, anxiety or total symptoms[2]. Another randomized study involving 32 women with PMS found that taking magnesium (360 mg per day) during the luteal phase of two cycles reduced premenstrual mood changes and total symptom scores. However, baseline symptom scores between the groups were significantly different, and a placebo effect was not seen, making the data questionable[3]. Another small trial involving 20 women with premenstrual migraine found that taking magnesium (360 mg per day) during the luteal phase of two menstrual cycles significantly reduced the number of days with headache compared with placebo[4].

Cerebral palsy: Analysis of six trials involving almost 4,800 women found that when women at risk of preterm delivery before 34 weeks' gestation were given magnesium sulphate supplements, the risk of cerebral palsy in their offspring was reduced by 31 per cent[5]. This was confirmed in another analysis involving over 6,000 babies which found that magnesium can also reduce muscle control problems[6]. How magnesium protects the brain from the damage that causes cerebral palsy is not certain, but it may involve improved neuron function and/or improved blood flow to the brain.

Dose

The old EU RDA for magnesium was 300 mg per day. The newly set EU RDA has increased to 375 mg. The UK RNI is 300 mg per day for men aged 19–50 years, and 270 mg for women. People who are

1. Sherwood RA et al. Ann Clin Biochem 1986; 23(Pt6):667–70
2. Walker AF et al. J Women's Health 1998;7:1157–1165
3. Facchinetti F et al. Obstet Gynecol 1991;78:177–181
4. Facchinetti F et al. Headache 1991;31(5):298–301
5. Conde-Agudelo A, Romero R. Am J Obstet Gynecol 2009; 200(6):595–609
6. Doyle LW et al. Cochrane Database Syst Rev 2009;(1):CD004661

physically active need more than those who are not, as large amounts are lost in sweat. The upper safe limit for long-term use from supplements is suggested as 400 mg per day.

Usual dose from supplements is 150–375 mg a day, taken with food to optimize absorption. Magnesium citrate is most readily absorbed, while magnesium gluconate is less likely to cause intestinal side effects such as diarrhoea at higher doses. If taking magnesium supplements, it is important to ensure a good intake of calcium.

Maitake
(Grifola frondosa)

Maitake is a rare, edible mushroom found in Japan growing on the trunks of deciduous trees. It forms large clusters that typically weigh around 20 pounds and is commonly known as cloud mushroom, monkey's shelf or the King of Mushrooms.

Maitake contains powerful immune-stimulating substances known as beta-glucans. Whereas most medicinal mushrooms contain a polysaccharide substance known as beta 1,3 glucan, that found in maitake is a unique, complex version known as beta 1,6 glucan (referred to as the D-fraction). This increases the activity of immune chemicals (lymphokines, interleukin-1 and interleukin-2) that help to control white blood cells, leading to increased activity of immune scavenger cells (macrophages) and natural killer cells.

Maitake is taken as a general health tonic, having many of the same adaptogenic actions as Korean ginseng, reducing the effects of stress and normalizing blood pressure and blood glucose levels. Maitake is also used as an immune stimulant against viral infection and cancer. When given during chemotherapy, it has been shown to reduce the dose of toxic drugs needed, and it is believed to be more effective at inhibiting tumours than either reishi or shiitake mushrooms.

Maitake is also used in the treatment of high blood pressure, diabetes, chronic fatigue syndrome, hepatitis B, glandular fever, and rheumatoid arthritis.

Benefits
Cancer: Cancer regression or significant symptom improvement has

been observed in patients with liver, breast or lung cancer. And, when taken in addition to chemotherapy, activity of immune cells was enhanced compared with chemotherapy alone[1]. Previous studies suggest that maitake may improve the side effects of chemo such as loss of appetite, nausea and low white blood cell count.

HIV: Laboratory studies suggest that maitake enhances the activity of T-helper cells to reduce their destruction when infected with HIV.

Dose
Extracts: 600 mg a day.

Dried mushroom: 1–4 g a day for general health, and 4–7 g to treat specific conditions.

Vitamin C improves absorption and effectiveness of maitake mushroom.

Should ideally be individually prescribed by a qualified medical herbalist.

Contraindications
As a food, maitake seems to have no toxic side effects, but none the less it is sensible to avoid taking it during pregnancy and breast-feeding.

Manganese

Manganese is an essential mineral involved in many metabolic functions, including the production of amino acids, carbohydrates, sexual hormones, blood-clotting factors, cholesterol and some brain transmitters. It also acts as an antioxidant.

Manganese is essential for normal growth and development, as it is needed for the synthesis of cartilage, collagen and structural molecules known as mucopolysaccharides. It is especially important for healthy bones, and women with osteoporosis have been found to have manganese levels that were four times lower than those who do not.

Foods containing manganese include black tea (one cup of tea

---

1. Kodama N et al. Altern Med Rev 2002;7(3):236–9

contains 1 mg manganese), wholegrains (although processing removes much of their manganese content), nuts, seeds, fruit, eggs, green leafy vegetables, offal, shellfish and milk.

Deficiency
The significance of manganese deficiency is currently unknown, but possible cases have been linked with reddening of body hair, scaly skin, poor growth of hair and nails, disc and cartilage problems, poor blood clotting, glucose intolerance, poor memory and worsening intellect. It may also contribute to reduced fertility.

Industrial workers exposed to inhalation of manganese dust have experienced toxicity with nervous system effects similar to Parkinson's disease.

Dose
The newly set EU RDA for manganese is 2 mg. Some researchers suggest that up to 7 mg are needed daily for optimum bone health. The upper safe level for long-term use from supplements (which takes average dietary intakes into account) is suggested as 4 mg.

Mastic gum
(Pistacia lentiscus)

Mastic gum is a white semi-transparent resin derived from pistachio-like trees that grow on the Greek island of Chios. It contains a number of unique constituents including masticonic, mastinininc and masticolic acids.

Mastic gum is used to maintain healthy digestion, and to overcome symptoms such as indigestion, heartburn and dyspepsia associated with *Helicobacter* infection. Laboratory studies have shown that mastic gum has a powerful antibiotic action against *H. pylori* (a stomach infection associated with peptic ulcers and gastric cancer) – even including the antibiotic-resistant strains.

Benefits
Helicobacter: In one study, seven strains of *H. pylori* (including three that were resistant to the antibiotic metronidazole) were

incubated with a dilute solution of mastic gum, which was found to kill the bacteria at low concentrations. In a clinical trial involving 38 people with duodenal ulcers, 20 were given mastic gum while 18 were given a placebo. Sixteen taking mastic and nine taking placebo obtained symptomatic relief, while at endoscopy, proven healing of the duodenal ulcers was shown to have occurred in 70 per cent taking mastic gum compared with only 22 per cent on the placebo which was highly statistically significant[1]. However, a later study involving eight people with *Helicobacter* infection found that taking 1 g mastic gum four times a day for 14 days had no effect on *Helicobacter* status with all remaining *H. pylori* positive[2].

Dental health: Chewing mastic gum for 15 minutes significantly decreases levels of bacteria in the mouth, including Streptococcus mutans, and may be useful in preventing dental caries[3].

Crohn's disease: Preliminary evidence suggests that mastic gum can reduce levels of inflammatory mediators in people with Crohn's disease[4].

Dose

1–4 g daily with water for two weeks at start of symptoms. Continue with maintenance dose of 500 mg nightly.

Milk thistle

(Silybum marianum)

Milk thistle seeds contain a powerful mixture of antioxidant bioflavonoids known as silymarin, of which the most active ingredient is the flavonolignan, silibinin. The seeds contain as much as 6 per cent silymarin by weight.

Silymarin can protect liver cells from the poisonous effects of excess alcohol and other toxins such as those produced by death cap mushroom and chemotherapy. It works as an antioxidant (and is at

1. Al-Habbal MG et al. Clin Exp Pharmacol Physiol 1984;11(5):541–4
2. Bebb JR et al. Antimicrob Chemother 2003;52(3):522–3
3. Aksoy A et al. Angle Orthod 2007;77(1):124–8
4. Kaliora AC et al. World J Gastroenterol 2007;13(5):748–53

least 200 times more potent than vitamins C or E), by inhibiting factors responsible for liver cell damage – free radicals and leukotrienes – and by maintaining levels of an important liver antioxidant enzyme, glutathione. Some studies suggest that it can boost glutathione levels by over 33 per cent. Silymarin also seems to alter the outer structure of liver cell walls so poisons do not penetrate as readily – this means the liver can process toxins at a steady pace, as they enter, rather than being overwhelmed all at once.

Silymarin has been shown to stimulate liver cells regenerated after viral or toxic damage by increasing the rate at which new proteins are made and by reducing fibrosis. In addition, it has recently been shown to have a protective effect on kidney cells. It is also being investigated as a possible protectant against ultraviolet-induced skin cancers and is helpful for reducing the excessive skin cell turnover seen in psoriasis.

Silymarin is mainly used to treat liver conditions such as hepatitis, cirrhosis, non-obstructive gallstones (by increasing bile flow) and to protect the liver in mushroom poisoning, after chemotherapy, and during detox programmes. In women with high oestrogen states such as endometriosis, it helps the liver metabolize oestrogen more efficiently which may reduce symptoms.

Benefits

Liver disease: A meta-analysis of data from 19 clinical trials found that silymarin could prolong survival in people with liver cirrhosis (mostly alcoholic), in whom total mortality was 16.1 per cent versus 20.5 per cent in those taking placebo. Liver-related mortality was 10 per cent in those on silymarin compared with 17.3 per cent in those taking placebo[1].

Dose

70–200 mg silymarin (standardized to at least 70 per cent silymarin), three times a day, preferably between meals.

It is best to start with a low dose and slowly increase. Liver function should start to show an improvement within five days and continue over at least the next three weeks.

---

1. Saller R et al. Forsch Komplementmed 2008;15(1):9–20

Side effects

The only reported side effect is a mild laxative one in some people, due to increased production of bile.

Minerals

The word mineral literally means 'mined from the earth'. Minerals can be divided into two main groups of elements: metallic and non-metallic.

Carbohydrates, fats, proteins and vitamins are all based on the element carbon, and are known as organic substances. Minerals do not contain carbon and are said to be inorganic. In nutritional terms, the word mineral refers to inorganic substances of which we need to obtain more than 100 mg per day from our diet. Those needed in amounts much less than 100 mg are referred to as trace elements.

Around 20 minerals and trace elements are essential for the biochemical reactions occurring in human metabolism. The average adult contains around 3 kg of minerals and trace elements, most of which are found in the skeleton.

Minerals in the diet

In general, the mineral content of foods depends on the soil in which produce is reared or grown. This is in contrast to the vitamin content of food, which is usually more similar wherever it comes from. Acid rain and food processing can also reduce the mineral content of foods enough to cause deficiency.

Although some vitamins can be synthesized in the body in tiny amounts, minerals and trace elements can only come from the diet. As a result, mineral deficiency is more common than vitamin deficiency, especially amongst slimmers, the elderly, pregnant women, vegetarians and those eating vegetables grown in mineral-poor soils.

Benefits

Minerals have a number of different functions in the body.

- They act as antioxidants, e.g. selenium, manganese.
- They are important structurally – calcium, magnesium and phosphate strengthen bones and teeth.

- They maintain normal cell function, e.g. sodium, potassium, calcium.
- They act as a co-factor for important enzymes, e.g. copper, iron, magnesium, manganese, molybdenum, selenium, zinc.
- They are involved in oxygen transport, e.g. iron.
- They are important for hormone function, e.g. chromium, iodine.

Some trace elements such as nickel, tin and vanadium are known to be essential for normal growth in only tiny amounts, although their exact roles are not yet fully understood.

See separate individual entries for all of the above.

Molybdenum

Despite its importance in plant and animal life, molybdenum is one of the world's scarcest trace elements. It acts as a co-factor for the function of three enzymes and is involved in the metabolism of iron, carbohydrate, fat and alcohol. It is also needed for the production of uric acid.

Molybdenum in the diet
Food sources include buckwheat (the richest source), wholegrains, meats, dairy products and dark green leafy vegetables.

Deficiency
Symptoms that may be due to lack of molybdenum include anaemia, poor general health, increased incidence of dental caries, irritability, impotence, rapid irregular pulse, hyperventilation, visual problems and even coma due to intolerance of sulphur-containing amino acids.

A high incidence of oesophageal cancer in China has been linked with a lack of molybdenum, and this is thought to be the indirect effect of a carcinogenic fungus that can attack molybdenum-deficient maize.

Molybdenum and copper interact with one another and high copper intakes increase the rate at which molybdenum is lost from the body.

Dose

There is currently no EU RDA for molybdenum and requirements are unknown. A to Z-style vitamin and mineral formulas tend to contain around 25 mcg.

MSM

Methyl-sulphonylmethane, or MSM, is a sulphur compound that is made naturally in the body from the amino acids, methionine, cysteine and taurine. It is a source of sulphur, which is essential to health and is the fourth most abundant mineral in the human body after calcium, phosphorus and magnesium. Sulphur is involved in the production of energy in body cells, and the formation of antibodies. It is needed for the formation of detoxification enzymes, and the production of glutathione, one of the most important antioxidants found in the body. It is also essential for repair of joint cartilage and connective tissues; cartilage production is known to be reduced when sulphur is in short supply.

MSM is found in some foods such as fruit, alfalfa, corn, tomatoes, tea, coffee and milk. MSM found in supplements is produced synthetically but is identical to that found in nature.

MSM is used to help a number of conditions, including allergies, acid indigestion, constipation, and degenerative bone diseases. Like glucosamine sulphate, another sulphur-containing substance produced in the body, MSM seems to be important for healthy joints, cartilage, tendons and ligaments. It is also vital for healthy connective tissue containing the structural protein, collagen. With increasing age, skin tends to lose its elasticity due to the formation of cross-linkages within collagen so it becomes more fibrous. Some researchers believe that MSM helps to maintain suppleness of tissues by blocking the formation of these abnormal cross-linkages.

Benefits

Osteoarthritis: Sulphur metabolism is naturally reduced in arthritic joints so sulphur containing supplements are not necessarily going to be effective on their own. However, a study involving 50 people with knee OA found that those receiving MSM (3 g, twice a day) showed significant improvements in joint pain and physical functioning at 12 weeks compared with those on placebo[1]. Researchers are unsure exactly how MSM works against arthritis, but it is thought to reduce pain and swelling due to inflammation in a similar way to aspirin.

Dose
There is no EU RDA for sulphur.

Usual recommended dose: 1–3 g a day in divided doses although larger amounts may be taken under supervision.

Excess
Toxicity is low, but excess may produce gastrointestinal side effects.

Muira puama
(Ptychopetalum olacoides)

Muira puama – also known as Marapuama and potency wood – is a small tree found in the Brazilian rain forest. Its roots, bark and wood are widely used by natives of the Amazon and Orinoco river basins to enhance sexual desire and combat impotence.

Researchers are unsure as to how it works but it is thought to stimulate sexual desire both psychologically and physically, through a direct action on brain chemicals (dopamine, noradrenaline and serotonin) by stimulating nerve endings in the genitals and by boosting production/function of sex hormones, especially testosterone.

Muira puama is also used as a general tonic for the nervous system, and is used to help treat exhaustion, neuralgia, anxiety, depression, pre-menstrual syndrome and menstrual cramps. Interestingly, it is also used to treat some types of baldness.

Benefits
Sex drive: Research carried out by me and Professor Jacques Waynberg of the Institute of Sexology, Paris, involved 202 women

1. Kim LS et al. Osteoarthritis Cartilage 2006;14(3):286–94

with low sex drive. After taking muira puama plus ginkgo biloba for one month, statistically significant improvements occurred in frequency of sexual desire, sexual intercourse and sexual fantasies, with improved satisfaction in excitement, ability to reach orgasm and intensity of orgasm[1].

Erectile dysfunction: A trial involving 262 males with low sex drive and erectile dysfunction found that muira puama was more effective than yohimbine (a pharmaceutical drug originally used to treat impotence); 62 per cent of subjects who complained of lack of sexual desire claimed that muira puama had a dynamic effect on their sex lives, while 51 per cent who had erectile dysfunction felt it was of benefit[2].

Dose
1–1.5 g a day for two weeks.

Myrrh

For 4,000 years, myrrh has been valued for its rich and enduring scent used in perfumes, incense and as a funeral herb in embalming. It is a gum resin produced by several species of *Commiphora*, collected mainly from wild trees in Africa, India and Arabia. The name comes from the Arabic, *murr*, meaning 'bitter'. It is also known in Asia as Guggul. When the bark is cut, myrrh oozes out to form yellow-red, irregular, often tear-shaped lumps, sometimes as big as walnuts, which were said to come from the tears of Horus, the falcon-headed sun god.

Myrrh is one of the oldest known medicines, widely used by the ancient Egyptians for mouth and throat problems, and in the Middle East for treatment of infected wounds and bronchial complaints. Ancient Greek soldiers never went to war without a pouch containing myrrh paste for first aid. It is used in traditional Indian medicine for menstrual problems, as an aphrodisiac, and to lower cholesterol levels.

1. Waynberg J, Brewer S. Adv Ther 2000;17(5):255–62
2. Waynberg J et al. Am J Nat Med 1994; 1(3):8

Myrrh's astringent, antiseptic and anti-microbial actions mean it is a popular topical treatment for mild inflammations of the mouth and throat (e.g. gingivitis, ulcers) and is often added to gargles and mouthwashes. It is one of the most effective herbal medicines worldwide for speeding the healing of sore throat, mouth ulcers and gum infections. It is also used for acne, boils, bronchial, digestive and menstrual problems, including irregular or painful periods.

Benefits
Cholesterol: Preliminary evidence suggests that taking myrrh extracts (2160 mg daily) can reduce total cholesterol and LDL-cholesterol, total/HDL-cholesterol ratio and triglyceride levels[1].

Dose
Gargle or rinse: add 5–10 drops of tincture to a little warm water.

Undiluted tincture 1:5 (g/ml): apply locally to affected areas of gums or mucous membranes of the mouth, twice or three times a day.

Capsules: 300 mg–1 g, twice a day.

N-acetyl cystine

N-acetyl cysteine (NAC) is an amino acid that boosts levels of a powerful antioxidant (glutathione) in the respiratory tract. Mucus dispersion can be boosted by supplements containing NAC and studies show that it can significantly reduce mucus production and associated cough in chronic respiratory conditions such as bronchitis, emphysema and sinusitis. It may also be helpful for ear infections and glue ear. Interestingly, research is currently under way to investigate observations that NAC can prevent some of the lung damage linked with lung cancer in smokers. NAC is also thought to interfere with viral replication and may be recommended to people with viral illness, including HIV.

Benefits
Trichotillomania: Chronic hair-pulling, or trichotillomania, affects

---

1. Nohr LA et al. Complement Ther Med 2009;17(1):16–22

between one and seven out of every 200 people. A recent study among 50 people with trichotillomania found that taking NAC (1200 mg daily for six weeks, then 2400 mg for another six weeks if no improvement) helped 56 per cent to stop pulling, compared with 16 per cent taking placebo[1].

NAC is believed to reduce compulsive behaviour through an effect on the brain neurotransmitter, glutamate.

Cardiac surgery: A meta-analysis of 13 trials involving over 1,300 people undergoing cardiac surgery found that NAC significantly reduced the risk of developing a post-operative abnormal heart rhythm (atrial fibrillation) by 36 per cent[2]. However, it may increase blood loss and the need for transfusion[3].

Lung disease: By thinning mucus, NAC can improve chronic obstructive pulmonary disease. A meta-analysis of data from eight trials involving over 2,200 people found that taking NAC significantly reduced the risk of experiencing an exacerbation of symptoms such as bronchitis by 51 per cent. The benefits were as great in active smokers as non smokers. Benefits were greatest in those not using inhaled corticosteroids[4].

Dose
300–500 mg, three to four times a day.

Contraindications
NAC should not be taken by people who have peptic ulcers.

Nettle
(Urtica dioica)

Stinging nettle roots contain beta-sitosterol and a variety of other sterols and are often used together with saw palmetto.

Nettle extracts are used to treat symptoms of male urinary

1. Grant JE et al. Arch Gen Psychiatry 2009;66(7):756–63
2. Baker WL et al. Eur J Cardiothorac Surg 2009;35(3):521–7
3. Wijeysundera DN et al. Crit Care Med 2009;37(6):1929–34
4. Sutherland ER et al. COPD 2006;3(4):195–202

retention due to an enlarged prostate gland. The ability to improve urinary symptoms of benign prostate enlargement without shrinking the gland is a relatively new finding. Nettle extracts seem to interfere with testosterone metabolism by lowering the amount bound to a blood protein (sex hormone binding globulin – SHBG) so that more testosterone is free and active in the circulation. This means that more testosterone is available for absorption into the prostate gland, so that congestion is relieved. Increased levels of freely circulating testosterone also increase sex drive.

Another possible way in which nettle extracts work is in reducing the flow of sodium and potassium ions in and out of prostate cells to reduce their metabolism and growth.

Benefits

Arthritis: Nettle stings are traditionally used to treat chronic osteoarthritis joint pain[1]. Oral nettle root extracts can also damp down inflammation by reducing production of inflammatory cytokines and they are used in the treatment of rheumatoid arthritis. A study involving 152 with rheumatic conditions found that taking 1.5 g nettle extract for three weeks produced improvement in 70 per cent of cases[2].

BPH: One trial involved 246 men with symptoms due to benign prostate enlargement who were treated with 459 mg stinging nettle root extracts or placebo for one year. The International Prostate Symptoms Score was significantly reduced in those on active treatment compared with placebo[3]. In a study involving 2,080 patients with benign prostatic hyperplasia (BPH), a combined extract containing saw palmetto berry and nettle root extracts improved both obstructive and irritative symptoms, with results described as 'very good' or 'good' in over 80 per cent of cases[4]. Less than 1 per cent of men developed mild side effects. Another interesting trial compared the activity of a combination of saw palmetto berry and nettle root extracts against the prescribed drug finasteride. A group of 431 men were treated for 48 weeks with either two capsules of

1. Randall C et al. Complement Ther Med 2008;16(2):66–72
2. Ramm S, Hansen C. Dtsch Apoth Ztg 1995;135(39):3–8
3. Schneider T, Rubben H. Urologe A 2004;43(3):302–6
4. Schneider T et al. Fortsch Med 1995;113(3):37–40

plant extracts or one capsule of finasteride daily. The results were similar in both groups with equivalent reductions in urinary flow rate, International Prostate Symptoms Score and increased quality of life[1]. The natural plant extracts proved superior when it came to side effects however, with fewer cases of erectile problems and headache.

Dose
250 mg extract twice a day, together with saw palmetto.

Side effects
Nettle extracts can cause mild gastrointestinal upsets. Avoid overdosage as this may cause temporary kidney problems.

Gynaecomastia (breast enlargement) has been reported in a man and milk production in a woman in which the only obvious factor identified was drinking nettle leaf tea.

Note: Men with prostate symptoms should continue to have a regular medical review of their condition.

Nickel

Nickel has only been recognized as important in human metabolism within the last thirty years. It acts as an antidote to the effects of stress hormones to help offset constricted blood vessels, increased heart rate and raised blood pressure. It may therefore be important in reducing the risk of stressrelated coronary heart disease.

Foods tend to contain nickel due to contamination from nickel alloys used in processing machinery and cooking utensils. Margarine is also a source where nickel is used as a catalyst during production.

In animals, nickel is also known to help the sugarlowering effects of insulin, to have an effect on fat metabolism and to stabilize genetic material. Nickel deficiency also leads to impaired iron absorption and anaemia in animals. It is not yet known whether similar effects occur in humans.

1. Sokeland J. BJU Int 2000;86(4):439–42

Dose
There is currently no EU RDA for nickel.

Oatstraw
(Avena sativa)

Extracts from the young, whole plant or unripe grain of oats are known as oatstraw or wild oats. These contain a variety of flavonoids, steroidal compounds, vitamins (especially B group) and minerals (especially calcium).

Benefits
Oatstraw is one of the most popular herbal remedies used as a restorative nerve tonic. It is used to help treat depression, nervous exhaustion and stress. It is a useful source of B group vitamins which are essential for energy production and which are needed in extra amounts during times of stress. Oatstraw soothes the nervous system and has a calming but spirited effect. It helps to reduce cravings and is helpful for those who are trying to stop smoking.

As oatstraw contains hormone building blocks, it is also recommended to women suffering from oestrogen deficiency and anyone with an underactive thyroid gland. Oat bran has been shown to help reduce high blood cholesterol levels and, taken regularly, can ease constipation.

Research in Australia found that athletes who followed an oat-based diet for three weeks showed a 4 per cent increase in stamina.

Dose
1 dropper fluid extract or tincture, twice or three times daily.

People who are sensitive to gluten (coeliac disease) should allow the tincture to settle, and decant the clear liquid for use.

Olive leaf
(Olea europaea)

The olive tree is well known around the Mediterranean where its fruits are eaten and used to make olive oil.

Olive leaf extracts have a powerful antibacterial, anti-viral, anti-fungal and anti-parasitic activity. Clinical studies involving 500 patients suggest that olive leaf is effective in treating 98 per cent of bacterial and viral infections – better than many prescribed antibiotics. The active ingredients appear to be iridoid substances such as oleuropein and R-calcium elenolate which give the leaves of certain strains of olive tree a characteristic bitter taste. The iridoids work together in synergy to kill microbial infections by interfering with the production of certain amino acids so that they cannot grow or reproduce properly. Olive leaf extracts can also inactivate bacteria by dissolving and weakening their outer coating.

Olive leaf extracts are used to treat candida and other fungal infections, sinusitis, common colds, influenza, herpes, parasitic infections, shingles, respiratory infections, tonsillitis, pharyngitis, urinary tract infections, fibromyalgia and chronic fatigue syndrome.

Benefits

Herpes simplex: A comparative trial of three products conducted by the Herpes Viruses Association (olive leaf extract versus the cactus, *Opuntia streptacantha*, and a combined lysine, pollen and propolis capsule) found that olive leaf extracts were the clear winner. Out of 45 members taking part, 78 per cent of those using olive leaf extracts were pleased with the results in treating and preventing attacks.

Blood pressure: Preliminary research suggests that olive leaf extracts can lower a raised blood pressure. When tested in 40 identical twins with borderline hypertension, one of each pair took either 500 mg or 1000 mg olive leaf extracts per day, while the other twin received diet and lifestyle advice. Blood pressure reduced significantly between pairs, with reductions of 11/4 mmHg in those taking 1000 mg extracts[1]. There were no reductions in the control group receiving diet and lifestyle advice. LDL-cholesterol levels also decreased in those taking the extracts.

Dose

500 mg, twice to four times a day, between meals. For persistent problems take 1 g, three times a day. As symptoms improve,

1. Perrinjaquet-Moccetti T et al. Phytother Res 2008;22(9):1239–42

reduce back to a maintenance dose of 500 mg twice a day as necessary.

Side effects
No toxic side effects have been reported even at doses several hundred times higher than those used therapeutically. However, a few people have developed a Herxheimer reaction due to large numbers of bacteria being killed at once, which releases bacterial toxins into the system. Symptoms include fever, headache, and worsening of any current symptoms. This is usually treated with paracetamol and drinking plenty of fluids, and will resolve within 24 to 48 hours. If it occurs, cut back on the dose you are taking. Similar reactions can occur with traditional antibiotics and most people are not affected.

Olive oil
(Olea europaea)

All olives start off green. These are the unripened fruit with firm skin and a slightly bitter taste. Olives intended for producing oil are picked when unripe. They taste bitter and are totally inedible. These have a low acid content which is crucial, as the lower the acidity, the better the oil.

Extra virgin olive oil is the best quality and has not been purified. Only around 10 per cent of oil produced is of this premium grade quality. It has a distinctive green hue and often hazes at room temperature. Its flavour is superb as it comes from the first pressing of the fruit and retains the fresh, olive aroma with less than 1 per cent acidity. It also has the highest antioxidant content (vitamin E, carotenoids and polyphenols). Virgin olive oil comes next in quality with an acidity level of not more than 1.5 per cent. Virgin olive oil is also a premium product as it is not purified and has a slightly more piquant taste. Pure olive oil is a blend of refined olive oil mixed with virgin oil to provide flavour and a quality suitable for cooking. Although the flavour is less pleasing, this is the most widely sold oil as it is less expensive.

As with other oils, oxidation occurs over time. As the oil matures, extra acidity is gained which detracts from the original flavour. Most oils are best used within one year of pressing. If left longer than this, stale or even rancid flavours can develop. All types of olive oil should therefore be kept somewhere cool and dark, and used fresh – buy from outlets where turnover is high, and avoid large containers (especially those made from tin or aluminium). It is best bought in small sizes, and frequently renewed.

Pure olive oil remains stable at elevated temperatures due to its high levels of monounsaturated fatty acids and natural antioxidant, vitamin E. Refined olive oil can therefore be heated up to 210°C before chemical changes take place. Virgin and extra virgin olive oils are less stable, however, due to their higher content of heat-sensitive components. Because of this, virgin olive oil may cause unwanted smells or taste changes if heated above 180°C. Pure olive oil should therefore be used for frying, and virgin or extra virgin olive oils be kept for steaming, braising and dressing. Discard any oil that begins to smoke or smell odd during use. Ideally, cooking oils should not be re-used.

Olive oil is native to the Mediterranean – an area with a low incidence of coronary heart disease. It is a rich source of mono-unsaturated fats, such as oleic acid, which make up 73 per cent of its oil content. Monounsaturated fats consist of chains of carbon atoms in which there is only one double bond, which makes it flexible. A diet high in monounsaturated fat may help to reduce your risk of atherosclerosis, high blood pressure, coronary heart disease, stroke and Type 2 diabetes. This is thought to explain some of the benefits of the so-called Mediterranean diet. Extra virgin and virgin olive oils also contain significant amounts of plant sterols and antioxidants such as polyphenols and vitamin E.

Benefits

Cholesterol: Olive oil contains sterols which help to reduce absorption of cholesterol. Oleic acid is processed in the body to slightly lower levels of total and 'bad' oxidized LDL-cholesterol while increasing desirable high-density lipoprotein (HDL) cholesterol[1]. These effects are less marked for pure olive oil than for virgin and extra virgin olive oils.

High blood pressure: Among 160 men with normal blood pressure, taking 25 ml olive oil per day lowered systolic blood pressure by

---

1. Corvas MI et al. Ann Inten Med 2006;145(5):333–41

around 4 mmHg, but did not affect diastolic BP[1]. This effect was seen in those from non-Mediterranean countries, but not in those from the Mediterranean region who already had a high olive oil intake. Among a group of elderly people with hypertension, enriching the diet with olive oil normalized systolic blood pressure (down to 136 mmHg) with no effect on those taking sunflower oil (remained in the region of 150 mmHg)[2]. Among people with Type 2 diabetes, an olive-oil enriched diet can lower day-time blood pressure by 6/6 mmHg and average 24 hour blood pressure by 4/3 mmHg compared with the normal carbohydrate based diabetic diet[3].

Coronary heart disease: In a study involving over 11,000 people who had had a heart attack, the following of a Mediterranean-style diet rich in olive oil, fish, fruit, vegetables and garlic reduced the risk of death over the subsequent 6.5 years by 49 per cent compared with those following a less healthy diet[4].

Diabetes: Monounsaturated fats can improve insulin sensitivity and fasting glucose levels in people with Type 2 diabetes[5].

Cancer: Studies looking at the link between diet and colon cancer suggest that populations with the highest intakes of olive oil have the lowest risks of bowel cancer. It is thought that the activity of a digestive enzyme, diamine oxidase, is reduced by olive oil so that less cancer-causing chemicals are released from the diet into the gastrointestinal tract. Following a Mediterranean-style diet can reduce the recurrence of colon adenoma by 50 per cent[6]. Following a low-fat diet enriched with extra virgin olive oil may reduce the risk of breast cancer[7].

Dose

At least 10 g daily, and preferably 30–40 g a day. For those who do not cook their own food, or who have little opportunity to include

1. Bondia-Pons I et al. J Nutr 2007;137(1):84–87
2. Perona JS et al. Clin Nutr 2004;23(5):1113–21
3. Rasmussen OW et al. Ugeskr Laeger 1995;157(8):1028–32
4. Barzi F et al. Eur J Clin Nutr 2003;57(4):604–11
5. Paniaqua JA et al. J Am Coll Nutr 2007;26(5):434–44
6. Cottet V et al. Eur J Cancer Prev 2005;14(1):21–9
7. Lipworth L et al. Prev Med 1997;26(2):181–90

extra virgin olive oil in their diet, extra virgin olive oil capsules are available as a supplement.

1 tablespoon olive oil contains 15 g total fat, 2 g saturated fat.

1 tablespoon butter contains 12 g total fat, 8 g saturated fat.

Oregano oil
(Oreganum vulgare)

Oregano is a popular herb used extensively in Mediterranean cooking. Oil of wild oregano contains essential oils (e.g. carvacrol, thymol, terpinenes, cymenes) that have powerful antimicrobial actions, and has been used to kill moulds, yeasts, bacteria and parasites even when diluted over a thousand times. It is also used to boost general immunity and to help cleanse the body during detox programmes.

Oregano oil may be used as a general immune tonic to increase resistance against infection, and to help improve symptoms due to upper respiratory tract infections, asthma, low blood pressure, tiredness, candida, irritable bowel syndrome, colitis, chronic fatigue, diarrhoea, constipation, cystitis, eczema and psoriasis.

It may also be used topically (dilute in olive oil if stinging occurs) to treat toothache, ringworm, athlete's foot, cold sores, psoriasis, eczema, warts, rosacea and wounds.

Dose
Only a small amount is needed, and doses range from 10–600 mg daily.

Pelargonium sidoides

Pelargonium sidoides is a Zulu herbal remedy known as Umckaloabo. It is traditionally used to treat respiratory tract infections such as colds, bronchitis and sinusitis, and to treat dysentry. It contains a number of unique substances, including coumarins and a diterpene called reniformin. Pelargonium sidoides root extracts have direct antibacterial activity against a spectrum of Gram-positive and Gram-negative bacteria and increase the activity of phagocytic immune cells that absorb and neutralize infecting microorganisms. Pelargonium sidoides also appears to inhibit adhesin molecules used by bacteria to stick to cell walls. Another interesting action is that it stimulates the rate of beating of hair-like projections (cilia) on the surface of respiratory tract cells which help clear mucus and infection.

Benefits

Respiratory tract infections: A systematic review identified three trials, involving almost 750 adults with acute bronchitis, and three trials involving over 800 children, in which Pelargonium sidoides was investigated. The review found significant treatment effects for Pelargonium sidoides, and the authors concluded that it may be effective in treating symptoms of acute rhinosinusitis and the common cold[1]. When the results of eight trials were considered, effectiveness was found in reducing cough, sputum production, headache and nasal discharge.

Bronchitis: A meta-analysis of data from four trials suggests that Pelargonium sidoides extracts are significantly more effective than placebo in treating acute bronchitis[2].

Common cold: A study involving 103 people with cold symptoms present for between 24 and 48 hours found that taking Pelargonium sidoides extracts produced significant improvements in symptoms. After ten days, 78.8 per cent of those receiving treatment were clinically cured, versus only 31.4 per cent taking placebo[3]. A review of eight trials confirms it can reduce sore throat, cough, runny and blocked nose.

Tonsillitis: A study involving 140 children with tonsillitis found that taking Pelargonium sidoides extracts was significantly better than placebo in treating acute tonsillopharyngitis. Treatment reduced the severity of symptoms and shortened the duration of sore throat by at least two days[4].

1. Timmer A et al. Cochrane Database Syst Rev 2008 (3):CD 006323
2. Agbabiaka TB et al. Phytomedicine 2008;15(5):378–85
3. Lizoqub VG et al. Explore (HY) 2007;3(6):573–84
4. Bereznov VV et al. Altern Ther Health Med 2003;9(5):68–79

Helicobacter pylori: Preliminary evidence suggests that Pelargonium sidoides is a potent inhibitor of the adhesin molecules needed by *Helicobacter* to stick to the stomach wall[1,2].

Dose
Tincture: 60 drops three times daily.
  Tablets: 20 mg three times a day.

Peppermint
(Menthe piperitae)

Peppermint is a popular culinary and medicinal herb. It contains an essential oil that has antiseptic and painkilling properties, and it is also widely used in the treatment of fevers, colds, headaches and the discomfort of cystitis, as well as relieving tension, itching and inflammation. The essential oil is obtained by steam distillation of peppermint's aerial parts (leaves, stems and shoots). The oil is rich in menthol which may make up to 50 per cent of the oil by volume.

It improves digestion by increasing gastric emptying, stimulating secretion of digestive juices and bile, and also relaxes excessive spasm of the smooth muscle lining the digestive tract. Peppermint is therefore taken to relieve indigestion, colic, intestinal cramps, flatulence, diverticulitis and irritable bowel syndrome (IBS). It may also help to dissolve gallstones. Inhaling menthol helps to relieve nasal congestion.

Benefits
Irritable bowel syndrome: While mild symptoms of IBS are helped by drinking peppermint tea, more severe symptoms benefit from taking peppermint oil capsules that are enteric-coated to prevent the release of peppermint oil until it has reached the large bowel. A meta-analysis of data from 12 trials, involving almost 600 people, explored the effectiveness of fibre, antispasmodics and peppermint oil in treating IBS[3]. The NNT (number needed to treat) to prevent

1. Wittischier N et al. Phytomedicine 2007;14(4):285–8
2. Beil W, Kilian P. Phytomedicine 2007;14(Suppl 6):5–8
3. Ford AC et al. BMJ 2008;337:a2313

one person having persistent symptoms for peppermint oil was 2.5, making it the most effective therapy. On average, 75 per cent of people with IBS who take peppermint oil experience a greater than 50 per cent reduction in symptoms compared with 38 per cent taking inactive placebo[1].

Dose
Mint tea: add 1 tablespoon mint leaves to a cup of boiling water and infuse for 20 minutes.

50–100 mg (enteric-coated capsules), three times a day, after each meal or as required.

Side effects
Treatment may produce a warm, tingling feeling in the back passage due to some of the essential oil not being absorbed. This is not harmful and will usually disappear if you cut back on the dosage you are taking.

Contraindications
• Peppermint should not be taken during pregnancy.

Perilla frutescens

Perilla frutescens is an annual plant native to Asia, which has either green or purple leaves. It is also known as Chinese basil, the purple mint plant or wild coleus.

The leaves, stems and seeds are a traditional Chinese herbal remedy used to help prevent food poisoning. In India, Perilla seed oil (similar to flaxseed oil) is often added to curries.

Perilla seed oil has a high content of linolenic acid which is processed in the body to produce anti-inflammatory effects similar to those of evening primrose oil.

Leaf extracts also contain a number of anti-allergy and anti-inflammatory substances, including elemicine, apigenen and beta-sitosterol. Leaf extracts are believed to reduce abnormal immune reactions by inhibiting tumour necrosis factor (TNF), inhibiting

1. Cappello G et al. Dig Liver Dis 2007;39(6):530–6

immunoglobulin E (IgE) production and function as well as having antioxidant activity.

Benefits
Hay fever: In a trial involving 29 people with hay fever, Perilla extracts significantly reduced itchy nose, watery eyes, itchy eyes and total symptoms compared with placebo. The number of allergy cells in nasal fluids was also reduced[1].

Asthma: Perilla seed oil was tested in 14 people with asthma. Those taking Perilla for four weeks showed significantly decreased production of inflammatory substances and improved lung function tests compared with those taking placebo[2].

Dose
200 mg once or twice a day.

Pfaffia
(Pfaffia paniculata)

Pfaffia – also known as suma, Brazilian ginseng and Brazilian carrots – is regarded as a panacea for all ills locally, where it is called *para todo* – 'for everything'. The dried golden root of pfaffia is a rich source of vitamins, minerals, amino acids, pfaffocides and plant hormones (up to 11 per cent by weight) such as stigmasterol and sitosterol (which have oestrogen-like actions and reduce high cholesterol levels) and beta-ecdysone which increases cellular oxygenation.

Benefits
Although pfaffia is unrelated to Chinese ginseng, it has similar adaptogenic properties and can help the immune system to adapt to various stresses including overwork, illness and fatigue. It improves resistance to stress, illness and fatigue and evens out hormone imbalances. Due to its oestrogenic nature, it is used to treat a variety

1. Takano H et al. Exp Biol Med (Maywood) 2004;229(3):247–54
2. Okamoto M et al. Intern Med 2000 39(2):107–11

of gynaecological problems linked with hormonal imbalances such as pre-menstrual syndrome and menopausal symptoms.

Pfaffia has been used as a female aphrodisiac for at least 300 years, and is also used to help treat male impotence and prostatitis. It is used to boost physical, mental and sexual energy levels as well as producing a general sense of wellbeing. Pfaffocides are also being used to improve sleep and to treat diabetes, chronic fatigue syndrome, joint problems, high cholesterol and gout.

An extract of the root, pfaffic acid, is in development as a treatment to inhibit the growth of skin melanoma cancer cells.

Dose
Extracts standardized to 5 per cent ecdysterones: 500 mg–1 g a day to combat physical and mental stress.

Note: Diabetics should monitor sugar levels closely as it seems to boost insulin production, normalizes blood sugar levels and may reduce insulin requirements.

Contraindications
- Pfaffia should not be taken by pregnant or breast-feeding women.
- Although plant-oestrogens may protect against oestrogen sensitive conditions such as endometriosis and gynaecological tumours (e.g. of the breast, ovaries and cervix), pfaffia should not be taken by women with a history of these problems except under specialist advice.

Phosphatidylserine

Phosphatidylserine is a phospholipid that occurs naturally in the body and is found in foods such as mackerel, herring, liver, kidneys and white beans. Supplements are produced commercially from soybeans.

Its molecular structure resembles an old-fashioned gipsy clothes peg, with a head at one end and two tails sticking down at the other. The head end attracts water, while the tail end repels water. Because of these attracting and repelling properties, the phospholipids naturally line up to form a two-layered membrane with the heads on the outside and the tails on the inside. The molecules tend to float around each other to form a membrane that is more fluid than solid. This fluidity helps to improve the speed at which electrical and chemical messages are passed from one brain cell to another. This beneficial effect is enhanced when the tails of the molecule consist of the omega-3 essential fatty acid, DHA.

Phosphatidylserine (PS) also acts as a co-factor for several enzymes, and regulates the release of nerve cell communication chemicals (neurotransmitters) such as acetylcholine, dopamine and noradrenaline.

Benefits

Cognitive function: Phosphatidylserine supplements can help to enhance memory and the ability to think straight (cognition), to improve age-related memory impairment. It is especially helpful for improving cognitive functions in older people, helping to improve learning, recall, recognition and concentration. For example, it can help to increase the recall of word lists. Researchers believe that phosphatidylserine supplements may improve cognitive functions in people experiencing the early stages of Alzheimer's disease. Some evidence suggests it helps to protect against the inflammatory effects of neuronal support cells (microglia) whose activation is linked with Alzheimer's.

ADHD: Phosphatidylserine may have a positive effect in children with attention problems. In a pilot study involving 15 children aged 6–12 years, a dose of 200 mg phosphatidylserine per day for two months significantly improved inattention, hyperactivity, impulsiveness and visual perception[1]. It should only be used in children with ADHD under medical supervision, however.

Exercise: Phosphatidylserine reduces exercise-induced stress by reducing production of the stress hormone, cortisol. This helps to protect muscles from the effects of exercise, improving the speed of recovery of post-exertion muscle soreness and to boost perceived well-being (including the 'high' you can get from exercise). It may also improve exercise capacity during high intensity activities such

1. Hirayama S et al. AgroFood 2006; 17(5):32–36

as cycling and running, making it a helpful supplement for sports training.

Dose
100–500 mg daily.

Phosphatidylserine is generally recognized as safe in older people at doses of up to 200 mg three times a day.

Phosphorus

Phosphorus is an essential mineral of which 90 per cent of the body's stores is found in the bones and teeth where it forms part of an important structural salt, calcium phosphate, which is also known as hydroxyapatite. The remaining 10 per cent of the body's stores serves a number of functions and is:

* Involved in the production of energy-rich molecules (ATP, ADP) in muscle cells
* Needed to activate the vitamin B complex which is also involved in energy production
* An important component of genetic material
* A co-factor for several metabolic enzymes and helps to keep blood slightly alkaline.

Phosphorus in the diet
Phosphorus is obtained from many food sources, including meats, eggs, dairy products, wholegrains, pulses, nuts, soft drinks such as colas, and yeast extract. Vitamin D is essential for the absorption of phosphorus from the gut and for its deposition, with calcium, into bones. Deficiency can develop in people using antacids containing aluminium hydroxide long term as these impair absorption of phosphates from the gut.

Benefits
As phosphate is so important for producing energy in the body, it is needed for optimum athletic performance. Research involving endurance athletes (such as cyclists) found that taking sodium phosphate supplements for three days before a competition

decreased lactic acid build-up in muscles, increased oxygen consumption by 11 per cent and prolonged the time to exhaustion by 20 per cent. Other studies suggest that sodium phosphate supplements can increase maximal power output by up to 17 per cent.

Deficiency

As phosphorus is widely found in the diet, deficiency is rare, although symptoms that may be due to phosphorus deficiency include general malaise, loss of appetite, increased susceptibility to infection, anaemia due to shortened life of red blood cells, muscle weakness, bone pain, joint stiffness and nervous system symptoms such as numbness, pins and needles, irritability and confusion.

Dose

The UK RNI for phosphorus is 550 mg per day for adults. The old EU RDA for phosphorus was 800 mg. The newly set EU RDA for phosphorus reduces this to 700 mg. The upper safe level for long-term use from supplements (which takes average dietary intakes into account) is suggested as 250 mg.

Few people are at risk of phosphorus deficiency, and single supplements are rarely needed, although low doses are included in most A to Z-style vitamin and mineral products.

Pine bark

Extracts from the bark of the French maritime pine (*Pinus maritima*, known commercially as Pycnogenol®) contain a rich blend of flavonoid proanthocyanidins which research suggests are 50 times more powerful than vitamin E, 20 times more powerful than vitamin C and 16 times more active than grapeseed extracts[1]. They are anti-inflammatory, and regulate the production of nitric oxide – a substance involved in blood vessel dilation. Together, these effects make it one of the most versatile supplements available.

---

1. Chida M et al. Ophthal Res 1999; 31(6):407–415

Benefits

Circulation: Pine bark extracts strengthen fragile capillaries and reduce abnormal blood clotting – even in smokers[1]. They help to reduce ankle swelling and are used to reduce the risk of developing a deep vein thrombosis (DVT) during long-haul air flights[2,3]. They have also been used medically to improve the blood-thinning action of aspirin[4]. Pine bark extracts can reduce cramp and muscular pain in those with impaired circulation to the legs[5]. They may also help to improve leg ulcers associated with poor blood flow through peripheral veins (chronic venous insufficiency)[6].

Blood pressure: By improving blood vessel dilation, pine bark extracts lower blood pressure, and can reduce the dose of antihypertensive medication needed[7].

Cholesterol: By increasing the antioxidant level of blood, pine bark extracts lower circulating levels of 'bad' LDL-cholesterol and raise 'good' HDL-cholesterol[8].

Memory: By improving circulation to the brain, pine bark extracts can improve memory and the ability to think straight. A recent double-blind, placebo-controlled study involving 101 people aged 60–85 years found significant improvements in working memory in those taking 150 mg pine bark extracts for three months[9].

Asthma: By stabilizing cell membranes, pine bark extracts inhibit the release of histamine from mast cells to reduce symptoms of hay fever and asthma. In a trial involving 60 asthmatic children aged 6–18, those taking pine bark extracts for three months showed significant improvements in peak flow and asthma symptoms compared with placebo, and reduced their need for inhalers[10].

1. Putter M et al. Thromb Res 1999; 95(4):155–61
2. Cesarone MR et al. Clin Appl Thromb Hemost 2005; 11(3):289–94
3. Belcar G et al. Clin Appl Thromb Hemost 2004; 10(4):373–7
4. Golanski J et al. Postepy Hig Med Dosw 2006; 60:316–21
5. Vinciquerra G et al. Angioloty 2006; 57(3):331–9
6. Belcaro G et al. Angiology 2005; 56(6):699–705
7. Liu X et al. Life Sci 2004; 74(7):855–62
8. Devaraj S et al. Lipids 2002; 37(10):931–4
9. Ryan J et al. J Psychopharmacol 2008; 22(5):553–62
10. Lau BH et al. J Asthma 2004; 41(8):852–32

Diabetes: Pine bark extracts can improve blood glucose control in people with Type 2 diabetes[1,2]. Fasting blood glucose levels lowered significantly in a dose-dependent fashion until a dose of 200 mg was reached then did not reduce further[3]. Haemoglobin A1c levels also decreased but insulin levels were not affected, suggesting that the effect is not due to stimulation of insulin secretion. Pycnogenol® has been shown in studies, involving over 1,200 people, to help seal leaky blood vessels in the retina, reducing the progression of retinopathy and improving visual acuity to help preserve vision[4]. It may also help to treat and even prevent diabetic foot ulcers[5].

Osteoarthritis: By reducing inflammation, pine bark extracts can improve pain, stiffness, walking distance and a reduced need for non-steroidal anti-inflammatory drugs in those with arthritic joints[6,7].

Menopause: Because pine bark extracts reduce blood vessel hyper-activity, they can improve menopausal flushing and night sweats. A study involving 200 menopausal women showed significant improvements in menopausal symptoms and menstrual pain in those taking 200 mg pine bark extracts daily, compared with placebo[8].

Dose
50–200 mg daily.

NB: If you have diabetes, monitor glucose levels carefully when taking any supplement that may affect blood glucose control.

As pine bark extracts enhance the effects of other antioxidants such as co-enzyme Q10, vitamin C and E, they are often combined in supplements.

1. Liu X et al. Life Sci 2004; 75(21):2505–13
2. Zibadi S et al. Nutr Res 2008;28(5):315–20
3. Liu X et al. Diabetes Care 2004;27(3):839
4. Schonlau F, Rohdewald P. Int Ophthalmol 2001; 24(3):161–71
5. Cesarone MR et al. Angiology 2006; 57(4):431–6
6. Cisar P et al. Phytother Res 2008; 22(8):1087–92
7. Belcaro G et al. Phytother Res 2008; 22(4):518–23
8. Yang HM et al. Acta Obstet Gynecol Scand 2007; 86(8):978–85

Plant sterols

Plant sterols, such as campesterol, sitosterol and stigmasterol, are natural plant substances that closely resemble the animal sterol, cholesterol. This similarity means they can block absorption of dietary cholesterol although they are not absorbed themselves. Plant sterols reduce absorption of cholesterol in the small intestines – both the cholesterol obtained ready-made in the diet, and the cholesterol that is made in the liver and secreted into the intestines via the bile. As a result, less cholesterol is absorbed and more is voided via the bowels.

Although diet should always come first, it's difficult to obtain optimum amounts of sterols from food sources alone. The average diet provides 180–460 mg sterols per day, with vegetarians obtaining the highest amounts. Sterols in plant foods are naturally bound to fibre, which limits their action, however. Functional foods fortified with sterols such as spreads and yoghurts, and supplements, have therefore been developed to boost intakes.

The cholesterol lowering drugs known as statins work in a different way from sterols. Statins inhibit an enzyme in the liver, so less cholesterol is made and released into your circulation. Because they work in a different way from statins, plant sterols can be combined with statin therapy to lower cholesterol levels even further[1]. In fact, adding sterols to statin medication is more effective than doubling the statin dose[2].

Benefits

Cholesterol: A large trial involving over 22,500 men and women living in Norfolk showed that people with the highest dietary intake of plant sterols have the lowest cholesterol levels[3]. Following a sterol-enriched diet can lower levels of harmful LDL-cholesterol by around 15 per cent[4] to significantly reduce your risk of cardio-vascular disease. They appear to be even more effective in people with Type 2 diabetes; one study showed they reduced LDL-choles-

1. Thompson GR. Am J Cardiol 2005;96(1A):37D–39D
2. Katan MB et al. Mayo Clin Proc 2003;78:965–978
3. Andersson SW et al. Eur J Clin Nutr 2004;58(10):1378–85
4. Patch CS et al. Vasc Health Risk Manag 2006;2(2):157–62

terol levels of 26.8 per cent in people with Type 2 diabetes, compared to a reduction of 15.1 per cent in those without diabetes[1].

Dose

1–3g per day.

For optimum benefits, intakes of 1–2 g per day are ideal, and this is the level used in trials that show the benefits of enriching the diet with sterol supplements. In addition, sterols in plant foods are naturally bound to fibre, which limits their action, unlike those found in supplements which are therefore more effective.

A panel of 32 experts who deliberated on the efficacy and safety of sterols concluded that present evidence is sufficient to promote their use for lowering LDL-cholesterol levels in people at increased risk for coronary heart disease[2].

The only recognized potential adverse effect is a reduced absorption of some dietary carotenoids. This is easily overcome by eating an additional serving of a carotenoid-rich (yellow or orange) fruit or vegetable per day[3] – something we should all be aiming to do anyway!

Pollen pistil

Extracts from flower pistils (the part that carries the pollen) contain hormone building blocks that help to reduce symptoms associated with female hormone imbalances.

Benefits

Menopause: In a study involving 64 menopausal women, pollen pistil extracts taken for three months reduced hot flushes by 65 per cent (versus 38 per cent with placebo). After three months, there was a 27 per cent greater reduction in hot flushes than with placebo[4]. Other studies suggest pollen pistil extracts can improve menopausal joint pains, sweating and irritability.

1. Lau VW et al. Am J Clin Nutr 2005;81(6):1351–8
2. Katan MB et al. Mayo Clin Proc 2003; 78: 965–78
3. Nestel PJ Med J Aust 2002;176 Suppl:S122
4. Winther K et al. Climacteric 2005;8(2):162–70

PMS: In a trial involving 101 women with premenstrual syndrome, taking pollen extracts for four menstrual cycles was shown to reduce symptoms in those for whom irritability was the main symptom[1]. Other studies have found that pollen pistil extracts significantly reduce tension, irritability, bloatedness and weight gain compared with inactive placebo.

Dose
160 mg twice a day

The pollen is treated to minimize risks of allergic reactions, so it doesn't cause any problems if you have hay fever.

Pomegranate
(Punica granatum)

Pomegranates are the fruit of a tree that is native to Asia and the Mediterranean. The fleshy aryls (seed casings) contain a ruby-coloured juice that contains vitamin C, carotenoids, unique anti-oxidant tannins called punicalgins, catechins, gallocatechins, ellagic acid and anthocyanins.

Laboratory studies suggest that pomegranate juice can reduce the development of atherosclerosis, lower blood pressure and has beneficial effects on the elasticity of arterial walls and against prostate cancer cells.

Benefits
Antioxidant: Although widely promoted as an antioxidant superfruit, the juice itself has a relatively modest ORAC score of 2,341 units (microTE per 100g)[2]. However, when 26 elderly people were given 250 ml of either apple juice or pomegranate juice, those taking pomegranate showed significantly improved antioxidant status[3].

Erectile dysfunction: In a cross-over trial involving 53 males with erectile difficulties, volunteers took either pomegranate juice or

1. Gerhardsen G et al. Adv Ther 2008; 25(6):595–607
2. www.oracvalues.com
3. Guo C et al. Nutr Res 2008;28(2):72–7

placebo for four weeks then, after a 'wash-out' period of two weeks, took the other preparation for another four weeks. Of the 42 men reporting improvements in sexual function, 25 improved when taking pomegranate juice compared with 17 while taking placebo. Although this was not statistically significant, further research is warranted[1].

Dental plaque: Research involving 60 people (aged 9–25 years) suggests that pomegranate fruit extracts have an inhibitory effect on the bacteria causing dental plaque and may help to reduce tooth decay[2].

Coronary heart disease: Forty-five people with ischaemic heart disease were given either 240 ml pomegranate juice or placebo per day for three months. Assessments of blood flow through their coronary arteries during stress testing showed significant improvements in those taking pomegranate but worsening in those on control juice. There were no changes in heart medication, blood glucose levels, weight or blood pressure in either group. The researchers concluded that daily consumption of pomegranate juice can improve stress-induced myocardial ischemia[3].

Chronic obstructive airways disease: COAD results from inflammation and structural damage to the lungs (chronic bronchitis, emphysema) which is usually related to smoking cigarettes. Although antioxidants will not affect loss of lung structure, they might be expected to reduce inflammation and improve bronchitis. But when 30 patients with stable COAD consumed either 400 ml pomegranate juice or a placebo for five weeks, no significant differences were found between either group in respiratory function or clinical symptoms[4].

Dose
250 mg–1 g daily.

1. Forest CP et al. Int J Impot Res 2007;19(6):564–7
2. Menezes SM et al. J Herb Pharmacother 2006;6(2):79–92
3. Sumner MD et al. Am J Cardiol 2005;96(6):810–4
4. Cerda B et al. Eur J Clin Nur 2006;60(2):245–53

Potassium

Potassium is the main positively charged ion found inside cells, where it is present in concentrations 30 times greater than those in the extracellular fluid surrounding each cell. It is actively pumped inside cells by ion-exchange pumps found in cell walls and, in exchange, sodium ions are pumped out to make room for it.

Benefits

Potassium is essential for muscle contraction (including the heartbeat), nerve conduction, maintenance of blood sugar levels and the production of nucleic acids, proteins and energy. The kidney regulates blood potassium levels and keeps them within a fairly narrow range.

Because the sodium-potassium exchange system in cells also occurs in the kidneys, a good intake of dietary potassium helps to flush sodium from cells into the urine for excretion from the body. As excess sodium is linked with high blood pressure in some people, following a diet that is relatively high in potassium and low in sodium is linked with a lower risk of hypertension and stroke. In one study, for example, over 80 per cent of people taking antihypertensive medication were able to halve their dose by just increasing their dietary intake of potassium.

Most people do not need potassium supplements, unless they exercise a lot (e.g. top athletes). Low levels of potassium commonly occur in people taking certain diuretics that do not have a potassium-sparing effect in the body. Symptoms that may be due to lack of potassium include poor appetite, fatigue, weakness, low blood glucose, muscle cramps, irregular or rapid heart beat, constipation, irritability, pins and needles, drowsiness and confusion.

Excess potassium levels are rare as the body usually controls blood levels well. They can occur in people with kidney problems, or those who take excess potassium supplements however, to produce symptoms such as irregular heartbeat, and muscle fatigue.

Potassium in the diet

Foods that contain potassium include seafood, fruit (particularly tomatoes, bananas), vegetables, wholegrains and low-sodium potassium-enriched salts.

Dose

The UK RNI for potassium is 3500 mg per day for adults. The newly set EU RDA for potassium is 2000 mg (ie 2 g). The upper safe level for long-term use from supplements is suggested as 3700 mg.

Potassium supplements should not be taken by anyone who is taking a type of medication called an ACE inhibitor or who has kidney disease, except under medical advice.

Probiotics

Probiotics is a term that literally means 'for life'. It is used to describe the use of live 'friendly' bacteria and yeasts (found in some fermented foods and supplements) which, when administered in adequate amounts, confer a health benefit on the host.

The most commonly used probiotic organisms are lactic acid bacteria (LAB) such as certain strains of Lactobacilli and Bifidobacteria. Because these are acid tolerant, a significant number survive passage through the stomach to reach and colonize the large intestines. Dietary sources of probiotic bacteria include live Bio yoghurts, fermented milk drinks, capsules, powders and tablets which are available in supermarkets, pharmacies and healthfood stores.

The gut contains around 11 trillion bacteria, weighing a total of 1.5 kg. Ideally, at least 70 per cent of these should be healthy 'probiotic' bacteria and only 30 per cent other bowel bacteria such as E. coli. In practice, however, the balance is usually the other way round. Probiotic bacteria play an important role in maintaining a healthy intestinal balance. They produce lactic and acetic acids which discourage the growth of potentially harmful bacteria, secrete natural antibiotics (bacteriocins) and stimulate production of anti-viral interferons. They also compete with harmful bacteria and yeasts for available nutrients, and for attachment sites on intestinal cell walls so that organisms that cause gastroenteritis are less likely to gain a foothold. LAB also produce short-chain fatty acids which, as well as decreasing flatulence, act as a major energy source for intestinal lining cells. These beneficial short-chain fatty acids are also absorbed from the colon and transported to the liver where they have a positive effect on cholesterol metabolism.

Prebiotics are non-digestible food ingredients that selectively stimulate the growth of prebiotic bacteria in the colon. They cannot be used as a food source by other, less beneficial bacteria, including E. coli. Prebiotics include substances known as fructo-oligosaccharides (FOS) which are found in some foods such as oats, barley, wheat, garlic, onions, bananas, honey and tomatoes. Probiotics and prebiotics are now increasingly used together, in a practice known as synbiotics[1].

Benefits

Gastroenteritis: Some LAB can inhibit the growth of harmful bacteria that cause gastroenteritis such as Salmonella, Shigella and Clostridium[2,3]. They can also reduce diarrhoea caused by taking antibiotics that reduce that level of natural LAB within the intestines[4,5]. They are especially helpful for people travelling abroad and to reduce antibiotic-associated diarrhoea.

Helicobacter pylori: Probiotic organisms can inhibit *Helicobacter pylori* to help protect against gastritis, peptic ulceration and possibly stomach cancer[6]. A meta-analysis of data from ten trials involving almost 1,000 people found that adding probiotics to the standard 14-day H. pylori treatment regime of antibiotics improves the eradication rate by 5 per cent to 15 per cent[7].

Irritable bowel syndrome: Alterations in the bowel bacterial balance have been suggested as a cause or contributing factor in IBS[8]. A meta-analysis of data from 14 trials suggests that replenishing the bowel population of LAB with probiotics for from four to 26 weeks can improve IBS symptoms when used alone or in combination with standard anti-spasmodic medications[9]. This is probably because of their ability to reduce the presence of gas-producing enterobacteria associated with IBS symptoms[10].

1. Gibson GR et al. Nutr Res Rev 2004; 17(2):259–75
2. Makras L et al. Res Microbil 2006; 157(3):241–7
3. Basu S et al. J Clin Gastroenterol 2007;41(8):756–60
4. Rohde CL et al. Nutr Clin Pract 2009; 24(1):33–40
5. Doron SI et al. J Clin Gastroenterol 2008;42 Suppl 2:S58–63
6. Lopez-Brea M et al. J Antimicob Chemother 2008; 61(1):139–42
7. Sachdeva A, Nagpal J. Eur J Gastroenterol Hepatol 2009; 21(1):45–53
8. Hawrelak JA, Myers SP. Altern Med Rev 2004; 9(2):180–97
9. Hoveyda N et al. BMC Gastroenterol 2009; 9:15
10. Nobaek S et al. Am J Gastroenterol 2000; 95:1231–1238

Inflammatory bowel disease: LAB produce butyrate, a short-chain fatty acid that acts as a 'food' for bowel lining cells (colonocytes). Abnormal metabolism of butyrate has been suggested as a possible cause of ulcerative colitis[1]. By helping to maintain butyrate levels, probiotic bacteria may have a beneficial role to play in inflammatory bowel disease to reduce relapses in colitis symptoms[2]. Unfortunately, not enough research is currently available to show whether or not taking probiotic supplements is beneficial for people with inflammatory bowel diseases[3].

Lactose intolerance: Because LAB ferment milk sugar (lactose) and convert it to lactic acid, they might be expected to improve symptoms associated with lactose intolerance. However, although some trials have shown benefit, others have not. A review of the evidence concluded that, in general, probiotic supplements do not appear to help overall[4].

Urinary tract infections: Urinary tract infections are linked with bowel bacteria that find their way into the bladder. By inhibiting these bacteria, probiotics may help women experiencing recurrent urinary infections. Most research shows encouraging results, but this is not yet definitely confirmed[5].

Candida: Probiotic LAB naturally found in the gut are believed to inhibit the growth of yeasts responsible for vaginal candida infections (thrush). A recent study shows that taking both probiotics and the anti-fungal drug, fluconazole, can significantly improve treatment response with less discharge and lower presence of yeasts[6].

Eczema: Probiotic supplements may reduce the development of allergic conditions such as eczema by stimulating the production of antibodies rather than allergic reactions[7]. As a result, probiotics appear to reduce the development of eczema during at least the first

1. Ahmad MS et al. Gut 2000;46:493–9
2. Hallert C et al. Inflammatory Bowel Diseases 2003;9:11–21
3. Butterworth AD et al. Cochrane Database Syst Rev 2008; 3:CD006634
4. Levi KM et al. J Fam Pract 2005; 54(7):613–20
5. Falagas ME et al. Drugs 2006; 66(9):1253–61
6. Martinez RC et al. Lett Appl Microbiol 2009; 48(3):269–74
7. Viljanen M et al. Pediatr Allergy Immunol 2005; 16(1):65–71

four years of life[1]. Infants should only receive probiotic supplements specifically designed for their age group, under medical supervision. It may be better to stimulate growth of their own natural LAB through the use of prebiotics which are now added to some baby milk formulas.

Colds: Vitamins, minerals and probiotics have a synergistic action. Probiotic bacteria have a natural immune-boosting action, while micronutrients such as vitamin E, iron and selenium are needed to boost the production of antibodies and other infection-fighting chemicals. One study found that taking probiotics plus multi-vitamins and minerals significantly reduced the duration of common cold and flu episodes by almost two days, compared with a similar group taking multivitamins and minerals alone. The researchers felt this was most likely through an effect on the activity of T-lymphocytes – the cells that regulate immune responses[2]. Another study found that taking a supplement containing both probiotics and vitamins and minerals (for at least three months in winter/spring) reduced the severity and – perhaps more importantly – the incidence of common colds. Those taking the combination supplement were 13.6 per cent less likely to develop cold and flu symptoms than those taking inactive placebo (no participants had been vaccinated against influenza). Symptom severity was also reduced by 19 per cent, and the number of days with fever was more than halved[3]. The researchers found that all immune cells (leukocytes, T-lymphocytes and monocytes) showed increased activity, suggesting that this combination of supplements can stimulate cellular immunity.

Dose

For optimum benefits, select a supplement supplying a known quantity of probiotic bacteria such as 1–5 billion colony-forming units (CFU) per dose. Supplements that are enteric coated, which improves the survival of probiotic bacteria as they pass through the stomach, can contain less (e.g. 10 million freeze-dried probiotic bacteria) and still provide beneficial effects.

1. Kalliomaki M et al. Lancet 2003; 361(9372):1869–71
2. De Vrese N et al. Vaccine 2006 24(44–46):6670–4
3. Winkler P et al. Int J Clin Pharmacol Ther 2005;43(7):318–26

Check the shelf life of the supplement – those close to their expiry date will contain fewer live probiotic bacteria than those with a longer shelf life. Also check whether the supplement needs to be refrigerated. Supplements containing freeze-dried bacteria which are held in suspended animation do not need to be kept chilled.

Taking oral probiotic supplements appears to be safe with few side effects reported[1]. Although they have been used in clinical trials involving people with reduced immunity, they should only be used under medical supervision in pregnant women, infants and in individuals with intestinal bleeding, pancreatitis, HIV infection and cancer. Some probiotic products do not contain strains proven to confer any health benefits.

Pumpkin seed
(Cucurbita pepo)

Pumpkin seeds are a popular snack food with a high oil and vitamin E content. The oil is used as a salad dressing, but due to its dark green colour and foaminess, it cannot be used for cooking.

Benefits
Anaemia: Pumpkin seeds are a good source of iron and can improve the iron status of women with iron-deficiency anaemia[2].

Prostate enlargement: Relatively little research seems to have been carried out on humans, although there is a long tradition of using pumpkin seeds for prostate problems. Some evidence suggests that pumpkin seed extracts can reduce bladder pressure and increase bladder compliance as well reducing pressure in the urethra which might help those with urinary voiding problems due to benign prostatic enlargement.

Urinary stones: Pumpkin seeds reduce the formation of calcium-oxalate crystals in the urine and increase levels of phosphorus, pyrophosphate, glycosaminoglycans and potassium[3]. By providing

1. Naidu AS et al. Crit Rev Food Sci Nutr 1999; 39(1):13–126
2. Naqhii MR, Mofid M. Biofactors 2007;39(1):19–26
3. Suphakarn VS et al. Am J Clin Nutr 1987;45(1):115–21

high phosphorus levels they may reduce the risk of kidney/bladder stone disease.

Dose

Raw seeds: 30 g daily.

Pumpkin seed oil: 160 mg three times a day.

Pumpkin seed extracts are often combined with other active ingredients such as saw palmetto and zinc in supplements designed to improve prostate health.

Rapeseed oil
(Brassica napus)

Rapeseed oil (also known as canola) is a nutritious and healthy oil that contains a high concentration of the monounsaturated fat, oleic acid (70 per cent) and the essential omega-3 fatty acid, alpha-linolenic acid (20 per cent ALA) plus a relatively low amount of the essential omega-6 fatty acid, linolenic acid (10 per cent). Its ratio of omega-6 and omega-3 fatty acids is around 2:1. It also contains a high concentration of plant sterols (see page 252) which lower cholesterol absorption from the intestines.

Population based studies in Finland found that, between 1972 and 1992, coronary heart disease mortality declined by 55 per cent in men and 68 per cent in women. Three-quarters of this decline was attributed to reduction in coronary risk factors such as cholesterol levels[1]. Much of this was due to a switch towards growing and using rapeseed oil.

The leaves and stems of oilseed rape are also edible and similar to kale.

Benefits

Cholesterol: Taking 75 g rapeseed oil per day for three days can reduce cholesterol absorption by 11 per cent compared with olive oil[2]. When 95 people with raised cholesterol levels followed a diet rich in rapeseed oil for three weeks, their total cholesterol fell by 15

1. Pietinen P et al. Prev Med 1996;25(3):243–250
2. Ellegard L et al. Eur J Clin Nutr 2005;59(12):1374–8

per cent, LDL-cholesterol by 16 per cent and HDL-cholesterol by 11 per cent.[1]

Dose
Oil: 1 teaspoon–1 tablespoon once or twice a day.
Best taken with food.

Raspberry leaf

Raspberry leaf is taken in the form of tea or tablets towards the end of pregnancy to help soften the neck of the womb in preparation for delivery. It seems to reduce the duration and pain of childbirth, and is thought to work by strengthening the longitudinal muscles of the uterus to increase the force of uterine contractions. It seems only to work on the pregnant rather than non-pregnant uterus, and research has not so far isolated the active ingredients. Women who have taken raspberry leaf extracts often confirm that their contractions were relatively pain-free and that their baby was born within just a few hours of the start of labour.

Raspberry leaf has also been used to reduce pain in endometriosis, and to relieve painful diarrhoea.

Benefits
Childbirth: A trial involving 192 women having their first baby looked at the effects and safety of using 1.2 g raspberry leaf tablets, twice a day, from the 32nd week of gestation (34 weeks of pregnancy) until labour. They found a significant shortening of the second stage of labour (pushing the baby out) of 9.59 minutes, and lower rate of forceps deliveries in those taking the supplements (19.3 per cent) compared with controls (30.4 per cent). It did not shorten the length of the first stage of labour (dilation of the cervix). No significant side effects were found.

Dose
1 cup raspberry leaf tea a day *or*
Tablets: 400–800 mg, two or three times a day with meals.

---

1. Gustafsson IB et al. Am J Clin Nutr 1994;59:667–74

Raspberry leaf should only be taken daily during the last six weeks of pregnancy (from 34 weeks). It should not be taken during early pregnancy and is best taken under the supervision of a qualified medical herbalist or a midwife.

RDAs and RNIs

Vitamins and minerals are micro-nutrients which, although essential for health, are only needed in tiny amounts. The quantities you need are measured in milligrams (mg) or micrograms (mcg).

1 milligram = one thousandth of a gram (1/1000 or 10^{-3} grams)
1 microgram = one millionth of a gram (1/1,000,000 or 10^{-6} grams)
1 milligram therefore = 1000 micrograms.

The UK has developed its own system of daily recommended intakes based on a unit called the Reference Nutrient Intake (RNI). For labelling purposes on supplement packs, the EU equivalent is used, which is termed the Recommended Daily Amount (RDA).

Everyone has different, individual needs depending on their age, weight, level of activity and the metabolic pathways and enzyme systems they have inherited. Some people need more vitamins and minerals, while some need fewer. The EU Recommended Daily Amount (EU RDA) is an estimated intake that is believed to supply the needs of most (up to 97 per cent) of the population.

The new EU RDAs (in force from 31 October 2009 for labelling purposes) suggest the following daily intakes of each vitamin and mineral:

Vitamins New EU RDA
Vitamin A (retinol) 800 mcg
Vitamin B1 (thiamine) 1.1 mg
Vitamin B2 (riboflavin) 1.4 mg
Vitamin B3 (niacin) 16 mg
Vitamin B5 (pantothenic acid)
  6 mg

Minerals New EU RDA
Calcium 800 mg
Chloride 800 mg
Chromium 40 mcg
Copper 1 mg
Iodine 150 mcg

Vitamin B6 (pyridoxine) 1.4 mg	Iron 14 mg
Vitamin B12 (cyanocobalamin) 2.5 mcg	Magnesium 375 mg
	Manganese 2 mg
Folic Acid 200 mcg	Phosphorus 700 mg
Biotin 50 mcg	Potassium 2000 mg
Vitamin C 80 mg	Selenium 55 mcg
Vitamin D 5 mcg	Zinc 10 mg
Vitamin E 12 mg	
Vitamin K 75 mcg	

See the table on page 16 for the full list of RNIs for adults aged 19–50 years, and for the suggested upper safe levels for long-term use of supplements that may be taken in addition to dietary intakes.

Red Clover
(Trifolium pratense)

Red clover is one of over 70 different species of clover native to Europe and Asia. Of all the clovers, red clover is the most popular for medicinal use. The flower heads are collected when newly opened in spring, and the leaves and roots are also edible.

Red clover contains three classes of oestrogen-like plant hormones, isoflavones, coumestans and lignans. Like soy, it contains all four isoflavones – genistein, daidzein, formononetin (methoxy-daidzein) and biochanin A (methoxy-genistein). It is also a source of antioxidant flavonoid glycosides. However, the isoflavone content of red clover is highly variable, so it is best to purchase a standardized supplement with a known quantity of named isoflavones for a consistent result[1].

Red clover is used to balance oestrogen levels – either where oestrogen levels are too high (by competing for stronger oestrogens in the body and diluting their effect) or by providing an additional oestrogenic boost where oestrogen levels are low. It is therefore widely used to treat pre-menstrual syndrome, endometriosis,

1. Wang SW et al. J Altern Complement Med 2008;14(3):287–97

fibroids and menopausal symptoms. It has also been shown to have activity at opioid receptors in the brain, which may also affect regulation of temperature, mood and hormone balance[1].

Benefits
Menopause: One study suggests that taking 80 mg red clover isoflavones can reduce the frequency of hot flushes by 44 per cent, more than the 16 per cent achieved with placebo[2]. Red clover extracts also appear to have a beneficial effect on vaginal cells, LDL-cholesterol levels and triglycerides[3]. A meta-analysis of data from five studies suggested that, overall, red clover isoflavones (40–82 mg daily) can reduce the number of hot flushes per day by 1.5 episodes compared with placebo. This was described as a marginally significant effect[4]. Another review concluded that, like soy isoflavones, red clover extracts may have a small but positive effect on cholesterol balance, bone mass density and cognitive function (ability to think straight)[5].

Sex hormones: A study involving 109 postmenopausal women compared the use of 80 mg red clover isoflavones per day versus placebo for 90 days. After a week of not taking any supplement, each woman then crossed over to the other group to take either the extracts or the placebo, so each woman acted as her own control. Interestingly, when taking the red clover extracts, significantly increased plasma testosterone levels were seen, along with reduced thickness of the endometrium (uterine lining)[6]. Oestradiol levels remained unchanged. This study confirms that red clover isoflavones do not cause unwanted stimulation of the uterine lining. It appears that the raised testosterone levels may benefit women with low sex drive after the menopause but this needs further investigation.

Dose
500 mg–1 g daily (standardized to provide 40–80 mg isoflavones).

1. Nissan HP et al. J Ethnopharmacol 2007;112(1):207–10
2. Van de Weijer PH, Barentsen R, Maturitas 2002;42(3):187–93
3. Hidalgo LA et al. Gynecol Endocrinol 2005;21(5):257–64
4. Coon JT et al. Phytomedicine 2007;14(2–3):153–9
5. Geller SE, Studee L. Climacteric 2006;9(4):245–63
6. Imhof M et al. Maturitas 2006;55(1):76–81

No serious side effects have been reported. It should not be taken during pregnancy or while breast-feeding. Red clover extracts have been found to lower levels of prostate specific antigen (PSA) by more than 30 per cent. This may make it unsuitable as a supplement for men having regular PSA level checks to screen for prostate cancer[1].

See also: **Isoflavones**.

Red vine leaf
(Vitis vinifera)

Red grapes are well known to contain beneficial antioxidants that have a powerful protective effect on the circulation. Less well known is that red vine leaf extracts are also beneficial. They contain a variety of antioxidants (flavonol-glycosides, glucuronides) and are thought to work by reducing inflammation, and by reducing the permeability of small blood vessels (capillaries) so that fluid cannot leak from capillaries into the tissues so easily[2]. They also promote repair of damaged vein linings. Recently, extracts from red vine bark (containing substances called vitisin A and B) were shown to inhibit HMG-coA – the same enzyme that is blocked by statin drugs to lower cholesterol levels. This activity may also be present in vine leaves.

Benefits
Varicose veins: In a placebo-controlled trial involving 257 people with varicose veins, one group took 360 mg red vine leaf extracts per day, one took 720 mg daily, while another took placebo for 12 weeks. For those treated with placebo, lower leg volume increased by an average of 34 g (weight of water displaced) after 12 weeks, while those taking active treatment experienced a reduction in lower leg volume. This was equivalent to a difference between the active and placebo groups of –76 g with the lower dose, and –100 g with the higher dose. Changes in calf circumference showed a similar

1. Engelhardt PF, Riedl CR. Urology 2008;71(2):185–90
2. Nees S et al. Arzneimittelforschung 2003;53(5):330–41

pattern and reductions in swelling were at least equivalent to those reported for compression stockings. There were also clinically significant reductions in symptoms such as tired, heavy legs, sensations of tension, tingling and pain[1]. Open studies have shown similar results with reductions in calf swelling, sensations of heaviness and pain[2,3].

Dose
360–720 mg daily.

Reishi
(Ganoderma lucidum)

Reishi is one of seven different varieties of *Ganoderma* mushroom, each of which has differing colours. Reishi is the red *Ganoderma lucidum* and is regarded as superior. The Japanese name 'reishi' means literally 'spiritual mushroom', while the Chinese call it 'ling zhi' ('the mushroom of immortality') and classify it as a superior herb equal in importance to ginseng. Reishi has been used medicinally for over 3,000 years. It is too woody and fibrous for culinary use, but is widely consumed in tablet form as a herbal supplement.

Reishi contains at least 100 different triterpenes, which have a four fused ring structure similar to steroid hormones. These include a unique group of ganoderic acids (e.g. ganoderic, ganoderenic, lucidenic, and ganolucidic acids). These triterpenoids possess adaptogenic and antihypertensive as well as anti-allergic properties.

It also contains lentinan and a nucleotide, adenosine, which forms part of the body's energy regulation and storage system.

Reishi is a powerful adaptogen, tonic and antioxidant. It is traditionally used to strengthen the liver, lungs, heart and immune system, to increase intellectual capacity and memory, boost physical and mental energy levels and to promote vitality and longevity. It is also used to speed convalescence, regulate blood sugar levels and to help minimize the side-effects of chemotherapy or radiotherapy.

1. Kiesewetter J et al. Arzneimittelforschung 2000;50(2):109–17
2. Monsieur R, Van Snick G. Praxis (Bern 1994); 2006:95(6):187–90
3. Schaefer E et al. Arzneimittelforschung 2003;53(4):243–6

Reishi has antibacterial, anti-viral, anti-histamine, anti-allergy, anti-inflammatory (equivalent to hydrocortisone) and anti-cancer properties. It also reduces blood clotting and can lower blood pressure and cholesterol levels. It has recently been shown to increase brain blood flow and oxygen uptake in Alzheimer's disease. It also enhances energy levels and gives a more restful night's sleep.

Benefits

Cholesterol: In the laboratory, cholesterol synthesis in human liver cell cultures is inhibited by reishi extracts, which inhibit conversion of lanosterol and lathosterol[1].

Reishi extracts have also been shown to significantly decrease blood cholesterol, LDL-cholesterol and triglycerides in animal experiments, and to increase levels of antioxidant enzymes (glutathione and SOD)[2]. A trend towards lower blood cholesterol levels was seen in a group of 18 healthy volunteers taking reishi for four weeks, together with increased antioxidant activity[3].

Prostate symptoms: Reishi has anti-androgen activity. A study involving 88 men with lower urinary tract symptoms related to benign prostate enlargement found that it was significantly better than placebo in improving the International Prostate Symptoms Score without affecting testosterone levels[4].

Immunity: When 40 male football players were exposed to physical stress associated with high altitude/low oxygen levels, reishi extracts helped to reduce the adverse effects of low oxygen levels on their relative numbers of circulating T-lymphocytes[5]. It has also been shown to enhance immune function in 34 volunteers with advance-stage cancer[6]. In two people with severe pain due to shingles and two with post-herpetic neuralgia, reishi extracts have been shown to 'dramatically' decrease pain[7].

1. Hajjaj H et al. Appl Environ Microbiol 2005 71(7):3653–8
2. Chen WQ et al. Chinese Journal of Materia Medica 2005; 30(17):1358–69
3. Wachtel-Galor S et al. Br J Nutr 2004;91(2):171-3
4. Noquchi M et al. Asian J Androl 2008;10(5):777–85
5. Zhang Y et al. Br J Sports Med 2008;42(10):519–22
6. Gao Y et al. Immunol Invest 2003;32(2):201–15
7. Hijikata Y, Yamada S. Am J Chin Med 1008;26(3–4):375–81

Stress: A study involving 132 people with 'neurasthenia' or stress-related low mood and fatigue found significant improvements in those taking reishi compared with placebo for eight weeks. The score for overall well-being increased to 38.7 per cent in those taking reishi compared with 29.7 per cent on placebo. Over half (51.6 per cent) taking reishi said they were more than minimally improved compared with less than a quarter (24.6 per cent) on placebo[1].

In one Chinese study it was found to relieve feelings of weariness in 78 per cent of patients, cold extremities in 74 per cent and insomnia in 78 per cent. In a Japanese study of over 50 patients with essential hypertension, taking reishi extracts for six months lowered average blood pressure from 156/103 to 137/93. Chinese studies involving over 2,000 people found that reishi extracts were helpful in treating bronchitis.

Dose
500 mg twice to three times daily.

The effects of reishi are enhanced by vitamin C which increases absorption of the active components.

There is no cross reaction with traditional 'button' mushrooms and can usually be taken by those allergic to field mushrooms.

No serious side effects have been reported even at 300 times the therapeutic dose. A few people have experienced diarrhoea (often disappears if tablets are taken with food), irritability, thirst, dry skin rash or mouth ulcers during the first week of taking the reishi. A few cases of hepatitis have occurred in people taking reishi powder in combination with other drugs, but whether or not reishi was the cause is not certain. In fact, reishi is traditionally used to treat hepatitis.

Although used as a food, it is sensible to avoid taking reishi during pregnancy and breast-feeding.

Only use under medical supervision if taking immunosuppressive drugs or anticoagulant medication.

1. Tang W et al. J Med Food 2005;8(1):53–8

Rhodiola
(Rhodiola rosea)

Rhodiola is an alpine plant that grows more than 3,000 metres above sea level. It is also known as golden or Arctic root and has been used as a medicine for over a thousand years.

Rhodiola contains a number of active constituents, including rosavin and rhodioflavonoside, which together have an adaptogenic action. It increases serotonin levels by as much as 30 per cent to improve low mood, and supports the actions of the adrenal glands, through a direct action on the hypothalamus gland, to reduce levels of stress hormones (cortisol, adrenaline).

Rhodiola rosea has been classed as an adaptogen by Russian researchers who consider it to be one of the most active adaptogenic herbs[1]. It increases resistance to a variety of physical and emotional stress and is particularly helpful when burn-out causes fatigue, reduced work performance, sleep difficulties, poor appetite, irritability, hypertension and headaches[2]. It enhances performance and can improve alertness, concentration, memory, stamina and sleep quality.

Benefits
Anxiety: In a small pilot study involving ten people with generalized anxiety disorder, taking 340 mg Rhodiola extract for ten weeks significantly improved anxiety and depression rating scores[3].

Depression: A trial involving 60 people with depression found that, compared with placebo, taking 340 mg Rhodiola per day significantly improved overall depression, insomnia, emotional instability and preoccupation with bodily symptoms[4]. Those taking placebo did not show improvements.

Fatigue: In a clinical trial involving 60 people with stress-related fatigue, taking 576 mg Rhodiola extracts per day significantly reduced cortisol responses to stress compared with placebo. It had

1. Perfumi M, Mattioli L. Phytother Res 2007;21(1):37–43
2. Kelly GS Altern Med Rec 2001;6(3):293–302
3. Bystritsky A et al. J Altern Complement Med 2008;14(2):175–80
4. Darbinyan V et al. Nord J Psychiatry 2007;61(5):343–8

an anti-fatigue effect that increased mental performance, particularly the ability to concentrate in those experiencing burnout fatigue[1]. A study involving 161 young cadets aged 19–21 found a pronounced anti-fatigue effect and ability to concentrate on mental work in those taking Rhodiola compared with placebo[2]. When 56 doctors took Rhodiola extracts, they experienced less fatigue and improved mental performance during night duty than when taking placebo[3]. Similar results were seen in a group of students during a stressful examination period, with those taking Rhodiola showing significant improvements in physical fitness, mental fatigue and muscle testing[4].

Sleep: A study involving 24 men living at high altitude for one year found that blood oxygen levels were significantly increased after 24 days' treatment and the time spent asleep with low oxygen levels of below 80 per cent was significantly reduced in those taking Rhodiola. Sleep architecture was also improved with more time spent in REM and deep sleep, and less waking during sleep[5].

Dose

400 mg once or twice a day.

Rosehip
(Rosa canina)

Rosehip syrup is a popular traditional tonic which was given to children in winter as a source of vitamin C during the Second World War. Rosehips also contain folic acid, carotenoids such as lycopene, and antioxidant flavonoids. Their anti-inflammatory action is said to help keep colds at bay, though there has been little research into this area. There is, however, mounting evidence that rosehip extracts can help osteoarthritis symptoms. Some of this activity is related to an aspirin-

1. Olsson EM et al. Planta Med 2009;75(2):105–12
2. Shevtsov VA et al. Phytomedicine 2003;10(2–3):95–105
3. Darbinyan V et al. Phytomedicine 2000;7(5):365–71
4. Spasov AA et al. Phytomedicine 2000;7(2):85–9
5. Ha Z et al. Zhonghua Jie He He Hu Xi Za Shi 2002;25(9):527–30

like ability to inhibit cycloxoygenase enzymes (COX-1 and COX-2)[1]. A galactolipid isolated from rose hips has also been shown to inhibit the activity of inflammatory white blood cells within the laboratory[2].

Benefits

Osteoarthritis: Several studies have investigated the effects of taking rosehip powder, versus placebo, in people with osteoarthritis. A review of two of these studies found that those taking rosehip powder had significantly improved hip flexion, compared with placebo, but no significant changes were seen in internal and external rotation of the hip joints, or in flexion of the knees[3]. One study reported significant reductions in pain after three months in those taking rosehip powder, although there were no differences in the use of analgesics between those taking rosehip and those on placebo. Another study showed reductions in pain, stiffness, disability and global severity of the disease, after three months, based on the Western Ontario and McMaster Universities (WOMAC) questionnaire. Those taking rosehip also consumed significantly less pain-relieving 'rescue' medication compared with those on placebo[4]. A meta-analysis of three studies pooled data from 287 people who took rosehip extracts for an average of three months. Significant improvements in pain scores were found and, compared with inactive placebo, those taking rosehip powder were twice as likely to show a beneficial response[5].

Dose

2.5–5 g daily.

Sage
(Salvia officinalis)

Sage is a well-known Mediterranean herb whose name, *Salvia*, comes from the Latin salvere which means 'to be saved'. It was

1. Jager AK et al. Phytother Res 2008;22(7):982–4
2. Larsen E et al. J Nat Prod 2003;66(7):994–5
3. Rossnagel K et al. MMW Fortschr Med 2007;149(11):51–6
4. Winther K et al. Scand J Rheumatol 2005;34(4):302–8
5. Christensen R et al. Osteoarthritis Cartilage 2008;16(9):965–72

known as *herba sacra* – sacred herb – by the Romans. Its leaves – especially those from the red purple-tinged varieties – contain a number of essential oils such as borneol and camphor.

Sage has antibacterial, anti-fungal, anti-viral, astringent and perspiration-inhibiting properties. It is a popular herbal remedy for menopausal hot flushes and night sweats. Other traditional uses include indigestion, as a gargle to reduce mouth inflammation, to reduce the flow of breast milk during weaning and to ease intestinal infections such as diarrhoea and vomiting.

It is also used as a mental stimulant to boost memory and concentration. These effects are due to its ability to inhibit cholinesterase – an enzyme that deactivates neurotransmitters in the brain. This activity may help people with Alzheimer's disease.

Benefits

Menopause: In a study involving 39 women, sage leaf extracts decreased the frequency of hot flushes by 56 per cent over a period of eight weeks, versus a 5 per cent increase in frequency among those taking inactive placebo[1]. Unfortunately, this study has not been published in an independent medical journal. However, a study in which 30 women with menopausal symptoms took a combination of safe leaf and alfalfa found that hot flushes and night sweats disappeared completely in 20 women and showed good improvement in another four[2]. There was no placebo group with which to compare results.

Memory: Among 20 volunteers, those taking 333 mg sage leaf extracts per day showed significant improvements in memory performance and accuracy when tested at 1, 2.5, 4 and 6 hours after treatment[3]. Those taking placebo showed a normal decline in performance over the day. In a study involving 30 healthy volunteers, taking 300 mg sage leaf extracts significantly improved mood and reduced anxiety, while taking 600 mg sage leaf extracts increased alertness, calmness and contentedness compared with placebo[4].

1. Bioforce Research Report Aug 2001
2. De Leo V et al. Minerva Gynecol 1998;50(5):207–11
3. Scholey AB et al. Psychopharmacology (Berl) 2008;198(1):127–39
4. Kennedy DO et al. Neuropsychopharmacology 2006;31(4):845–52

Alzheimer's: A study involving 42 people with mild to moderate Alzheimer's disease found that taking sage leaf extract for four months produced significantly better effects on cognitive function than placebo[1].

Dose

Sage tea: add 1 tablespoon sage leaves to a cup of boiling water and infuse for 20 minutes.

Extracts: 400–2000 mg daily.

Contraindications

• Sage stimulates uterine contractions, and should therefore be avoided during pregnancy, although small amounts are safe for use in cooking. It should not be used during breast-feeding other than for its ability to dry up milk.

• Sage should be avoided by those with epilepsy.

St John's Wort
(Hypericum perforatum)

St John's Wort is a common plant found in many parts of the world. When held up to the light, numerous pinpoint red dots are seen in the yellow petals – these are glands containing the fluorescent red dye, hypericin.

St John's Wort contains a number of substances that have a natural, antidepressant action. These include hypericin and pseudohypericin but especially hyperforin and adhyperforin. These chemicals do not inhibit the same transmitter binding sites on the transporter proteins as the prescribed SSRIs (serotonin re-uptake inhibitors) antidepressants. Taking St John's Wort therefore doesn't just increase levels of the brain neurotransmitter, serotonin. Instead, it affects the sodium gradient which leads to a more generalized action, inhibiting the neuronal uptake of serotonin plus noradrenaline, dopamine, gamma-aminobutyric acid (GABA) and L-glutamate. No other antidepressant shows such a broad inhibitory profile[2].

1. Akhondzadeh S et al. J Clin Pharm Ther 2003;28(1):53–9
2. Muller WE, Pharmacol Res 2003;47(2):101–9

It is currently being investigated for beneficial effects against viral infections and to support withdrawal in smoking cessation, alcohol and drug addiction. Early studies suggest it is also a promising treatment for premature ejaculation and for compulsive behaviour.

Benefits

Depression: A 2009 meta-analysis compared the effectiveness and tolerability of St John's wort in the treatment of major depression against SSRI drugs. Pooled data from 13 trials found that, compared with placebo, SSRIs were 22 per cent more likely to be effective. When compared with St John's Wort, no significant differences were found, suggesting that the herb is as effective as SSRIs in treating major depression[1]. A rigorous meta-analysis of data from 29 trials, involving almost 5,500 patients (who took St John's Wort for between four and 12 weeks), confirmed that St John's Wort was better than placebo in treating major depression, was of similar effectiveness to standard antidepressant drugs, and caused fewer side effects than prescribed drugs[2]. Analysis of symptoms suggests that St John's Wort speeds the recovery from depression in a general manner, improving all investigated symptoms and signs associated with low mood[3]. Taking St John's Wort starts to lift mood within two weeks and the optimum effect is reached within six weeks. Three out of four people show a marked improvement after only five weeks, with one in three becoming symptom-free.

Seasonal affective disorder: Field trials suggest that standardized extracts are as effective in treating seasonal affective disorder (SAD) when used alone as when combined with light box therapy[4,5,6].

Menopause: Research in Germany involving 111 peri-menopausal women (aged 45–65 years) showed that taking St John's Wort extracts improved psychological and physical symptoms of

1. Rahimi R et al. Prog Neuropsychopharmacol Biol Psychiatry 2009;33(1):118–27
2. Linde K et al. Cochrane Database Syst Rev 2008;(4):CD000448
3. Kasper S, Dienel A. Psychopharmacology (Berl); 2002:164(3):301–8
4. Wheatley D. Curr med res opin 1999;15(1):33–7
5. Kasper S. Pharmacopsychiatry 1997;30 (Suppl 2):89–93
6. Martinez B et al. J Geriatr Psychiatry Neurol 1994;7(Suppl 1):S29–33

menopause such as low mood, low sex drive and exhaustion. After three months, 60 per cent with low sex drive became interested in sex again, and enjoyed or even initiated sex with their partner. Eighty-two per cent also suffered less irritability, anxiety, low mood, hot flushes, sweating and disturbed sleep. Before the trial, 60 per cent said they were too exhausted for sex. At the end of the trial, none of them felt that way. They also reported increased self-esteem, as well as a marked increase in self-confidence and self-respect[1].

Pre-menstrual syndrome: PMS is often associated with low mood, and a pilot study of 19 women found a significant improvement in all outcome measures with overall premenstrual syndrome scores reducing by 51 per cent[2]. In a study involving 25 women with severe PMS, there was a reduction in the incidence of crying of 92 per cent, low mood reduced by 85 per cent and nervous tension by 71 per cent compared with baseline premenstrual scores. Although a third still suffered from some symptoms of PMS, all women in the study reported great improvement. A similar study of 169 women with recurrent PMS found a trend towards improvement with St John's Wort but the finding was not statistically significant[3].

Dose
Extracts standardized to contain at least 0.3 per cent hypericin or 3 per cent hyperforin: 300 mg, three times a day; one-a-day formulas supplying 900 mg are also available.

St John's Wort is best taken with food, and alcohol should be avoided.

Side effects
All studies have confirmed the good tolerability of St. John's wort extract and the very low frequency of adverse events. Those reported include indigestion, allergic reactions, restlessness and tiredness/fatigue each in fewer than 1 per cent of people. Side effects are significantly less likely than with standard anti-depressants.

Some drug interactions have been found to occur with St. John's

1. Grube B et al. Adv Ther 1999;16(4):177–86
2. Stevinson C, Ernst E; BJOG 2000;107(7):870–6
3. Hicks SM et al. J Altern Complement Med 2004;19(6):925–32

wort extract, a number of which are clinically important. If you are taking prescribed medications, it is important to check with a pharmacist for possible drug interactions before starting to take St John's Wort. This includes the oral contraceptive pill, although recent research suggests that usual doses (250 mg twice a day) of St John's Wort extracts (0.2 per cent hypericin; but with a low hyperforin content of less than 0.2 per cent) does not affect the pharmacokinetics of low-dose oral contraceptives[1].

Those who are sun-sensitive or on medications that cause photosensitivity (e.g. tetracycline, chlorpromazine) should avoid direct skin exposure to sunlight, especially if fair-skinned. There are no reports of skin sensitivity on exposure to sunlight (photosensitization) in therapeutic doses.

Sarsaparilla
(Smilax officinalis, S. sarsaparilla)

Sarsaparilla – also popularly known as *Smilax* – belongs to a group of climbing perennial vines found in tropical and subtropical parts of the world. Its dried, thick rhizomes and slender roots contain a wide range of hormone-like steroids (including sarsapogenin, smilagenin) and glycosides (e.g. sarsaponin) that have been used commercially as the basis for synthesizing sex hormones, particularly testosterone. Because of this, it is used by many males – especially body builders – to improve virility, vitality and energy levels. No studies have shown sarsaparilla to have an anabolic effect that increases muscle mass in humans, however, and the reactions needed to convert these plant steroids into testosterone are unlikely to occur in the body. It is therefore not as virilizing as one might expect – it is even used to treat acne which is a condition usually associated with increased androgen activity.

Sarsaparilla is mainly used as a tonic. It also acts as a diuretic and promotes sweating and expectoration of catarrh. It is said to hasten regeneration and to have anti-inflammatory properties. It is used to treat cystitis, psoriasis, eczema, acne, rheumatism, arthritis and gout,

1. Will–Shahab L et al. Eur J Clin Pharmacol 2009;65(3):287–94

as well as infections such as syphilis, herpes, gonorrhoea and the common cold.

Sarsaparilla is used to increase low sex drive in males and to help overcome impotence and infertility. It is also used in lower doses in women to boost a low sex drive and to improve menopausal symptoms.

Benefits

Laboratory studies suggest sarsaparilla extracts have anti-cancer, anti-viral and anti-fungal activity. More research is needed in these areas.

Dose

Capsules: 250 mg, three times a day.

Some dried roots labelled Mexican sarsaparilla may actually contain so-called Indian sarsaparilla, which is a different type of plant (*Hemidesmus indicus*) with entirely different uses. *Hemidesmus* is dark brown and smells of vanilla, while dried Smilax roots have a light colour (often orange-tinged) and are odourless.

No serious long-term side effects have been reported, although sarsaparilla can cause indigestion and, if excess is taken, may temporarily impair kidney function.

Because of its possible testosterone-boosting properties, some practitioners caution against its use in women with a tendency towards excessive unwanted hair.

Saw palmetto
(Serenoa repens; Sabal serrulatum)

The saw palmetto is a small palm tree native to North America and the West Indies. Its fruit contains a variety of fatty acids and hormone-like sterols that are widely used as a male tonic and sexual rejuvenator.

Saw palmetto is a popular and effective herbal remedy for benign prostatic hyperplasia (BPH) – a condition in which the number of cells in the male prostate gland starts to increase in middle age. As the gland increases in size, it often constricts the flow of urine as it passes through the middle of the gland. This causes a variety of obstructive and irritative lower urinary tract symptoms (LUTS) in men such as urinary hesitancy, frequency, urgency and poor flow.

While saw palmetto fruit extracts do not alter the circulating level of androgen hormones, they appear to block the action of a prostate enzyme, 5-alpha-reductase, which converts the male hormone, testosterone, to another more powerful hormone, dihydrotestosterone (DHT) within prostate gland cells. In prostate biopsies from men who have taken saw palmetto extracts, this effect is most noticeable in prostate tissues in the centre of the gland, directly surrounding the urinary tube (urethra). Selective shrinking of this central portion of the prostate may explain why studies do not show appreciable shrinking of the whole gland despite significant improvements in urinary flow and obstructive symptoms. Saw palmetto also appears to interact with alpha receptors in the prostate, relaxing smooth muscle cells and reducing spasm.

Benefits

BPH: In 1998 a meta-analysis published in the *Journal of the American Medical Association* pooled the results from 18 clinical trials, involving almost 3,000 men, and found that saw palmetto was significantly better than placebo for improving LUTS and produced similar improvements in the International Prostate Symptoms Score (IPSS) to finasteride – the main drug used to treat BPH at the time[1]. In 2004 a meta-analysis looking at the results of 14 trials, involving 4,200 men, confirmed that saw palmetto was significantly better than placebo for improving peak urinary flow rate, night-time urination (nocturia), and produced a 5 point reduction in the IPSS[2]. Noticeable relief is generally considered to be a decrease of 3 points in the symptoms score. However, five years later, in 2009, a meta-analysis of 30 trials involving over 5,200 men with LUTS (who took saw palmetto for between four and 60 weeks) found that *Serenoa repens* was significantly better than placebo at treating nocturia, but it was not more effective, overall, for improving other symptoms of the IPSS[3]. It is probable that some of the new trials were too short, at four weeks, to show a benefit. The authors state that more well-designed trials are needed, with a minimum follow-up of one year, to confirm or deny the effectiveness of saw palmetto fruit extracts.

1. Wilt TJ et al. JAMA 1998;280:1604–1609

2. Boyle P et al. BJU Int 2004;93(6):751–6

3. Tacklind J et al. Cochrane Database Syst Rev 2009;(2):CD001423

Prostate cancer: Saw palmetto fruit extracts have been shown to inhibit 5-alpha-reductase activity of human prostate cancer cell lines. It does this without affecting circulating levels of prostate specific antigen (PSA) which is used as a marker for prostate cancer. It therefore does not mask the development or recurrence of prostate cancer[1,2]. The authors of one study state: '...we confirm the therapeutic advantage of *Serenoa repens* over other 5-alpha-reductase inhibitors as treatment with the phytotherapeutic agent will permit the continuous use of PSA measurements as a useful biomarker for prostate cancer screening and for evaluating tumour progression.'[3]

Dose

Fruit extracts: 150 mg–3 g a day in divided doses.

Products standardized for 85–95 per cent fat-soluble sterols: 320 mg a day.

A beneficial effect is usually noticeable within six weeks.

Saw palmetto is often combined with pumpkin seed and/or nettle root extracts.

Saw palmetto is sometimes prescribed to women with polycystic ovary syndrome, due to its ability to inhibit the formation of dihydrotestosterone, which plays a role in this condition. Its use in women should only occur under the supervision of an experienced medical herbalist.

NB: Avoid cheap versions of saw palmetto which may contain inactive extracts from the leaves rather than the fruit.

Schisandra

(Schisandra chinensis)

Schisandra – also known as magnolia vine – is a Chinese tonic herb also known as wu wei zi or five-flavoured fruit as it simultaneously tastes salty, sweet, bitter, sour and pungent. Its dried berries contain lignans such as schizandrin, phytosterols and several antioxidants.

1. Fagelman E, Lose FC. Rev Urol 2001;3(3):134–138
2. Djavan B et al. World U Urol 2005;23(4):253–6
3. Habib FK et al. Int J Cancer 2005;114:190–194

Schisandra chinensis is used as an antioxidant and adaptogen in both Asia and Russia.

Like ginseng, Schisandra helps the body to adapt and cope during times of stress. It has been found to increase oxygen uptake of cells and improves mental clarity, irritability, forgetfulness and prevents emotional and physical fatigue. It is regarded as a calming supplement and also boosts liver function, enhances immunity and heart function and improves allergic skin conditions such as eczema.

Schisandra is a well-known sexual tonic that reputedly increases secretion of sexual fluids in men and vaginal lubrication in women. It has also been used to treat high blood pressure, influenza, sinusitis, pneumonia, and a variety of digestive disorders.

Benefits
Stress: Clinical trials have demonstrated a beneficial effect in treating asthenia (essentially fatigue linked with stress burn-out), neurosis, depression, schizophrenia and alcoholism[1]. Russian research is said to confirm it has a beneficial effect on the central nervous system, hormone balance, immune function and circulation. In healthy volunteers it has been shown to increase endurance, co-ordination, mental performance and working capacity. During times of stress, it lowers levels of the stress hormone, cortisol.

Dose
250–500 mg, once to three times daily.

Schisandra is traditionally taken for 100 days to boost sexual energy, vitality and produce radiant skin.

Selenium

Selenium is a trace element named after Selene, Greek Goddess of the Moon. Its importance in human health was only realized around 50 years ago, and it is now considered the most important trace element in our diet. This is underlined by the fact that selenium is the only trace element whose incorporation into proteins – as seleno-

---

1. Panossian A, Wikman G. J Ethnopharmacol 2008;118(2):183–212

cysteine, the twenty-first amino acid – is under direct genetic control. It is coded for by the RNA triplet, UGA which during protein formation acts either as a 'stop' signal or as the code to insert the amino acid, selenocysteine. Quite how the protein-building machinery (known as ribosomes) knows which way to translate this codon remains unknown.

Selenocysteine is found in at least 25 human proteins. Those whose function has been determined have structural, transport or antioxidant roles. The selenoenzymes, which have selenocysteine within their active centre, include at least five different glutathione peroxidase enzymes (powerful antioxidants) and three different iodothyronine deiodinases which are vital for the interconversion and deactivation of thyroid hormones.

Selenium is needed for normal cell growth and immunity. It helps to protect against a wide variety of degenerative diseases such as hardening and furring up of the arteries, emphysema, liver cirrhosis, cataracts, arthritis, stroke and heart attack. Selenium also enhances the action of a liver enzyme (P450) involved in detoxifying cancer-causing chemicals (carcinogens), and is involved in the repair of damaged genes (DNA).

In parts of the world where soil selenium levels are low, the incidence of cancer increases by two- to six-fold. Those with the lowest selenium intakes have the highest risk of developing leukaemia or cancers of the colon, rectum, breast, ovary, pancreas, prostate gland, bladder, skin and lungs. These risks seem to be even higher if intakes of vitamin E and vitamin A are also low. Selenium has been shown to prevent the growth of cancer cells in the laboratory, and some evidence suggests it is involved in triggering programmed cell death (apoptosis) of abnormal cells.

The best food sources of selenium are Brazil nuts, fish, poultry, meats (especially game), wholegrains, mushrooms, onions, garlic, broccoli and cabbage. Although diet should always come first, lack of selenium in our food is a growing cause for concern. The mineral content of crops depends on the soils in which they are grown. During the last Ice Age, selenium was leached out of the soil in many parts of Europe, including the UK. While we used to obtain good amounts from wheat imported from America and Canada, our wheat is now mainly sourced from Europe, and our selenium intake fell dramatically between 1978 and 1994 from 60 mcg per day to

34 mcg per day[1]. As a result, UK blood selenium concentrations also fell by around 50 per cent between 1974 and 1991 as intakes were only half the reference nutrient intake[2].

Benefits

Immunity: Selenium stimulates the production of natural killer cells which fight viral and bacterial infections, and is also needed for antibody synthesis. The production of antibodies, increases up to thirty-fold if supplements of selenium and vitamin E are taken together. Increased oxidative stress due to dietary lack of selenium and other antioxidants alters host immune responses[3,4,5,6,7,8]. Lack of selenium reduces the activity of T-lymphocytes and decreases antibody production[9]. This reduced immunity makes it more likely that a viral infection will survive long enough within the body for mutation to a more virulent genotype to occur. Lack of selenium also affects the way respiratory epithelial cells respond to influenza virus exposure[10]. People taking 100 mcg per day selenium supplements have shown a significantly better immune response when immunized with live polio virus vaccine, and cleared the virus from their system more quickly, than those taking placebo[11].

Influenza: Lack of selenium is now recognized as a 'driving force' for viral mutations[12], which may explain why so many new, pathogenic influenza viruses emerge from Asia, where selenium intakes are among the lowest in the world. Symptoms of influenza are also more severe in selenium deficient hosts and lung pathology persists for longer[13]. Influenza viruses recovered from selenium-deficient hosts consistently show genetic changes in the genes coding for viral matrix

1. Rayman MP. BMJ 1997;314:387–8
2. Brown KM et al. Clin Sci (Lond) 2000;98(5):593–9
3. Beck MA, Levander OA. Annu Rev Nutr 1998;18:93–116
4. Beck MA et al. FASEB J 2001;15:1481–3
5. Beck MA et al. Ann NY Acad Sci 2000;917:906–12
6. Grimble RF. Proc Nutr Soc 2001;60:389–97
7. Bhaskaram P. Nutr Rev 2002;60:S40–S45
8. Field CJ et al. J Leukoc Biol 2002;71:16–32
9. Arthur JR et al. J Nutr 2003;133:1457S–1459S
10. Jaspers I et al. Free Radic Biol Med 2007;42(12):1826–37
11. Broome CS et al. Am J Clin Nutr 2004;80(1):154–62
12. Beck MA et al. Trends Microbiol 2004;12(9):417–23
13. Beck MA et al. FASEB J 2001;15:1481–3

proteins. In one study, influenza viruses isolated from three different hosts showed identical mutations in 29 different nucleotide positions, seven of which would result in the insertion of a different amino acid from the original[1]. The changed amino acid sequences in the matrix proteins are thought to increase the virulence of the influenza virus by allowing more rapid uncoating of viral RNA from its associated nucleoproteins; the faster the genes are uncoated, the quicker the virus can start replicating, and the rate of viral production increases[2,3].

Cancer: Selenium has powerful antioxidant actions that help to protect against cancer, and may also reduce tumour progression by inducing programmed cell death (apoptosis) of abnormal cells and through effects on key cell-signalling enzymes. Low levels of selenium have been linked with an increased risk of developing certain cancers, including those of the oesophagus, stomach and prostate gland. In one intervention trial involving over 1,300 people, 200 mcg selenium per day was associated with a 52 per cent lower risk of cancer death and significant reductions in the incidences of lung, colorectal, prostate and total cancers compared with placebo. The incidence of prostate cancer fell by 63 per cent, colorectal cancer by 58 per cent, lung cancer by 46 per cent. The blinded phase of this trial was therefore stopped early as it was considered unethical to withhold selenium from the placebo group[4,5].

Brain health: Selenoenzymes have a vital antioxidant role within the brain and the brain receives a priority selenium supply when intakes are low. Selenium may reduce the risk of cerebrovascular disease by reducing oxidation, vasoconstriction and platelet clumping. Research involving over 1,110 males found that those with the lowest selenium levels were almost four times more likely to die from a stroke than those with the highest levels[6]. Selenium may also protect against senility and Alzheimer's disease[7]. Low plasma

1. Nelson HK et al. FASEB J 2001;15:1846–8
2. Lamb RA, Choppin PW. Annu Rev Biochem 1983;52:467–506
3. Smeenk CA, Brown EG. J Virol 1994;68:530–7
4. Clark LC et al. JAMA 1996;276(24):1957–63
5. Clark LC et al. Br J Urol 1998;81(5):730–4
6. Virtamo J et al. Am J Epidemiol 1985;122(2):276–82
7. Chen J, Berry MJ. J Neurochem 2003;86(1):1–12

selenium levels in the elderly are significantly associated with accelerated cognitive decline while brain selenium concentrations in Alzheimer's disease are 60 per cent lower than in controls[1,2]. When children with intractable epilepsy were given selenium supplements, the incidence of epilepsy decreased[3,4].

Coronary heart disease: Atherogenesis is an inflammatory process, and selenium is an antioxidant that reduces platelet clumping. An inverse association between selenium intakes and the incidence of heart attack has been found in population comparisons, but results are conflicting Whether or not selenium protects against coronary heart disease remains uncertain, although it is possible that selenium may reduce the risk of non-fatal heart attack[5].

Asthma: Asthma is a chronic inflammatory disease of the lungs that has been associated with low selenium levels. Activity of the selenoenzyme, glutathione peroxidase, is also reduced, although whether this is a cause or result of the inflammatory process is uncertain. Taking 100 mcg selenium supplements per day has been shown to significantly increase selenium levels, glutathione peroxidase activity and improve clinical symptoms in people with intrinsic asthma[6].

Fertility: Selenium is important for both male and female fertility. Low levels of selenium have been linked with miscarriage[7] and pre-eclampsia[8] in pregnant women. Taking selenium supplements can increase sperm motility and improve paternity rates in some men[9].

Thyroid function: The thyroid gland has the highest concentration of selenium in the body. This is because enzymes containing selenium (thyroxine deiodinases) are needed to regulate the production of the

1. Hawkes WC, Hornbostel L. Biological Psychiatry 1996;39:121–128
2. Berr C et al. J Am Geriat Soc. 2000;48:1285–1291
3. Weber GF et al. Lancet 1991;337:1443–1444
4. Ramaekers VT et al. Neuropediatrics 1994;25:217–223
5. Yoshizawa K et al. Am J Epidemiol 2003;158(9):852–60
6. Hasselmark L et al. Allergy 1993;48(1):30–6
7. Barrington JW et al. Br J Obstet Gynaecol 1996;103(2):130–2
8. Rayman MP et al. Am J Obstet Gynecol 2003;189(5):1343–9
9. Scott R et al. Br J Urol 1998;82(1):76–80

active form of the thyroid hormone, tri-iodothyronine. The reactions occurring within the thyroid gland continually generate dangerous chemical fragments (free radicals) within thyroid cells. Selenium acts as the main protective antioxidant against these, and if selenium is in short supply, thyroid cells become damaged and die to be replaced by scar tissue (fibrosis) if iodine intakes are high enough to allow normal thyroid gland activity. Selenium levels are significantly lower in people with an enlarged multinodular thyroid goitre compared with those whose thyroid gland is of normal size. Where selenium and iodine intakes are both low, there is a high risk of severely underactive thyroid function (myxoedema). Low selenium levels also increase the risk of thyroid cancer.

Rheumatoid arthritis: RA is a chronic inflammatory disease that has been associated with low levels of selenium. Those with the highest selenium levels appear to have a greater than 80 per cent lower risk of developing RA than those with low levels[1]. However, taking 200 mcg selenium per day has not been shown to significantly improve symptoms[2].

Deficiency
Problems that may be due to selenium deficiency include age spots, pale finger nail beds, increased susceptibility to infection, premature wrinkling of skin, poor growth, subfertility, arthritis, high blood pressure, coronary heart disease, cataracts, pancreatitis, muscle weakness, hypothyroidism and some cancers. Selenium is important for healthy muscle fibres, including those found in the heart. In parts of China, selenium intakes are low enough to cause a form of heart failure (Keshan Disease) and an unpleasant, deforming type of arthritis known as Kashin-Beck disease. These risks seem to be even higher if intakes of the antioxidant vitamins A, C and E are also low.

Dose
100–200 mcg daily.

Supplements are a good way to boost a selenium shortfall, but for

1. Knekt P et al. Epidemiology 2000;11(4):402–5
2. Peretz A et al. Scand J Rheumatol 2001;30(4):208–12

maximum absorption it is best to obtain it in a body-ready form, already incorporated into the amino acid, selenocysteine. The best quality supplements therefore contain selenium-enriched yeasts. This form has the greatest bioavailability, and has been shown to increase the activity of antioxidant selenoenzymes more effectively than inorganic chemical sources such as selenium selenite. That's why all the published, placebo-controlled, cancer prevention studies have used selenium-yeast supplements[1].

Selenium-enriched yeast supplements are notoriously 'smelly', but look out for low-odour products which, thanks to new coating technology, are more pleasant to take.

The new EU RDA for selenium is 55 mcg. The UK RNI for selenium is 75 mcg for adult males and 60 mcg for women. The upper safe level for long-term use from supplements is suggested as 350 mcg per day. The minimum daily intake to obtain full anti-cancer protection is between 75–125 mcg per day[1].

Safety
Intakes above 800 mcg can cause toxicity, leading to a garlic odour on the breath (from dimethyl selenide), fragile or black fingernails, a metallic taste in the mouth, dizziness, nausea and hair loss.

Shiitake
(Lentinus edodes)

Shiitake is a golden brown, umbrella-shaped Chinese mushroom found growing on fallen tree trunks. It is a popular gourmet mushroom whose medicinal use dates back over 600 years.

Shiitake contains a powerful immune-stimulating substance, lentinan, which is believed to boost the body's defences against cancer, viral and fungal infections. It increases production of the body's anti-viral substance, interferon, and increases activity of a powerful, antioxidant enzyme known as superoxide dismutase (SOD).

Shiitake is traditionally used to treat raised cholesterol levels,

---

1. Rayman MP. Br J Nutr 2004;92:557–73

gallstones, stomach ulcers, diabetes, the common cold and as a general tonic to increase the life-force energy known in traditional Chinese medicine as *chi*.

Benefits

In Japan, lentinan is extracted and given by injection to treat upper respiratory tract problems, poor circulation, liver disease, and chronic fatigue. To date, most research has been in laboratory cell cultures. Anecdotal reports suggest it may improve survival of patients with advanced and recurrent cancers and people with viral hepatitis or HIV infection, but much more research is needed.

Dose

Extracts: 400 mg, three times a day.

Dried mushroom: 5–15 g a day.

No serious side effects have been reported at standard doses. Larger doses may cause diarrhoea and bloating. Contact dermatitis and hypersensitivity pneumonitis have been described in shiitake growers exposed to the spores.

Note: Shiitake should only be prescribed by a qualified medical herbalist if used to treat serious medical conditions.

Siberian ginseng
(Eleutherococcus senticosus)

Siberian ginseng is a deciduous shrub native to eastern Russia, China, Korea and Japan. It has been used as an adaptogen for over 2,000 years and has similar actions to that of Korean and American (*Panax*) ginsengs, although it is not closely related.

Siberian ginseng contains triterpenoid saponins known as eleutherosides, some of which are similar in structure to the saponins in Korean ginseng. Comparative studies suggest that there is little qualitative difference between the two, but *Eleutherococcus* has the advantage of being more abundant, easier to cultivate, and therefore cheaper. Although Siberian ginseng is often regarded as an inexpensive substitute for Korean ginseng, many researchers consider it to be the more remarkable adaptogen with a higher activity and wider range of therapeutic uses. Some users prefer it to Korean ginseng as they find it more stimulating, while others find it too strong and prefer to take the gentler American ginseng.

Some practitioners maintain that Siberian ginseng is best for women, while Korean is better for men, but it is really a question of trial and error as to which suits who the best.

Siberian ginseng has oestrogen-like activity and may help to relieve hot flushes, vaginal dryness, night sweats and anxiety. It is also said to improve fertility by enhancing overall vitality and by normalizing levels of sex hormones.

Benefits

Stress: Most research was carried out in the Soviet Union during the 1960s and 1970s and included 70 clinical trials involving over 4,500 people. However, they did not have placebo control groups with which to compare results. According to the World Health Organization monograph, uses supported by clinical data include 'as a prophylactic and restorative tonic for enhancement of mental and physical capacities in cases of weakness, exhaustion, tiredness and during convalescence'. Some research suggests there is a stress threshold below which Siberian ginseng may increase cortisol production and above which it decreases the stress response[1].

Immunity: Russian research suggests that as a result of boosting immunity, those taking it regularly have 40 per cent fewer colds, flu and take a third fewer days off work due to health problems than those not taking it. However, this research did not involve a placebo group for comparison. It is, however, supported by a study involving 36 volunteers who received Siberian ginseng extract or placebo, three times a day, for four weeks. Researchers recorded a 'dramatic' increase in total numbers of immune cells, especially T-lymphocytes, compared with placebo[2].

Endurance: Siberian ginseng is popular among athletes who claim it can improve performance and reaction times. Some research suggests that it increases glycogen storage in muscles and decreases

1. Gaffney BT et al. Life Sci 2001;70(4):431–42
2. Bohn et al. Arzneimittelforschung 1987;37(10):1193–6

lactic acid build-up. Three small studies have suggested that athletes taking Siberian ginseng have increased their total exercise duration by up to 23 per cent compared with only 7.5 per cent for those taking a placebo. However, a review of five more rigorous studies suggests no benefit from Eleutherococcus on cardiorespiratory fitness, fat metabolism or endurance performance[1].

Quality of life: Among 20 older people with hypertension and heart problem, taking 300 mg Siberian ginseng extract per day for four weeks significantly improved quality of life compared with placebo, although these differences did not persist when taken for eight weeks[2].

Colour perception: Russian research suggests that taking Eleutherococcus extracts may improve light and colour perception by increasing retinal sensitivity[3].

Dose
1–3 g a day or equivalent concentrated extracts.

Choose a brand that is standardized to contain more than 1 per cent for eleutherosides. Start with a low dose in the morning at least 20 minutes before eating. If increasing the dose, work up slowly and take two or three times per day.

As with *Panax ginseng*, Siberian ginseng is best taken cyclically by those who are generally young, healthy and fit. It should be taken daily for two to three months, then left for a month. Most people begin to notice a difference after around five days, but it should be continued for at least one month for the full restorative effect. Older people, and those who are unwell, may take their doses continuously.

Siberian ginseng should be taken on an empty stomach unless its effects are too relaxing, in which case it can be taken with meals.

Side effects
No serious side effects have been reported. Unlike *Panax ginseng*, Siberian ginseng does not seem to produce overstimulation or a

1. Goulet ED, Dionne JJ. Int J Sport Nutr Exerc Metab 2005;15(1):75–83
2. Cicero AF et al. Arch Gerontol Geriatr Suppl 2004;(9):69–73
3. Arushanian EB, Shikina IB. Eksp Klin Farmakol 2004;67(4):64–6

stress-like syndrome in excess. A few people do find Siberian ginseng too strong, however, and it may interfere with sleep. If this is the case, the last dose of the day should be taken before the midday meal.

Siberian ginseng should not be used (except under medical advice) if you have high blood pressure, a tendency to nose bleeds or heavy periods, insomnia, rapid heartbeat, high fever or congestive heart failure. Like most other supplements, it should not be taking when pregnant or breast-feeding.

See also: **Ginseng**.

Silicon

Silicon in its pure form is biologically inactive, but it is now recognized as an essential trace element. In its soluble (colloidal) state it forms silicic acid, which is vital for normal growth. The highest concentration of silica (silicon oxide) is found in connective tissues, cartilage and skin, where it strengthens collagen and elastin fibres and contributes to tissue elasticity. The silica acid content of skin and bones decreases with age as tissues become increasingly inelastic and brittle.

Foods containing silicon include rice bran, wholegrains, green leafy vegetables, potatoes, capsicum peppers, parsnips, nuts and seeds. The herb horsetail (*Equisetum arvense*) is also a rich source.

Symptoms that may be due to lack of silicon include premature skin ageing, brittle hair and nails, hardening of arteries, abnormal bone formation and osteoporosis.

Supplements containing silica strengthen bone by cross-linking collagen strands. Silica has been shown to increase mineralization in growing bones, especially in people whose calcium intakes are low. It is also needed for the formation of cartilage.

Benefits
Hair, Skin and Nails: Silica supplements are widely taken to boost hair, skin and nail growth. A supplement containing orthosilicic acid or placebo was given to 48 women with fine hair, at a dose equiva-

lent to 10 mg silicon per day, for nine months. Positive effects on tensile strength of hair, improved elasticity, increased break load and thickness of hair were noted in those taking the supplements. In those on placebo, hair quality continued to deteriorate[1]. A supplement containing orthosilicic acid or placebo was given to 50 women with photo-damaged skin, at a dose equivalent to 10 mg silicon per day, for 20 weeks. Skin roughness increased in the placebo group but significantly decreased in those receiving silicon. Significant improvements were also noted in hair and nail quality with reduced brittleness[1].

Dose
There is currently no EU RDA for silicon. Intakes of 10–30 mg a day have been suggested.

Sodium

Sodium is obtained in the diet as common table salt, known chemically as sodium chloride. Salt is widely added to food to enhance its flavour, act as a stabilizer, retain moisture and help products last longer on the shelf. It is also used to preserve foods such as fish and meats, as bacteria and moulds that would spoil these foods cannot grow in very salty environments. In fact, salt was so highly valued in fridge-free, Ancient Rome, that soldiers received a salt allowance as part of their pay. They were literally 'worth their salt'.

Salt dissolves in water to form two types of electrically charged particles (ions): positively charged sodium (Na^+) and negatively charged chloride (Cl^-). Most sodium in the body is found outside our cells in the surrounding tissue fluids. Very little sodium is present inside our cells. This is because millions of salt pumps in our cell membranes force sodium out of each cell in exchange for potassium ions (K^+) which are forced inside the cells.

1. Wickett RR et al. Arch Dermatol Res 2007;299(10):499–505
2. Barel A et al. Arch Dermatol Res 2005;297(4):147–53

Location	Sodium ions (Na⁺)	Potassium ions (Ka⁺)
Amount found inside cells	9 per cent	90 per cent
Amount found outside cells	91 per cent	10 per cent

The sodium-potassium pump transports three positively charged sodium ions out of a cell for every two positively charged potassium ions it transports in. It is therefore an electrogenic (electricity-producing) pump as it produces a net movement of positive charge out of each cell. As a result of these ion changes, the inside of the cell is negatively charged compared with the outside of the cell, and there is a potential difference across the membrane of all living cells. The electrical charge across cell membranes, known as the membrane potential, is given a negative sign (–) by convention, and varies from –9mV to -100 mV in different tissues. It averages around –70 millivolts (mV) in human nerve cells.

Concentration of various ion inside and outside a spinal nerve cell

ION	Concentration inside cell	Concentration outside cell
Sodium (Na+)	15 mmol/l	150 mmol/l
Potassium (K+)	150 mmol/l	5.5 mmol/l
Chloride (Cl-)	9 mmol/l	125 mmol/l
Resting membane potential = –70mV		

This small, negative electric charge across our cell membranes is vital for life. It is what allows nerve and brain cells to conduct electrical signals, and muscle cells – including those in the heart – to contract.

When a nerve cell is activated, ions quickly flow in opposite directions so that the inside of the cell becomes positive and the outside of the cell negative. This condition – known as depolarization – only lasts for a short time before the cell returns to its original resting state with the inside of the cell negatively charged compared with the outside. This is accompanied by the flow of a substantial electric current through the active cell membrane. While human cells only generate small bioelectric potentials measured in millivolts, specialized electric cells in the electric organ of some fish can generate voltages as large as 1,000 volts which they use to stun or even kill their prey.

The movement of positive and negatively charged ions in and out of cells means that every cell acts like a mini battery to produce a minute electric current. Because moving electric charges produce a magnetic field, the flow of ions in and out of every cell in the body also contributes to our magnetic field.

Interestingly, the active transport of sodium and potassium ions in and out of our cells is one of the main energy-using metabolic processes occurring within the body. It is estimated to account for 33 per cent of energy (in the form of glucose fuel) used by cells overall, and 70 per cent of energy used by nerve cells alone.

A certain amount of sodium is therefore essential as, without it, our nerve and brain cells couldn't pass messages to one another, and heart muscle cells would not be able to contract. It's when we obtain too much salt from our diet that health problems occur.

Food sources of sodium include table salt, salted crisps, bacon, salted nuts, tinned products (especially those canned in brine), cured, smoked or pickled fish/meats, meat pastes, pâtés, ready-prepared meals, packet soups and sauces, stock cubes and yeast extracts.

Dangers of excess salt

We evolved on a diet providing less than 1 g salt per day[1]. Salt is now used as a flavour enhancer and preservative, with consumption around 9–12 g salt per day. This ten-fold rise in sodium intake is responsible for the age-related rise in blood pressure (BP) seen in Westernized populations, as the kidneys of many people are unable to excrete the additional salt load[2]. The retained salt stimulates thirst and causes fluid retention, which causes BP to rise[3].

High blood pressure: Populations with salt intakes of less than 3 g per day do not show increased BP with increasing age[4]. Yanomamo

1. de Wardener HE, MacGregor GA. Curr Opin Cardiol. 2002;17(4):360–7
2. de Wardener HE. Arch Mal Coeur Vaiss Spec 1996; 4:9–15
3. de Wardener HE et al. Kidney Int 2004;66(6):2454–66
4. de Wardener HE, MacGregor GA. Curr Opin Cardiol 2002;17(4):360–7

Indians with a salt intake of less than 1 g daily have an average BP of 96/60 mmHg and do not develop hypertension[1,2,3].

A meta-analysis of data from 28 randomized trials assessing realistic sodium reductions (equivalent to cutting out 4.6 g salt per day) over at least four weeks showed blood pressure (BP) fell by an average of 4.96/2.73 mmHg in those with hypertension and by 2.03/0.97 mmHg for those with normal BP. Reducing salt intake by 6 g salt per day was predicted to lower BP by 7.11/3.88 mmHg in hypertensives and 3.57/1.66 mmHg for normotensives[4]. Other studies have also shown that restricting salt intake reduces BP and the need for medication[5,6,7,8,9]. New research indicates that people whose high blood pressure does not respond to multiple medications are likely to be eating too much salt, and that sodium restriction can produce sharp reductions in blood pressure in these cases of up to 22.7/9.1 mmHg[10].

Heart and circulation: Dietary salt intake is strongly correlated with left ventricular mass and wall thickness, independently of BP, and reducing salt intake has been shown to reduce left ventricular hypertrophy[11,12,13]. In people with hypertension, a high sodium intake decreases the diameter and increases the stiffness of conduit arteries, independent of effects on BP and atherosclerosis[14]. It also thickens and narrows small arteries (arterioles)[15]. It is estimated that reducing salt intake by 3 g per day (for example, from 12 g down to 9 g) would reduce the incidence of stroke by 13 per cent and of coronary

1. Mancilha-Carvalho JJ et al. J Hum Hypertens 1989;3(5):309–14
2. Carvalho JJ et al. Hypertension 1989; 14(3):238–46
3. Mancilha-Carvalho Jde J, Souza e Silva NA. Arq Bras Cardiol 2003;80(3):289–300
4. He FJ, MacGregor GA. J Hum Hypertens, 2002;16(11):761–70
5. Forte JG et al. J Hum Hypertens 1989;3(3):179–84
6. Weinberg MH et al. JAMA 1988; 259:2561–2565
7. MacGregor GA et al. Lancet 1989; 2(8674):1244–1247
8. Stamler J. Am J Clin Nutr 1997;65(2 Suppl):626S–642S
9. Elliott P et al. BMJ 1996;312(7041):1249–53
10. Pimenta E et al. Hypertension 2009; 54(3):475–81
11. Schmieder RE et al. J Hypertens Suppl. 1988;6(4):S148–50
12. Schmieder RE et al. Circulation 1988;78(4):951–6
13. Messerli FH et al. Arch Intern Med 1997;157(21):2449–52
14. Safar ME et al. Cardiovasc Res 2000;46(2):269–76
15. Simon G et al. Am J Hypertens 2003;16(6):488–93

heart disease by 10 per cent. Restricting salt intake to 6 g per day could double this, while restricting salt intake to 3 g daily might triple the benefits, reducing strokes by a third and coronary heart disease by a quarter[1].

Dose

The UK RNI for sodium for adults aged 19–50 years is 1600 mg (equivalent to 4 g salt) daily but most people obtain more than twice this amount from their diet.

Target maximum intakes suggested by the Food Standards Agency are as follows:

Age	Target Salt Intake (g per day maximum)
0 to 6 months	less than 1 g daily
7–12 months	1 g per day
1–3 years	2 g per day
4–6 years	3 g daily
7–10 years	5 g daily
from age 11	6 g daily (as for adults)

NB: Although 6 g has been selected as a realistic adult target to aim for, the recommended intake is no more than 4 g based on the sodium RNI.

Most dietary salt (around 75 per cent) is in the form of hidden salt, added to processed foods including canned products, ready-prepared meals, biscuits, cakes and breakfast cereals.

When reading labels, those giving salt content as 'sodium' need to be multiplied by 2.5 to give table salt content: e.g. a serving of soup containing 0.4 g sodium contains 1 g salt (sodium chloride). Some foods are more salty than sea water which provides a mere 2.5 g salt per 100 g water. Checking labels of bought products, and avoiding those containing high amounts of salt is vital to influence your salt intake.

A good general rule is that, per 100 g food (or per serving if a serving is less than 100 g):

1. He FJ, MacGregor GA. Hypertension 2003;42(6):1093–9

0.5 g sodium or more is **a lot** of sodium
0.1 g sodium or less is **a little** sodium

To cut back on salt intake avoid:

- Adding salt during cooking or at the table
- Obviously salty foods such as crisps, bacon, salted nuts
- Tinned products, especially those canned in brine
- Cured, smoked or pickled fish/meats
- Meat pastes, pâtés
- Ready prepared meals
- Packet soups and sauces
- Stock cubes and yeast extracts.

And:

- Check all labels and select brands with the lowest salt content.

Where salt is essential, use mineral-rich rock salt rather than table salt, or use a low-sodium, higher-potassium brand of salt sparingly. Potassium helps to flush excess sodium from the body via the kidneys, and a diet that is lacking in potassium is linked with a higher risk of high blood pressure and stroke, especially if your diet is also high in sodium. In one study, people taking medication for high blood pressure were able to reduce their drug dose by half (under medical supervision) after increasing the potassium content of their food. Good sources of potassium include seafood, fresh fruit, vegetables, juices and wholegrains.

Salt is easily replaceable with herbs and spices as it doesn't take long to retrain your taste buds. Adding lime juice to food stimulates tastes buds and decreases the amount of salt you need, too.

Tribulus terrestris

Tribulus terrestris is an Indian plant – also known as ci ji li – used in Ayurvedic medicine. Its fruit contains furostanol saponins that are widely used to treat male genito-urinary problems, low sex drive and impotence. Some researchers have claimed that taking Tribulus for five days can increase testosterone levels in healthy men by around 30 per cent to improve low sex drive, lethargy, fatigue and lack of interest in daily activities. However this has not been confirmed in other studies.

Benefits

Testosterone: Tribulus is said to increase production of testosterone and other androgens in the body, although this is controversial[1]. A study involving 21 healthy males who took either Tribulus extracts or placebo for four weeks found no differences between the two groups for blood levels of testosterone, androstenedione, or luteinizing hormones, suggesting that Tribulus does not, either directly or indirectly, increase androgen production in the body[2]. A similar, earlier study also found that supplementation with Tribulus does not enhance body composition or exercise performance in males undergoing resistance training[3].

Athletic training: When 22 elite rugby players took either Tribulus or placebo for five weeks during pre-season training, no differences were found in muscle strength, lean muscle mass or urinary testosterone levels between the two groups[4].

Angina: In China, Tribulus is used to dilate coronary arteries and improve myocardial ischemia (angina). When 406 people with angina were treated with Tribulus saponins, or placebo, Tribulus produced remission in 82.3 per cent and improvement in ECG readings in 52.7 per cent (versus 67.2 per cent and 35.8 per cent with placebo)[5].

Dose

250 mg capsules standardized to contain 40 per cent furostanol saponins: 1–2 capsules a day.

Using Tribulus has been reported to affect urinary drug test screening in athletic competitions.

1. Saudan C et al. Forensic Sci Int 2008;178(1):e7–10
2. Neychev VK, Mitev VI. J Ethnopharmacol 2005;101(1–3):319–23
3. Antonio J et al. In J Sport Nutr Exerc Metab 2000;10(2):208–15
4. Rogerson S et al. J Strength Cond Res 2007;21(2):348–53
5. Wang B et al. Zhong Xi Yi He Za Zhi 1990;10(2):85–7, 68

Tribulus has been reported to cause gynaecomastia (benign breast enlargement) in a body builder using it as an alternative to anabolic steroids.

Turmeric
(Curcuma longa)

Turmeric is native to Asia, where its orange-yellow spicy root is widely used in curry dishes. It is also a traditional Ayurvedic and Chinese herbal medicine.

Turmeric contains an anti-inflammatory antioxidant, curcumin, that stimulates secretion of bile and boosts liver function by increasing levels of two liver enzymes: glutathione-s-transferase and glucuronyl transferase. It also supports liver regeneration, increases bile flow, relieves bloating and indigestion, reduces blood clotting and has been used to help lower raised cholesterol levels.

Recent research has found that curcumin inserts itself into cell membranes to stabilize them and improve the cell's resistance to infection and malignancy[1].

Benefits
Cholesterol: Despite its traditional use, when 36 older people consumed curcumin or placebo daily for six months, no significant effects were found on total LDL-cholesterol, HDL-cholesterol or triglycerides[2].

Gall bladder: Turmeric is widely used to treat right upper abdominal pain due to gall bladder/biliary dysfunction. It has been confirmed to induce contraction of the gall bladder[3]. Participants in a pilot trial with colicky gall-bladder pain were given either turmeric (with celandine) extracts or placebo for three weeks. Those receiving the extracts showed more rapid reduction in pain during the first week of treatment[4].

1. Barry J et al. J Am Chem Soc 2009;131(12):4490–8
2. Baum L et al. Pharmacol Res 2007;56(6):509–14
3. Rasyid A et al. Asia Pac J Clin Nutr 2002;11(4):314–8
4. Niederau C, Gopfert E. Med Clin (Munich) 1999;94(8):425–30

Irritable bowel syndrome: In one study, 207 people with IBS symptoms were given turmeric extracts daily for eight weeks. In those taking 1 g per day, IBS symptoms decreased by 53 per cent, and in those taking 2 g daily, symptoms improved by 60 per cent[1]. Placebo controlled trials are needed to confirm its effectiveness, however.

Ulcerative colitis: 89 people with ulcerative colitis who were in remission took either 1 g curcumin twice a day or placebo, in addition to their usual medication (sulfasalazine or mesalamine) for six months. During this period, 2 out of 43 (4.6 per cent) taking curcumin relapsed, compared with 8 out of 39 (20.5 per cent) taking placebo. Curcumin also improved the findings on endoscopy, suggesting that it is an effective treatment for this condition.

Dose
Two level teaspoons of powder twice a day, or as capsules 500–1200 mg a day, standardized to 95 per cent curcuminoids.

It may be combined with pineapple extracts (bromelain) to improve absorption.

Turmeric increases urinary excretion of oxalates and may increase the risk of kidney stone formation in some people[2].

Valerian
(Valerian officinalis)

Valerian is a common herb with pink or white flowers that grows throughout Europe and Asia. It is one of the most calming herbs available. Its roots have been used as a sedative since mediaeval times to calm nervous anxiety, reduce muscle tension, stimulate appetite and promote a refreshing night's sleep.

Valerian contains a number of unique substances (such as valeric acid, valepotriates) that are thought to act together in synergy to produce significant, positive effects on stress and anxiety. Valerian appears to work in a number of ways. It raises levels of an inhibitory

1. Bundy R et al. J Altern Complement Med 2004;10(6):1015–8
2. Tang M et al. Am J Clin Nutr 2008;87(5):1262–7

brain chemical, gamma-aminobutyric acid (GABA), to damp down the over-stimulation occurring during anxiety. Its sedative effect occurs through a direct inhibition of enzymes that break GABA in the brain. Valepotriates themselves act as prodrugs and are transformed into the sedative, homobaldrinal. Valerian roots also contain appreciable amounts of GABA but it is uncertain whether these can be absorbed or cross the blood-brain barrier to produce a direct effect. They also contain a lignan, hydroxypinoresinol, which has been shown to react with the same benzodiazepine receptors as drugs such as diazepam.

Benefits
Sleep: Some studies have shown that valerian root extracts are an effective aid to sleep, while others have shown only a weak effect. A meta-analysis of results from 16 studies involving almost 1,100 people found that most studies had significant design problems and the doses used and length of treatment varied considerably. The outcome of six acceptable studies showed a statistically significant benefit with sleep improved by 80 per cent compared with placebo. The authors concluded that valerian might improve sleep quality without producing side effects. More research is needed to confirm these positive findings[1]. In general, those taking valerian extracts fall asleep more quickly and wake up less frequently during the night than those taking placebo. Interestingly, in a trial comparing the effects of taking a valerian extract (600 mg) or the prescribed hypnotic drug, oxazepam, for six weeks, both treatments showed similar improvements in feelings of refreshment after sleep, exhaustion in the evening, duration of sleep and dream recall. More patients taking valerian assessed their treatment as very good (82.8 per cent) compared with those on the prescribed drug (73.4 per cent)[2]. The authors concluded that valerian extracts were as effective as the sleeping tablet, oxazepam for treating insomnia. Importantly, valerian extracts do not have a negative effect on reaction times, daytime alertness or concentration the morning after intake[3].

1. Bent S et al. Am J Med 2006;119(12):1005–12
2. Ziegler G et al. Eur J Med Res 2002;7(11):480–6
3. Kuhlmann J et al. Pharmacopsychiatry 1999;32(6):235–41

Anxiety disorder: Trials involving people with emotional symptoms due to stress showed that it helped to overcome low mood, loss of initiative, feeling unsociable, irritability, anxiety and difficulty in sleeping. A small trial of 36 people which compared valerian extracts with the prescribed anxiolytic drug, diazepam (a benzodiazepine), and placebo, found that both valerian and diazepam produced significant reductions in the part of the Hamilton anxiety scale, suggesting that valerian has an anxiolytic effect[1]. The trial was too small to draw firm conclusions, however. Interestingly, in people withdrawing from benzodiazepine use, who experience rebound insomnia, using valerian can subjectively improve sleep better than placebo due to its mild anxiolytic effect[2].

Restless legs syndrome: When 37 people with restless legs syndrome were given either 800 mg valerian extracts or placebo for eight weeks, those receiving the extracts showed significant improvements in leg symptom and a reduction in daytime sleepiness compared with those taking placebo[3].

Dose
250–800 mg, two or three times a day.

Select standardized products containing at least 0.8 per cent valeric acid.

Valerian is often used together with other calming herbs such as lemon balm and hops to ease nervous anxiety, insomnia and to help avoid a panic attack. It may also be used together with St John's Wort for depression.

Valerian is non-addictive, and does not produce a drugged feeling or hangover effect, as it promotes a natural form of sleep whose architecture is preserved. However, it may cause mild drowsiness which will affect your ability to drive or operate machinery.

Valerian should not be taken by anyone using prescribed sleeping tablets.

1. Andreatini R et al. Phytother Res 2002;16(7):650–4
2. Poyares DR et al. Prog Neuropsychopharmacol Biol Psychiatry 2002;26(3):539–45
3. Cuellar NG, Ratcliffe SJ. Altern Ther Health Med 2009;15(2):22–8

Vitamins

Vitamins are naturally occurring substances that are essential for life, although they are only needed in tiny amounts. There are 13 major vitamins that must all be obtained from the diet as most cannot be synthesized in the body (e.g. vitamin C) or can only be made in minute amounts (e.g. vitamin D, niacin), too small to meet our needs.

Vitamins are involved in all the body's metabolic reactions from digestion, energy production and immunity to cell division, growth, tissue repair, hormone secretion and reproduction. They are involved in the transportation of oxygen and wastes in the circulation, vision, sensory perception and mental alertness.

Lack of vitamins is common, and if intakes are consistently below recommended levels, a variety of nonspecific ailments may appear including dry, itchy skin with poor wound-healing properties, tiredness, lack of energy, lowered immunity and difficulty in conceiving.

How quickly a particular vitamin deficiency will cause problems depends on how much is stored in the body, and how quickly supplies run out. In general, vitamins that are fat-soluble are stored more easily in the body (e.g. in the liver) than those that are water-soluble and easily lost in the urine. The highly fat-soluble vitamins are A, D, E and K, and the water-soluble vitamins are the B group and C whose levels (with the exception of vitamin B12) must be continually replenished from the diet.

Lack of water-soluble folic acid may develop quite quickly (e.g. during pregnancy, to cause certain developmental abnormalities in the foetus), while in contrast, stores of the more fat-soluble vitamin B12 are large, and it can take years for deficiency to develop into pernicious anaemia.

Vitamin A

Vitamin A is a fat-soluble vitamin that is stored in the liver. We obtain vitamin A from two main sources: as retinol (pre-formed vitamin A) found only in animal foods, and from carotenoids – yellow-orange plant pigments – some of which can be converted into vitamin A . (See page 86.)

Foods containing pre-formed vitamin A (retinol) include:

- Animal and fish liver
- Meat
- Oily fish and cod liver oil
- Dairy products
- Eggs
- Milk and dairy products
- Butter and margarine (fortified by law to contain as much vitamin A as in butter).

Vitamin A is easily destroyed by exposure to light and heat. Boiling or frying, for example, reduces a food's vitamin A content by 40 per cent after one hour and by 70 per cent after two hours.

Benefits

Vitamin A has a number of important functions in the body. It is a powerful antioxidant in both the water-soluble (as carotenoids) and fat-soluble (as retinol) phases of the body. It also binds to special receptors in the cell nucleus to regulate the way in which genes are read. This makes it vital for the production of a number of proteins, including many important enzymes. As so many genes are controlled by this hormone-like action of vitamin A, it is essential for normal growth and development, sexual health and fertility. It maintains healthy skin, teeth and bones, and keeps mucous membranes moist, such as those lining the eyes, nose, mouth and lungs. It is also important in the healing of sores, wounds, and burns. Vitamin A derivatives are also used medically to treat severe forms of acne, psoriasis and sun damage (photoageing) including wrinkles.

In the eye, vitamin A is converted into a pigment known as visual purple (rhodopsin). When exposed to light, this pigment absorbs photon energy which induces a change that stimulates nerve endings in the back of the eye (retina). This triggers sensory messages that are relayed to the brain for interpretation by the visual cortex to form visual images. This was one of the first functions of vitamin A to be recognized – hence its common name of retinol.

Vitamin A also plays an important role in maintaining immunity and strengthening resistance. It is needed in higher amounts during times of infection and is involved in the production of immune cells needed to line the mucus membranes of the respiratory and intestinal tracts – two of the body's front line defences against infection. Because of its role in immunity, optimum intakes of vitamin A help to protect against viral sore throats, the common cold, influenza, warts, conjunctivitis, cold sores, acute bronchitis and possibly shingles. It is also thought to have a protective action against inflammatory bowel disease, peptic ulcers, candida yeast infections and in reducing allergies.

Several studies have suggested that natural dietary intakes of vitamin A and some carotenoids are important in reducing the risk of coronary heart disease and a number of cancers (e.g. ovarian, endometrial, stomach, prostate, breast and possibly colon cancers). These studies assessed dietary intakes, for example from eating fruit and vegetables. There is no convincing evidence that vitamin A supplements may protect against cancer. In fact, taking high dose betacarotene supplements has been linked with an increased risk of lung cancer in smokers, and in those with previous occupational exposure to asbestos.

Deficiency

Vitamin A deficiency is uncommon in developed countries, but relatively common in poorer parts of the world. One of the first signs of lack of vitamin A is loss of sensitivity to green light, followed by difficulty in adapting to dim light (night blindness), hence the old adage that 'carrots help you see in the dark'.

More severe deficiency leads to dry, burning, itchy eyes, hardening of the cornea (the transparent part of the front of the eye), followed by corneal ulceration – a condition known as xerophthalmia. Lack of vitamin A also increases the risk of cataracts. It is estimated that as many as half a million people worldwide go blind from vitamin A deficiency each year.

Other symptoms of vitamin A deficiency include increased susceptibility to infection, scaly skin with raised, pimply hair follicles and flaky scalp; dull, brittle hair, inflamed gums and mucous membranes, loss of appetite and possibly kidney stones.

Supplements containing vitamin A are best taken with food as dietary fat aids absorption. It is most effective taken in conjunction with other antioxidants such as vitamins C, E, carotenoids and mineral selenium.

Dose

The UK RNI for vitamin A (retinol) is 700 mcg for adult males aged 19–50 years, and 600 mcg for adult women. The EU RDA is 800 mcg. The upper safe level for long-term intake from both diet and supplements is suggested as 1500 mcg (5000 IU).

1 International Unit (IU) vitamin A = 0.3 mcg retinol
1 mcg vitamin A = 3.33 IU

Children should ideally take a supplement providing vitamins A, D and E (at doses appropriate for their age) up until at least the age of five unless their diet is known to provide sufficient amounts of these important micronutrients.

Toxicity

It is important not to exceed the recommended dose of any supplement containing vitamin A. It has a narrow therapeutic window and intakes of just double the recommended daily amount may cause problems – especially during pregnancy.

Cases of vitamin A toxicity are usually associated with taking supplements at doses above 30,000 mcg (100,000 IU) daily.

As it is fat-soluble, vitamin A enters the central nervous system more easily than most other vitamins. Excess causes symptoms of retinol poisoning which include liver and nerve damage, headache, irritability, blurred vision, nausea, weakness, fatigue, dry skin, hair loss, itchy eyes, bone and joint pain, bone loss, bleeding gums and skin sores. In the long term, excess vitamin A may increase the risk of liver cirrhosis. Avoid eating polar bear liver, which is said to contain so much retinol that consuming just 100 g is lethal.

Avoid vitamin A supplements during pregnancy

High intakes of vitamin A during pregnancy may increase the risk of birth defects. In a study of over 22,700 pregnant women, those with total intakes (from both food and supplements) of more than 15,000 IU (4500 mcg) of pre-formed vitamin A (retinol) daily were three and a half times more likely to deliver a baby with congenital defects than those whose intakes were 5000 IU (1500 mcg) daily[1]. In those

1. Rothman KJ et al. N Engl J Med 1995;333(21):1369–73

women whose vitamin A intake came mainly from supplements, those obtaining 10,000 IU (3000 mcg) daily were almost five times more likely to deliver a baby with congenital abnormalities. The researchers concluded that, among the women taking more than 10,000 IU vitamin A per day, one infant in 57 had abnormalities due to the supplement. The most dangerous time to take excess vitamin A during pregnancy seems to be within the first seven weeks.

Pregnant women are therefore advised not to take supplements containing pre-formed retinol, or to eat foods that have a high vitamin A content, such as liver and liver products. You should also avoid cod liver oil, which contains high quantities of vitamin A.

As vitamin A is vital for normal healthy development in the womb, the safest way to obtain vitamin A during pregnancy is in the form of natural carotenoids (see page 86), that can be converted into retinol when needed.

See also: **Carotenoids**.

Vitamin B1

Vitamin B1, also known as thiamin or thiamine, is a water-soluble vitamin that is needed for the production of energy from glucose, for transmission of electrical messages in nerve and muscle cells, including the heart, and for the production of red blood cells. It is needed for the synthesis of some important amino acids and plays a role in digestion. It is also involved in the transport of glucose within cells, and in the function of pancreatic beta-cells (which produce insulin hormone), making it important for people with diabetes.

Vitamin B1 is readily lost from the body through the kidneys, and most people only have stores sufficient to last one month. A regular dietary supply is therefore essential. Food sources include whole-grains, oats, soy flour, pasta, meat – especially pork and duck – seafood, nuts and pulses. Brewer's yeast and yeast extracts are also good sources.

Vitamin B1 is easily lost by food processing, e.g. chopping, mincing, liquidizing, canning and preserving. Boiling reduces the thiamin content of foods by half as it is so water-soluble. It is also destroyed by high temperatures and adding baking powder. Toasting bread can lose almost a third of its vitamin B1 content. In addition, freezing meats reduces their vitamin B1 content by up to 50 per cent while cooking meat at 200°C lowers its vitamin B1 content by another 20 per cent.

Benefits

Tiredness: Many older people have low intakes of thiamin – supplements may help them to increase feelings of general well-being, reduce fatigue and boost appetite. In one trial, 10 mg helped people over the age of 65 to enjoy better quality sleep, increased energy levels and lower blood pressure than those taking a placebo.

Mood: Vitamin B1 may have beneficial effects on mood, promoting calmness, clear-headedness and elation. People with low levels of vitamin B1 are less likely to feel composed or self-confident and more likely to suffer from depression than those with higher levels. Among healthy young females, low thiamin status was associated with poor mood and an improvement in thiamin status after three months' supplementation was associated with improved mood[1].

Arterial disease: Vitamin B1 appears to have a protective effect against over proliferation of artery linings which is linked with atherosclerosis. Laboratory evidence involving cell cultures suggests that good intakes of vitamin B1 may delay hardening and furring up of the arteries associated with elevated glucose levels in people with Type 2 diabetes[2].

Retinopathy: Laboratory evidence suggests that vitamin B1 may help to prevent diabetic retinopathy[3]. These findings need to be investigated in humans[4].

Painful periods: A trial involving 556 teenage girls with painful periods compared a dose of 100 mg thiamin hydrochloride with placebo for 90 days. Among those taking vitamin B1, 87 per cent

1. Benton D et al. Neuropsychobiology 1995;32(2):98–105
2. Avena R. Ann Vasc Surg 2000;14(1):37–43
3. Obrenovich ME, Monnier VM. Sci Aging Knowledge Environ 2003;10:PE6
4. Hammes HP et al. Nat Med 2003;9(3):294–9

were 'cured', 8 per cent had pain relieved and 5 per cent showed no effect. After a further two months without treatment, the results were the same suggesting long-term effectiveness of the treatment.[1]

Deficiency

In some under-developed countries, thiamin deficiency is common especially where the main dietary staple is polished rather than brown rice. This causes a disease known as 'beri-beri', meaning 'extreme weakness'. Dry beri-beri produces heaviness, weakness, numbness and pins and needles in the legs, while wet beri-beri causes severe fluid retention. In those with a high alcohol intake, lack of thiamin is associated with Wernicke-Korsakoff syndrome which, if left untreated, leads to irreversible dementia.

Dose

The old EU RDA for thiamin was 1.4 mg per day. The newly set EU RDA has decreased to 1.1 mg. The UK RNI for adults aged 19–50 years is 1 mg for men and 0.8 mg for women. The upper safe level for long-term use from supplements is suggested as 100 mg per day.

In general, the more carbohydrate you eat, the more thiamin you need. People drinking large amounts of coffee or tea – which destroy the vitamin – may become thiamin deficient. Other common causes of thiamin deficiency include stress – which quickly uses up available thiamin stores – and drinking too much alcohol, which interferes with thiamin metabolism.

Side effects

Vitamin B1 is relatively non-toxic as excess is readily lost in the urine. High daily doses (5000 mg thiamine hydrochloride or more) may cause headache, nausea, irritability, insomnia, rapid pulse and weakness. These symptoms are reversible once supplements are stopped.

Vitamin B2

Vitamin B2 – also known as riboflavin – is a water-soluble vitamin that plays an important role in the production of energy and the

1. Gokhale LB. Indian J Med Res 1996; 103:227–31

metabolism of proteins, fats and carbohydrate. It acts as a building block for the production of a substance called flavin adenine dinucleotide, which is needed for the optimum activity of a number of metabolic enzymes. One of these, glycerophosphate dehydrogenase, plays a key role in the way insulin-producing B-cells detect the presence of glucose within the pancreas. It has been suggested that lack of vitamin B2, or its abnormal metabolism, is linked with the development of Type 2 diabetes. Certainly people with Type 2 diabetes tend to have lower blood levels of B2 than similar groups of people without diabetes. Vitamin B2 is also needed for production of thyroid hormones and red blood cells.

As it is water-soluble, vitamin B2 cannot be stored in the body, and a regular dietary intake is essential. Food sources include yeast extract, wholegrains, eggs, dairy products, green leafy vegetables and beans. Fortified cereals are another good source, and children who eat them for breakfast are less likely to have inadequate intakes of vitamin B2 compared with those who do not eat fortified cereals. Although milk is a rich source, its vitamin B2 content is quickly destroyed when exposed to light. The riboflavin content of milk is reduced by 90 per cent after two hours' sun exposure, so buy milk in cartons rather than bottles. Boiling milk also reduces its vitamin B1 content by up to 25 per cent. Vitamin B2 is also readily lost from vegetables into cooking water, to colour it yellow. In addition, freezing meat reduces its vitamin B2 content by up to 50 per cent.

Vitamin B2 acts as an antioxidant, and helps to maintain immunity as it is involved in the production of antibodies. It helps to keep skin, hair, eyes and mucus membranes healthy, and is important for brain function. Those with good intakes of vitamin B2 are more likely to show high scores in tests of mental functioning than those with low levels.

Vitamin B2 is often included in nutritional supplements designed to improve the symptoms of pre-menstrual syndrome as it is needed to convert vitamin B6 into its active form. It may also help to reduce migraine attacks, including those associated with menstruation, and is often recommended to reduce the facial redness that occurs in rosacea.

Benefits

Homocysteine: Vitamin B2 has a homocysteine-lowering action in people who have inherited two copies of a particular gene associated with reduced activity of an enzyme (methylenetetrahydrofolate reductase) needed for homocysteine metabolism[1].

Congenital defects: Vitamin B2 may provide some protection against certain congenital abnormalities (neural tube defects e.g. spina bifida) during early pregnancy in addition to that given by folic acid and vitamin B12.

Cataracts: Vitamin B2 appears to play an essential role in protecting against cataract formation. It acts as a building block for the production of flavin adenine dinucleotide – a co-factor needed for optimum activity of an antioxidant enzyme, glutathione reductase[2]. In a study involving 1,380 people attending an ophthalmology outpatient clinic, regular use of multivitamin supplements decreased the risk of developing cataracts by 37 per cent, with dietary intake of riboflavin, among other nutrients, decreasing the risk[3]. Studies suggest that people with good intakes of vitamin B2 are around a third less likely to develop lens opacities (cataracts) than those with low intakes.

Migraine: A study involving 55 people with migraine found that, for 59 per cent of people taking 400 mg riboflavin daily, the frequency of attacks and number of headache days was reduced by 50 per cent (compared with a similar improvement in only 15 per cent of those taking placebo)[4]. This effect is thought to be related to mitochondrial energy metabolism. However, a similar trial involving a dose of 200 mg riboflavin versus placebo in 48 children with migraine found no significant benefits[5].

Deficiency

Older people with low vitamin B2 levels may have reduced immunity due to sub-optimal antibody production and are also at

1. McNulty H et al. Circulation 2006;113(1):74–80
2. Head KA. Altern Med Rev 2001;6(2):141–66
3. Leske MC et al. Arch Ophthalmol 1991;109(2):244–51
4. Schoenen J et al. Neurology 1998;50(2):466–70
5. MacLennan SC et al. J Chil Neurol 2008;23(11):1300–4

higher risk of developing cataracts.

People with chronic fatigue syndrome often benefit from taking B group supplements and preliminary research suggests their level of B vitamin activity – including that of vitamin B2 – is low. Vitamin B2 deficiency may be a cause of recurrent aphthous mouth ulcers in some people.

Severe lack of vitamin B2 (ariboflavinosis) is rare in Western countries, but is occasionally seen in vulnerable groups such as the elderly and those with anorexia or alcohol dependency. Symptoms include weakness, sore and swollen throat and tongue, cracking and sores at the corners of the mouth (angular cheilosis), skin irritation and anaemia. Other signs that may be due to lack of vitamin B2 include eyes that are bloodshot, red, tired and which feel gritty or sensitive; cataracts, sores and cracks at the corner of the mouth, a red, inflamed tongue and lips, hair loss, a scaly eczema-like skin rash (seborrhoeic dermatitis), especially on the face and nose as well as trembling, dizziness, difficulty sleeping and poor concentration or memory.

Dose

The old EU RDA for vitamin B2 was 1.6 mg per day. The newly set EU RDA has decreased to 1.4 mg. The UK RNI for adults aged 19–50 years is 1.3 mg for men, and 1.1 mg for women. The upper safe level for long-term use from supplements is suggested as 40 mg.

People who are physically active need more vitamin B2 than those who take little regular exercise. Recent studies also suggest that metabolism changes with age, so older people need to obtain more B2 from their diet to maintain blood levels of this vitamin.

Side effects

Excess is excreted in the urine, and when taking supplements containing vitamin B2, urine colour becomes noticeably more yellow. High intakes may cause skin itching, numbness and pins and needles.

Vitamin B3

Vitamin B3 is a water-soluble vitamin, also known as niacin, which exists in two forms – as nicotinic acid and nicotinamide. Vitamin B3 can be made in the body in small amounts from the essential amino acid tryptophan (60 mg tryptophan produces 1 mg niacin). Because of this, many foods and supplements may describe their vitamin B3 content in the form of 'niacin equivalents' which are equal to the amount of nicotinamide and nicotinic acid they contain plus one-sixtieth of their tryptophan content. Dietary sources of vitamin B3 include wholegrains, fortified breakfast cereals, nuts, meat and poultry, oily fish, eggs, dairy products, dried fruit and yeast extract. Eggs and cheese are some of the richest dietary sources of tryptophan.

Vitamin B3 combines with the mineral, chromium, to form the Glucose Tolerance Factor (GTF). This is essential for the action of the hormone, insulin, in controlling the way glucose is taken up into body cells. Lack of vitamin B3 has been associated with impaired glucose tolerance which may lead to diabetes.

Like other B group vitamins, it also plays an important role in metabolism, enzyme function and energy production. It is essential for releasing energy from muscle sugar stores (glycogen) and for the uptake and use of oxygen in cells. Vitamin B3 works together with vitamins B1 (thiamin) and B2 (riboflavin) for these tasks, and also works on its own to maintain healthy skin, nerves, intestines and intellectual function.

Benefits

Cholesterol: Vitamin B3 is prescribed medically to lower abnormally high cholesterol levels and can reduce the risk of a heart attack by as much as 30 per cent. It can lower total cholesterol, harmful low-density lipoprotein (LDL) cholesterol, and triglycerides as well as being one of the few treatments that can lower a harmful type of fat particle known as apolipoprotein (apo) B, and of another fat, apoA[1]. It seems to work in the liver to reduce production of triglycerides and apoB, while also blocking the reactions that break down HDL-cholesterol to increase levels by as much as 20 per cent. As a result, niacin is now recognized as the most effective treatment available to increase levels of beneficial high-density lipoprotein (HDL) cholesterol[2]. A once daily slow-release preparation was shown in a 16-week trial, involving 148 people with diabetes, to increase beneficial HDL-cholesterol levels

1. Pan J et al. Metabolism 2002; 51(9):1120–7
2. Malik S, Kashyap ML. Curr Cardiol Rep 2003;5(6):470–6

by 19–24 per cent compared with placebo, and to lower triglyceride levels by 13–28 per cent with no significant changes to glucose control or haemoglobin A1c levels. Four people stopped treatment due to flushing (including one receiving placebo)[1]. A new drug that combines niacin with an agent to reduce flushing (laropiprant) is now available. Flushing can also be reduced by using aspirin[2].

Cataracts: Good dietary intakes of vitamin B3 may reduce the development of cataracts[3].

Deficiency

Lack of vitamin B3 produces a rare deficiency disease known as pellagra which classically produces symptoms of dermatitis, diarrhoea and dementia. This occurs in parts of Africa where the diet contains large quantities of maize whose niacin is in a non-usable form of niacytin. In central America, maize for cooking tortillas is soaked overnight in calcium hydroxide which releases the niacin content.

Dose

The old EU RDA for vitamin B3 was 18 mg per day. The newly set EU RDA has decreased to 16 mg. The UK RNI for adults (aged 19–50 years) is 17 mg for men and 13 mg for women. The upper safe level for long-term use from supplements is suggested as 500 mg.

People who are physically active need more niacin than those with a sedentary lifestyle. When used for medicinal purposes, higher doses of 50 mg niacin a day may be taken. Doses as high as 1500 mg nicotinamide may be prescribed daily for certain medical disorders. Therapeutic use of high-dose niacin usually needs regular blood liver function tests.

Side effects

High-dose vitamin B3 (especially in the form of nicotinic acid) can produce a red flush and warming of the skin similar to blushing. People who blush easily seem to be more sensitive to this effect. For those who are very sensitive, a low dose of aspirin (75–300 mg)

1. Grundy SM et al. Arch Intern Med 2002; 62(14):1568–76
2. Thakkar RB et al. Am J Cardiovasc Drugs 2009;9(2):69–79
3. Leske MC et al. Arch Ophthalmol 1991;109(2):244–51

taken half an hour before the dose of niacin can reduce this effect.

Symptoms of niacin toxicity can occur at very high doses, including thickening and darkening of patches of skin (acanthosis nigricans), palpitations, worsening of pre-existing conditions such as diabetes and peptic ulceration. Gout and liver inflammation (hepatitis) can also be triggered.

Contraindications
High dose vitamin B3 (above 30 mg) should only be used under medical supervision.

Vitamin B5

Vitamin B5, also known as pantothenic acid or pantothenate, is a water-soluble vitamin widely found in foods such as wholegrains, beans, vegetables, nuts, eggs, meats and yeast extract. One of the richest supplementary sources is royal jelly.

It is easily destroyed by food processing. Cooking, for example, destroys up to 50 per cent of B5 in meats, and an additional 30 per cent is lost into cooking juices. Up to 75 per cent of B5 in vegetables is lost during processing. Freezing causes a slow destruction of this vitamin, too.

Like other B group vitamins, vitamin B5 is vital for many energy-yielding metabolic reactions involving carbohydrates, fats and protein. It is particularly significant in the synthesis of glucose and fatty acids which are both important fuels for muscle cells and may even improve athletic performance, although this is far from proven. It has also been suggested that supplements containing vitamin B5 may help during weight-loss diets by ensuring that fatty acids released from body fat stores are fully broken down. This is believed to reduce the formation of ketones and hunger pangs but more research is needed to confirm this.

Vitamin B5 plays a role in the production of adrenal gland hormones during times of stress and in maintaining a healthy nervous system. It is also taken to reduce nasal congestion, increase resistance to stress, to help overcome chronic fatigue and indigestion and as an aid in giving up smoking.

Vitamin B5 can stimulate cell growth in healing tissues by increasing the number and speed of cells moving into wounds, increasing the rate at which these cells divide and improving protein synthesis. This encourages stronger scar tissue formation, helps to rejuvenate ageing skin and to reduce skin mottling. Its boost to healing processes may also explain why vitamin B5 derivatives (calcium pantothenate and pantotheine) have been helpful in treating viral hepatitis A. When given to 156 patients with this relatively common infection, their liver function tests improved and blood antibody levels increased as did the activity of white blood cells. Pantotheine produced the most pronounced therapeutic effect.

Benefits

Rheumatoid arthritis: Vitamin B5 may improve symptoms of rheumatoid arthritis. The evidence relating to this claim is intriguing. Nearly forty years ago, researchers noted that young rats who were deficient in vitamin B5 showed abnormal growth and development of bone and cartilage. These defects were reversed by vitamin B5 supplements, suggesting that symptoms were part of a deficiency disease. Several years later, blood levels of vitamin B5 were shown to be significantly lower in people with rheumatoid arthritis (RA). When 20 people with RA were given daily injections of 50 mg calcium pantothenate, their blood levels of vitamin B5 rose and symptoms improved. When the injections were discontinued, however, their joint problems gradually returned. With the exception of a 1963 study attributing relief from symptoms of osteoarthritis in a small number of patients given vitamin B5, no further studies were carried out until 1980. A double-blind study conducted by the US General Practitioner Research Group reported significant effects for oral calcium pantothenate in reducing the duration of morning stiffness, degree of disability, and severity of pain in people with rheumatoid arthritis, compared with those receiving placebo. The dose used in this study was 500 mg daily for two days, increasing to 1 g daily for three days, followed by 1.5 g daily for four days, and 2 g daily thereafter (in divided doses). The calcium/vitamin B5 supplement was only found to be effective against RA, not other forms of arthritis such as osteoarthritis. Further trials are needed.

Deficiency
Symptoms that may be caused by a lack of vitamin B5 include weakness and fatigue, headache, difficulty in coping with stress, poor muscle co-ordination and muscle cramps, numbness and tingling sensations, loss of appetite, nausea, indigestion, abdominal cramps, painful and burning feet, increased susceptibility to infection, poor wound healing, possibly joint degeneration, difficulty in sleeping and depression.

Dose
The EU RDA for vitamin B5 is 6 mg per day. No UK RNI has been set, but an intake of around 4–7 mg is believed to be adequate. The suggested upper safe level for long-term use from supplements is 200 mg.

Side effects
High doses may cause diarrhoea.

Vitamin B6

Vitamin B6 is not just one substance, but a group of water-soluble compounds that includes pyridoxine, pyridoxal and pyridoxamine. All are converted into the most active form, pyridoxine, in the body. As it is water-soluble, it is readily lost in the urine, so regular intakes are essential. Food sources of vitamin B6 include wholegrains, liver, meat, oily fish, soy products, bananas, nuts (especially walnuts), green leafy vegetables, avocado and egg yolk. Yeast extract and royal jelly are also good sources.

Pyridoxine is an essential co-factor for the action of over 60 enzymes involved in the synthesis of genetic material, amino acids, proteins and the metabolism of carbohydrate and essential fatty acids. It is especially important for the health of rapidly dividing cells such as those found in the gut, skin, hair follicles and marrow as well as those involved in immunity. It increases production of antibodies and the number and activity of T4-helper lymphocytes.

Benefits

Homocysteine: Vitamin B6 is involved in the break down of homocysteine – an amino acid which, when allowed to build up in the circulation, is an important risk factor for the development of atherosclerosis, coronary heart disease and stroke. Homocysteine is formed in the body from the breakdown of the dietary amino acid methionine. Normally, its level is tightly controlled by three different enzymes that convert homocysteine to cysteine – a safe end product used by cells for growth. When certain B vitamins are lacking, including vitamin B6, this conversion cannot occur so efficiently and potentially harmful levels of homocysteine build up in the circulation. Taking supplements of B group vitamins (folic acid plus vitamins B6 and B12) has been shown to lower homocysteine levels where they are raised – especially in older people, although B6 is less effective than folic acid or B12. Supplementation with folic acid (1 mg daily), vitamin B12 (400 mcg daily) and vitamin B6 (10 mg per day) for six months following percutaneous coronary intervention (angioplasty) significantly reduced the risk of major adverse events (2.6 per cent heart attacks versus 4.3 per cent with placebo; 9.9 per cent needed repeat vascular surgery versus 16 per cent on placebo)[1].

Neuropathy: Vitamin B6 is involved in the synthesis of brain chemicals such as serotonin and GABA, which are important for nerve cell function in the central and peripheral nervous systems. Deficiency may be a factor in the development of neuropathy in people with diabetes who can experience pain, burning and pins and needles as a result. Some studies suggest that people with diabetic neuropathy have lower levels of vitamin B6 than people with diabetes who do not have neuropathy, but other studies have found no significant differences. Taking 50 mg B6 three times a day had no greater effect than placebo in 18 people with diabetic peripheral neuropathy[2].

Retinopathy: It has also been suggested that vitamin B6 may help to reduce retinopathy in people with diabetes. This followed observa-

1. Schnyder G et al. JAMA 2002;288(8):973–9
2. Levin ER et al. Diabetes Care 1981;4(6):606–9

tions in 18 people with diabetes who were followed for periods of up to 28 years that those who took vitamin B6 supplements did not develop retinopathy[1]. The researchers described this discovery as 'monumental' and it needs further investigation.

Carpal tunnel syndrome: Lack of vitamin B6 has also been linked with carpal tunnel syndrome. However, when vitamin B6 levels were measured in 13 people with both diabetes and carpal tunnel syndrome, no significant differences were found between those with carpal tunnel syndrome, those without neuropathy, and normal subjects. Although supplements are not effective in everyone, some people respond to high doses of vitamin B6. Preliminary evidence also suggests that people with chronic fatigue syndrome may respond to taking B group vitamins, including vitamin B6.

PMS: Anecdotal evidence suggests vitamin B6 may improve PMS in some women, possibly through its role in synthesizing neurotransmitters and in regulating the function of sex hormones. However, the vitamin B6 status of women with PMS does not differ significantly from matched controls, and many researchers now believe that B6 deficiency is unlikely to contribute to the cause of PMS[2,3].

Kidney stones: Vitamin B6 supplements may protect against kidney stones as it decreases the production of a chemical, oxalate, that is found in many kidney stones.

Cancer: Research involving almost 15,000 people suggests that vitamin B6 (from diet or supplements) may halve the risk of developing cancer of the colon/rectum by 50 per cent[4].

Deficiency
Lack of vitamin B6 can cause recurrent mouth ulcers (aphthous ulceration), split lips, red, inflamed tongue, burning skin, anaemia and headache. Deficiency has also been linked with carpal tunnel syndrome, and symptoms similar to those occurring in PMS

1. Ellis JM et al. Biochem Biophys Res Commun 1991;179(1):615–9
2. van den Berg H et al. Hum Nutr Clin Nutr 1986;40(6):441–50
3. Ritchie CD, Singkamani R. Hum Nutr Clin Nutr 1986;40(1):75–80
4. Lee JE et al. Cancer Epidemiol Biomarkers Prev 2009;18:1197–1202

such as anxiety, irritability, mild depression, bloating and tender breasts.

Dose

The old EU RDA for vitamin B6 was 2 mg per day. The newly set EU RDA has decreased to 1.4 mg. The UK RNI for adults aged 19–50 years is 1.4 mg for men, and 1.2 mg for women. In general, the more protein you eat, the more vitamin B6 you need.

The upper safe level for long-term use from supplements is suggested as just 10 mg. Higher doses of 50–200 mg may be used short term under medical supervision for the treatment of carpal tunnel syndrome and premenstrual syndrome.

Side effects

There is some evidence that prolonged high doses may cause reversible nerve symptoms such as pins and needles (sensory neuropathy)[1].

High doses may case headache, acne, skin reactions, nausea, abdominal pain, loss of appetite and abnormal liver function tests.

Vitamin B12

Vitamin B12, also known as cobalamin, is a water-soluble substance that contains cobalt – the only known requirement for this metal in the human body. Unlike most water-soluble vitamins, B12 can be stored in the liver with enough stocks to last for several years.

Food sources of vitamin B12 include liver, kidney, oily fish – especially sardines – red meats, white fish, eggs and dairy products. Around 20 per cent of the B12 present in these foods leaches out into juices during cooking.

Vegetarians, especially vegans, are at risk of vitamin B12 deficiency since it is mainly found in animal based foods. The only plant products to contain consistent amounts of vitamin B12 are blue-green algae and fortified breakfast cereals. Vitamin B12 is also made by bacteria, and supplements containing B12 derived from bacterial and algae sources are available for use by vegetarians.

Vitamin B12 is absorbed in the lower part of the small intestine,

1. Bendich A, Cohen M. Ann NY Acad Sci 1990;585:321–330

but only if a special carrier protein, intrinsic factor, is present. Intrinsic factor is made by the acid-producing parietal cells in the stomach lining. Vitamin B12 deficiency can develop if insufficient intrinsic factor is produced, or if a bowel disease such as Crohn's disease, ulcerative colitis, or coeliac disease affects absorption in the lower intestines. Lack of intrinsic factor can occur as a result of auto-immune attack, in which the body makes antibodies against the factor or the cells producing it, and when ageing parietal cells slow their production of both stomach acid and intrinsic factor. Lack of stomach acid (hypochlorhydria) is common in later life and results in reduced absorption of several nutrients, including other B vitamins.

Interestingly, absorption of vitamin B12 (attached to intrinsic factor) is dependent on the presence of calcium, and some evidence suggests that calcium supplements can improve vitamin B12 absorption[1].

Lack of vitamin B12 has also been associated with infection of the stomach with *Helicobacter pylori*, a motile form of bacteria that burrows into the stomach lining to trigger inflammation. Although it doesn't cause symptoms in everyone, infection can lead to peptic ulceration and has also been linked with gastric cancer.

Vitamin B12 is needed together with another vitamin, folic acid, when new genetic material (DNA) is made during cell division. It is most needed by cells with a rapid turnover such as those lining the gut (shed every three days on average), cells in hair follicles and in the marrow, which is continually producing new red blood cells.

Benefits

Homocysteine: A raised blood level of the amino acid, homocysteine, is now recognized as an important risk factor for developing coronary heart disease and stroke. Homocysteine is formed in the body from the breakdown of the dietary amino acid, methionine. Normally, its level is tightly controlled by three different enzymes that convert homocysteine to cysteine – a safe end product used by cells for growth. When certain B vitamins are lacking,

---

1. Bauman WA et al. Diabetes Care 2000; 23;9:1227–31

including vitamin B12, this conversion cannot occur so efficiently and potentially harmful levels of homocysteine build up in the circulation. Taking supplements of B group vitamins (folic acid plus B12) has been shown to lower a raised homocysteine level – especially in older people. Data from 25 trials show that taking 400 mcg vitamin B12 per day can reduce homocysteine levels by 7 per cent, in addition to the effects of folic acid supplements[1].

Congenital defects: Together with folic acid, vitamin B12 seems to protect against some congenital developmental disorders (neural tube defects) such as spina bifida, increasing the level of protection that occurs when taking folic acid supplements alone.

Retinopathy: Raised levels of homocysteine are linked with an increased risk of proliferative retinopathy in people with diabetes[2]. In one early study, vitamin B12 (100 mcg added to insulin injections) was given to 15 people with retinopathy associated with Type 1 diabetes[3]. A year later, the retinopathy was said to have disappeared in seven of the subjects. Similar results were also reported in another study from the same year[4]. Macular degeneration – another leading cause of blindness – is also associated with raised homocysteine levels and taking supplements containing folic acid and vitamin B12 may protect against this, too.

Deficiency
Low vitamin B12 levels are common in the elderly both because of reduced dietary intake and reduced absorption from the gut (malabsorption) linked with reduced production of hydrochloric acid in the stomach.

Lack of vitamin B12 causes production of cells that are larger than they should be. In the case of red blood cells, this leads to a particular form of anaemia known as pernicious anaemia. As this creeps up slowly, symptoms are often not recognized until it is

1. Homocysteine lowering trialists' collaboration: Am J Clin Nutr 2005; 82(4):806–12
2. Looker HC et al. Diabetologia 2003; 46;6:766–72
3. Kornerup T, Strom L. Acta Paediatr 1958; 47:646–51
4. Cameron AJ, Ahern GJ. Br J Ophthalma1 1958; 42:686–93

advanced. People with other auto-immune conditions such as Type 1 diabetes, and auto-immune thyroid disease, have a higher chance of developing pernicious anaemia than usual.

Vitamin B12 is also needed for healthy nerve function and if not recognized and treated, deficiency can damage nerves in the spinal cord, leading to a rare condition known as sub-acute, combined degeneration of the cord.

Other symptoms that may be due to vitamin B12 deficiency include a smooth, sore tongue, tiredness, exhaustion, menstrual disorders, numbness, tingling, trembling, clumsiness, difficulty walking, especially in the dark when you can't see where you are going, poor memory, lack of concentration, confusion and depression.

Because the symptoms are so variable, vitamin B12 deficiency should be considered in all spinal cord, nerve and psychiatric disorders. Many people who are lacking in B12 do not develop obvious symptoms for several years, however.

B12 is needed to make antibodies after vaccination, or infections and, in people who are HIV positive, those with the highest levels of B12 seem to progress to AIDS more slowly than those whose levels are low.

Dose

The old EU RDA for vitamin B12 was 1 mcg per day. The newly set EU RDA has more than doubled to 2.5 mcg. The UK RNI for adults aged 19–50 years is 1.5 mcg for both men and women. The upper safe level for long-term use from supplements is suggested as 2000 mcg (2 mg).

Although vitamin B12 supplements to treat pernicious anaemia are traditionally given as regular injections, it can be given sublingually in very high doses. Absorption through the mucus membranes of the mouth overcomes the body's inability to produce intrinsic factor or to absorb B12 in the lower intestines, which is the root cause of this condition.

Vitamin B12 supplements are best taken together with folic acid (folate) supplements.

Excess

As excess B12 is excreted in the urine, there are no known toxic side effects from high doses. Itchy rash and diarrhoea have been reported, however.

Vitamin C

Vitamin C (ascorbic acid or 2-oxo-L-threo-hexono-1,4-lactone-2,3-enediol) is a water-soluble vitamin which cannot be stored in the body, so a regular intake is essential. Vitamin C is an important antioxidant in all body tissues, and is needed for at least 300 metabolic reactions including the production of collagen, a major structural protein in the body. It is necessary for proper growth and repair and for healthy skin, bones, teeth and reproduction. It is also involved in the metabolism of stress hormones. Some evidence suggests that vitamin C acts as a natural antihistamine and may help to damp down allergic reactions. It also has anti-viral and anti-bacterial actions and is used to treat or prevent common colds and influenza.

Perhaps the most important role of vitamin C is as an antioxidant. It is also vital for regenerating other antioxidants, such as vitamin E. Studies show that men and women with the highest dietary intakes of vitamin C have a lower risk of developing coronary heart disease and stroke. It also protects genetic material from oxidation and mutation and may also help to protect against cancer.

Another useful role for vitamin C is its ability to increase absorption of dietary iron. People taking iron supplements for anaemia should ideally wash down their tablets with a glass of fresh orange juice.

Most animals make their own vitamin C, but humans and other primates lack the enzyme (L-gulonolactone oxidase) needed for its synthesis. The goat, for example, which weighs around the same as a man, normally produces between 2 and 13 g of vitamin C per day and synthesis dramatically increases during times of physical stress and illness. Quite why we humans have either lost or never acquired the ability to synthesize our vitamin C requirements remains one of the greatest mysteries of human biochemistry. It is thought to have resulted from a genetic accident millions of years ago. As a result, some scientists have suggested that we all suffer from a genetic disease, named hypoascorbaemia, of which the final and potentially fatal result is scurvy. This genetic defect also increases our risk of a number of other common illnesses such as viral infections, raised cholesterol levels, coronary heart disease and cancer as well as reducing our ability to cope with the effects of stress.

Because our primitive ancestors ate a vegetarian diet full of vitamin C-rich plants such as purslane (just 100 g of which contained 12 mg vitamin E, 27 mg vitamin C and 2 mg betacarotene), their vitamin C intake was much higher than ours and has been estimated at 392 mg a day. This high dietary intake meant that humans were able to survive since the vitamin C they failed to make was adequately replaced by their diet. Vitamin C is found in most fruit and vegetables including citrus, berries, blackcurrants, capsicum peppers, kiwi fruit and green leafy vegetables.

Benefits

Diabetes complications: When blood glucose levels are raised, some glucose is converted to a substance called sorbitol inside cells. The amount of sorbitol that builds up in cells contributes to the complications of diabetes, especially those affecting the eyes (retinopathy, cataracts) and nervous system (peripheral neuropathy). Vitamin C reduces sorbitol formation by blocking one of the enzymes needed to convert glucose to sorbitol (aldose reductase). Taking 1 g vitamin C per day for just two weeks can reduce the amount of sorbitol within red blood cells by over 12 per cent[1], while taking 2 g vitamin C daily reduces the build-up of sorbitol in red blood cells by 44.5 per cent in people with diabetes[2]. Smaller amounts of vitamin C supplements (100 or 600 mg daily) can normalize red blood cell sorbitol levels in people with diabetes within 30 days, and this reduction is not affected by how good the person's diabetic control is[3]. Vitamin C has been shown to improve blood vessel dilation and blood flow in people with diabetes[4]. This is an important finding as blood flow is often impaired in people with diabetes – probably due to free radical damage and inactivation of the mechanism that dilates blood vessels[5]. This mechanism involves nitric oxide, raising the possibility that vitamin C may act in a similar way to another drug that acts through nitric oxide – sildenafil (Viagra). Whether or not

1. Wang H et al. Diabetes Res Clin Pract 1995;28:1–8
2. Vinson JA, Staretz ME, Bose P, et al. Diabetes 1989; 38:1036–41
3. Cunningham JJ et al. J Am Coll Nutr 1994;13:344–50
4. Timimi FK et al. J Am Coll Cardiol 1998;31(3):552–557
5. Ting HH et al. J Clin Invest 1996;97:22–8

vitamin C supplements are helpful for men with diabetes who have erectile dysfunction remains to be seen.

Glucose control: In a trial involving 40 people with Type 2 diabetes and raised cholesterol levels, taking vitamin C (1 g daily) for four months significantly improved glucose tolerance, lowered total and LDL-cholesterol levels and decreased free radical damage. The percentage increase in plasma vitamin C was directly related to the percentage fall in LDL-cholesterol and the authors concluded that vitamin C has an important role to play in management of Type 2 diabetes[1]. Similar improvements in glucose control and cholesterol have also been shown in other studies[2].

Cholesterol: As an antioxidant, vitamin C protects cholesterol in the blood stream from oxidation. As only oxidized cholesterol is linked with hardening and furring up of the arteries (atherosclerosis), vitamin C has the potential to help protect against heart attack and possibly stroke. Taking 500 mg vitamin C per day for 12 months can significantly lower cholesterol levels and triglyceride levels compared with placebo[3]. The researchers thought that vitamin C helped to improve the liver's ability to flush cholesterol from the body through its conversion into bile acids.

Cardiovascular disease: Lack of vitamin C is now recognized as a risk factor for developing heart attack or stroke[4]. In a study involving over 6,600 men and women, those with the highest vitamin C levels enjoyed a 27 per cent lower risk of coronary heart disease and a 26 per cent lower risk of stroke than those with low levels[5]. A meta-analysis of the results of 15 trials suggests that people with the highest intake of vitamin C, from both diet and supplements, have a 16 per cent lower risk of coronary heart disease than those with the lowest intakes[6]. Vitamin C may also play a role

1. Paolisso G et al. J Am Coll Nutr 1995;14:387–92
2. Eriksson J, Kohvakka A. Ann Nutr Metab 1995;39:217–23
3. Ginter E et al. Int J Vitam Nutr Res 1978;48:368–73
4. Gale CR et al. BMJ 1995; 310:1563–1566
5. Simon JA et al, Epidemiology1998; 9(3):316–21
6. Ye Z, Song H. Eur J Cardiovasc Prev Rehabil 2008;15(1):26–34

in preventing symptoms in those with existing coronary artery disease[1] and low levels are significantly linked with an increased risk of developing angina[2]. A recent study in Norfolk, UK, involving over 19,000 adults aged 45–79 years found that circulating levels of vitamin C were inversely related to death from all causes over the four year study period[3]. New findings suggest that vitamin C is linked with levels of fibrinogen – a circulating protein that increases the likelihood of blood clots. The researchers concluded that even relatively small increases in vitamin C concentrations may have a measurable effect on risk of a fatal heart attack; for example, eating an orange a day was estimated to reduce the risk of coronary heart disease by as much as 10 per cent[4].

Cataracts: Vitamin C is an important antioxidant in the eye, and the level of vitamin C in the lens is 60 times that found in the circulation. In one study, those taking 300 mg vitamin C daily were 70 per cent less likely to develop cataracts than similar patients not taking supplements[5]. The Nurses Health Study found that 60 per cent of early cataracts occurred in women who had not taken vitamin C supplements. Those who had taken vitamin C for at least ten years had a 45 per cent decreased risk of developing cataracts than those who had not taken supplements[6]. Interestingly, those not taking vitamin C supplements still had a naturally high dietary intake of vitamin C averaging 130 mg – twice as high as the EU RDA – but only those taking additional vitamin C seemed to obtain a benefit. These findings were confirmed when women who took vitamin C supplements for at least ten years were found to have a 77 per cent lower risk of early lens opacities, and an 83 per cent lower risk of moderate lens opacities compared with women who did not use vitamin C. These studies suggest that long-term consumption of vitamin C supplements may substantially reduce the development of age-related cataracts[7].

1. Jacob RA. Nutr Rev 1998;56(11):334–7
2. Riemersma RA et al. Lancet 1991;337:1–5
3. Khaw K-T et al. Lancet 2001;357:657–63
4. Khaw K-T, Woodhouse P. BMJ 1995; 310:1559–63
5. Robertson J McD et al, Am J Clin Nutr 1991; 53:346S–51S
6. Hankinson S et al BMJ 1992; 305:335–9
7. Jacques PF et al. Am J Clin Nutr 1997; 66(4)911–6

Pneumonia: A meta-analysis of data from three trials involving 2,335 people found a statistically significant (80 per cent or greater) reduction in the incidence of pneumonia in military recruits and boys[1]. Some evidence also suggested a beneficial treatment effect in those developing symptoms.

Colds: Vitamin C is one of the most popular supplements to prevent or treat the common cold. It has an anti-viral action which suppresses the activation of viral genes. It seems the virus cannot survive in cells containing high dose vitamin C so symptoms are less likely to develop. Studies involving school children and students[2] suggest that vitamin C can reduce the risk of catching a cold by as much as 30 per cent. For men doing heavy physical exercise, and who are more likely to develop respiratory infections, vitamin C supplements have also been shown to provide protection. Military troops under training and participants in a 90 km running race were found to have half the risk of developing cold symptoms[3] when taking 600 mg to 1 g vitamin C per day. Researchers also believe that the powerful antioxidant action of vitamin C also mops up inflammatory chemicals produced during a viral infection, so that supplements can improve symptoms and hasten healing[4] even after a cold develops. Some researchers found that vitamin C at a dose of 1–6 g daily reduced the duration of a cold by over 20 per cent[5]. A meta-analysis of data from 30 trials involving 11,350 people showed a consistent treatment benefit representing a reduction in the duration of a cold by 8 per cent for adults and 13.6 per cent for children[6]. They found no evidence to support its effect in prevention of colds.

Herpes simplex: Vitamin C plus bioflavonoids (1800 mg complex) has also been shown to reduce the duration of recurrent Herpes simplex (cold sore) attacks by over half. The sores of those taking

1. Hemila H, Louhiala P. Cochrane Database Syst Rev 2007;(1):CD005532
2. Hemila H. Br J Nutr 1997;77(1) 59–72
3. Hemila H. Int J Sports Med 1996;17(5) 379–83
4. Hemila H. Br J Nutr 1992; 67(1)3–16
5. Hemila H, Herman ZS. J Am Coll Nutr 1995;14(2)116–23
6. Douglas RM et al. Cochrane Database Syst Rev 2007;(4):CD000980

the vitamin C/bioflavonoids healed within 4.5 days compared with 10 days for those taking inactive placebo[1].

Cancer: Some, but not all, studies suggest that people with the highest intakes of vitamin C are least likely to develop certain cancers, including breast, cervical, colorectal, oesophageal, lung, pancreatic, prostate, salivary gland, and stomach cancers, and leukaemia and non-Hodgkin's lymphoma and if already diagnosed may improve the prognosis – especially when vitamin C supplements are taken together with vitamin E and mineral selenium[2]. However, a meta-analysis of data from 38 studies found scant evidence that vitamin C prevents cancer or benefits survival[3].

Macular degeneration: A recent prospective study indicated that an above-median intake of antioxidants, including vitamin C (114 mg per day) was associated with a 35 per cent reduced risk of age-related macular degeneration during an average follow-up of eight years in people older than 55 years (independent of supplement use).

Gallstones: Vitamin C affects the breakdown of cholesterol to bile acids, and it seems that in women a good vitamin C intake may reduce the risk of symptomatic gallstones. A similar relationship was not found for men, however[4].

Gout: Taking 500 mg vitamin C per day significantly reduces serum uric acid levels to reduce the risk of gout[5]. A study involving almost 47,000 males measured vitamin C levels every four years for 20 years. Compared with men who had vitamin C intakes of less than 250 mg per day, those with intakes of 500–999 mg per day were 17 per cent less likely to develop gout; those with intakes of 1000–1499 mg per day were 34 per cent less likely to develop gout, and those with intakes of 1500 mg per day or more were 45 per cent less likely to experience gout[6].

1. Terezhalmy GT et al. Oral surgery, Oral medicine, Oral Pathology 1978; 45:56–62
2. Head KA. Altern Med Rev 1998 3 (3) p174–86
3. Coulter ID et al. J Gen Intern Med 2006;21(7):735–44
4. Simon JA, Hudes ES. Am J Public Health 1998;88(8)1208–12
5. Huang HY et al. Arthritis Rheum 2005;52(6):1843–7
6. Choi HK et al. Arch Intern Med 2009;169(5):502–7

Asthma: Increased vitamin C intakes are associated with improved lung function. Conversely, low intakes of vitamin C seem to be as harmful for lung function as smoking cigarettes for five years[1]. Some studies suggest that taking vitamin C for two weeks can reduce asthma attacks by a quarter compared with those taking placebo. As a result, it can reduce the dose of corticosteroids needed to control asthma symptoms. It also appears to protect against exercise-induced asthma when taken 30 minutes beforehand. However, a recent meta-analysis of data from nine studies, involving 330 people, concluded that there is insufficient evidence to recommend vitamin C in the treatment of asthma[2]. Further trials are needed.

Osteoporosis: Vitamin C (ascorbic acid) is essential for the synthesis of collagen, a major structural protein that makes up 30 per cent of bone volume. Vitamin C is therefore vital for healthy growth and repair of all tissues, including bone. Vitamin C has been found to stimulate bone-building cells (osteoblasts), enhance vitamin D activity and boost calcium absorption from the gut. Not surprisingly, therefore, researchers have found evidence of a positive association between dietary vitamin C intake and bone density at the hip[3]. This link seems to be strongest in women aged 55–64 years who have used vitamin C supplements for at least ten years and among women who have never used oestrogen hormone replacement therapy[4].

Osteoarthritis: Vitamin C may reduce the risk of cartilage loss and disease progression in people with osteoarthritis. Those with medium to high intakes of vitamin C had a 70 per cent lower risk of cartilage loss, 70 per cent lower risk of developing knee pain and – for those who already had knee disease – a three-fold reduction in knee osteoarthritis progression[5].

Helicobacter pylori is a motile bacterium that lives in the stomach of at least 20 per cent of the younger population and 50 per cent of

1. Britton JR et al. Am J Respir Crit Care Med 1995;151(5):1383–7
2. Kaur B et al. Cochrane Database Syst Rev 2009;21(1):CD000993
3. Wang MC et al. Osteoporos Int 1997;7(6):533–8
4. Leveille SG et al. J Epidemiol Community Health 1997;51(5):479–85
5. 1995 American College of Rheumatology meeting

those aged over 50. High levels of vitamin C are found in the normal stomach lining and gastric juices, and it is thought that it may play a protective antioxidant role during digestion – especially in protecting against stomach cancer[1]. H. pylori increases the risk of indigestion and peptic ulcers by burrowing into the mucous lining of the stomach and exposing the stomach wall to acid attack. It survives exposure to gastric acid by producing an enzyme, urease, which converts urea into a bubble of ammonia gas. This alkaline bubble coats the bacterium and protects it. At the same time, the ammonia acts as another irritant to inflame the stomach wall. H. pylori is now known to be the main cause of gastritis, peptic ulcer disease and stomach cancer. Researchers have found that vitamin C levels are significantly lower in the gastric juices of people with H. pylori infection compared with those who are H. pylori negative, and this finding is reversed when infection is eradicated with antibiotics[2]. This suggests that vitamin C is consumed locally by the H. pylori bacteria and/or the inflammatory process/free radicals associated with the infection. High doses of vitamin C have now been shown to inhibit the growth of H. pylori[3]. Research suggests that adding 500 mg vitamin C to the eradication regime (triple therapy) can improve eradication rates and reduce the dose of antibiotic needed.

Hay fever: Vitamin C has an antihistamine action and, in a small study, was found to reduce bronchial responsiveness to inhaled histamine at a dose of 2 g. There is some evidence that vitamin C may help to reduce symptoms linked with pollen allergy, but this has not been well studied.

Sperm health: Vitamin C is actively secreted into semen and is present at concentrations eight times higher than those found in the blood. It plays two roles in protecting sperm health – it stops sperm from clumping together and also acts as a powerful antioxidant to protect the genetic material (DNA) of sperm against the oxidizing reactions of free radicals. Both of these actions are important in

1. Schorah CJ. Acta Gastroenterol Belg 1997;60(3):217–19
2. Banerjee S et al. Gut 1994;35(3):317–22
3. Zhang HM et al. Cancer 1997;80(10):1897–903

maintaining sperm quality and the power to fertilize an egg. Taking 1 g vitamin C twice a day for two months has been shown to increase average sperm count from 14.3 x10^6 per ml to 32.8 x 10^6 per ml; the number of sperm with normal morphology from 43 per cent to 66.7 per cent and the number of sperm with normal motility from 31.2 per cent to 60.1 per cent[1].

Skin damage: When ultraviolet light strikes the skin, it generates free radicals which set up an inflammatory reaction known as helio-dermatitis. This damages skin structures and interferes with normal cell division. As a result of this 'photo-ageing', skin cells are unable to regenerate normally and collagen fibres – which make up 70 per cent of skin structure – become matted, branched and twisted. Skin that has been exposed to the sun over a long period of time eventually becomes dry, inelastic, thickened, yellow, scaly, mottled and wrinkled with a coarse, pebbly, leathery, rough texture. Skin exposure to solar ultra-violet radiation also increases the risk of skin cancer. Vitamin C protects skin during UV exposure to reduce the sunburn effect when taken at a dose of 2 g per day (plus 1000 IU vitamin E)[2]. This is not a sunscreen effect as vitamin C does not absorb light in the UV wavelength. Vitamin C is thought to help to neutralize free radicals as well as being needed for the production of new collagen. It is now added to many cosmetic creams designed to slow the visible signs of skin ageing.

Dementia: Alzheimer's disease may result from oxidation of fatty proteins (lipoproteins) in the brain which causes brain cells to die[3]. By acting as an antioxidant and reducing free radical damage to brain cells, vitamin C may help to reduce the risk of senile dementia, including Alzheimer's disease. When vitamin C intake of over 1,000 elderly individuals was assessed, taking vitamin C supplements was associated with a lower risk of severe cognitive impairment even when other factors such as age, sex, smoking and education were taken into account, which suggests that vitamin C is protective[4].

1. Akmal M et al. J Med Food 2006;9(3):440–2

2. Eberlein-Konig B et al. J Am Acad Dermatol 1998;38:45–48

3. Draczynska-Lusiak B, Doung A, Sun AY. Mol Chem Neuropathol 1998;33(2):139–48

4. Paleologos M et al. Am J Epidemiol 1998;148(1):45–50

Deficiency

Mild deficiency of vitamin C is associated with non-specific symptoms (sometimes known as pre-scurvy syndrome) such as frequent colds and other infections, lack of energy, weakness and muscle and joint pain.

More severe lack of vitamin C leads to scurvy. A minimum daily intake of 10 mg vitamin C is needed to prevent this, although 20 mg per day is needed for normal wound healing. In scurvy, reduced conversion of the amino acid proline to hydroxyproline (an important component of collagen) results in:

- Poor wound healing
- Dry, rough, scaly skin
- Broken thread veins in skin around hair follicles
- Easy bruising
- Scalp dryness
- Misshapen, tangled, corkscrew, brittle hair
- Hair loss
- Dry, fissured lips
- Inflamed, spongy, bleeding gums and loose teeth
- Bleeding skin, eyes and nose
- Weakness.

Dose

The old EU RDA was 60 mg per day The newly set EU RDA has increased to 80 mg. The UK RNI for adults aged 19–50 years is just 40 mg, but this is widely regarded as out-dated. An expert scientific panel in the US has suggested that the intake needed to meet the requirement of half the healthy individuals in a population is 100 mg per day, with a safety margin giving a proposed daily amount of 120 mg per day. The recommendation is 100 mg per day in Austria, Germany and Switzerland. The upper safe level for long-term use from supplements is suggested as 1000 mg.

Absorption and metabolism of vitamin C varies depending on the amount consumed. At intakes of up to 200 mg per day as a single dose, absorption of vitamin C is almost complete through an active transport process. At single doses of over 500 mg, it is also absorbed through a process of diffusion, but efficiency of absorption declines so that only half of a 1.5g dose is absorbed (i.e. 750 mg), and only

16 per cent of a 12 g dose (i.e. just under 2 g is absorbed).

Metabolism of vitamin C also decreases at higher doses, while urinary reabsorption becomes saturated so that more vitamin C is excreted as intakes increase. To achieve optimum vitamin C absorption and retention, supplements are best taken spread over several doses per day.

Excess

Large doses of vitamin C have been associated with increased formation of oxalate kidney stones. However, in the Harvard Prospective Health Professional Follow-Up Study of 1997, those in the highest 20 per cent of vitamin C intake (higher than 1500 mg per day) were found to have a lower risk of kidney stones than those in the lowest 20 per cent of vitamin C intake. It is therefore accepted that high doses of vitamin C do not increase the risk of calcium oxalate kidney stones in normal individuals[1]. Those known to be recurrent stone formers, however, and people with renal failure who have a defect in ascorbic acid or oxalate metabolism, should restrict daily vitamin C intakes to approximately 100 mg.

High doses can cause indigestion and have a laxative effect. These are largely due to the acidity of vitamin C itself and are not a sign of toxicity. When vitamin C enters the alkaline environment of the lower digestive tract, so called Acid Rejection Syndrome occurs which triggers inflammation, flatulence, diarrhoea and discomfort as well as reduced vitamin C absorption. Some people are more sensitive to the acidity of vitamin C than others. If indigestion occurs, it can usually be overcome by taking buffered vitamin C, or the non-acidic form, ester-C. Timed-release supplements may also help.

Note
- If you are taking high doses of vitamin C and you need to have a urine test inform your doctor that you are taking supplements as it can affect laboratory results.
- Some urine test kits used by diabetics are also affected by high dose vitamin C – use a kit that is not affected.
- High-dose vitamin C may mask the presence of blood in stool tests – inform your doctor if you are advised to have one of these.
- People with iron-storage disease (haemochromatosis) should only take vitamin C supplements under medical advice.

1. Gerster H. Ann Nutr Metab 1997;41(5):269–82

- Recurrent stone formers and sufferers of renal failure who have a defect in ascorbic acid or oxalate metabolism should restrict daily vitamin C intakes to approximately 100 mg.
- Anyone who is taking a very high-dose supplement and needs to reduce their vitamin C intake should do this slowly over a few weeks rather than stopping suddenly, in order to avoid a so-called 'rebound scurvy' effect. A sudden reduction in blood vitamin C concentration means that enzymes activated by high levels of vitamin C are suddenly deprived of the extra vitamin C they need to work properly, and this can produce temporary symptoms of vitamin C deficiency.

Vitamin D

Vitamin D is a fat-soluble vitamin that occurs in five different forms, the most important of which are vitamin D2 (ergocalciferol), derived from plants, and vitamin D3 (cholecalciferol), derived from animals. These two forms are collectively known as calciferol. Food sources of vitamin D3 include oily fish, fish liver oils, animal liver, fortified margarine, eggs, butter and fortified milk.

We can make some vitamin D3 in our skin from a reaction between 7-dehydrocholesterol and UVB ultraviolet sunlight (290–15 nm spectrum). This only occurs when the UV index is greater than 3 which, in the UK, is achieved during spring and summer. We cannot produce enough vitamin D to meet our needs during autumn and winter, when our blood levels of vitamin D naturally tend to fall.

Vitamin D is a prohormone. After it is consumed in the diet, or made in the skin, it enters the circulation (mostly bound to vitamin D binding protein) and is converted into the active hormone, calcitriol (1α,25-cholecalciferol), within kidney cells. Some conversion is also thought to occur in prostate, colon, skin and bone cells.

Calcitriol has a number of actions in the body. It:

- Regulates the absorption of calcium and phosphorus in the small intestines
- Promotes the reabsorption of calcium in the kidneys so less is lost in urine

- Reduces the secretion of parathyroid hormone from the parathyroid glands (to reduce the release of calcium from bones)
- Helps to maintain the balance between production and breakdown of bone and joint connective tissues such as collagen and elastin during bone growth and remodelling
- Stimulates the production of new cartilage building blocks (proteoglycans) within joints
- Boosts the activity of immune cells that fight infection and target cancer cells
- Plays a role in brain health
- Plays a role in cardiovascular health.

We can make vitamin D3 in our skin on exposure to sunlight. To balance adequate production of vitamin D against skin cancer risk, the usual advice is to obtain 10 to 15 minutes' sun exposure to face, arms, hands or back, two or three times a week, without sunscreen. Longer exposures do not provide additional benefit, as vitamin D is rapidly degraded by excess UV radiation. Used properly, a sunscreen with a sun protection factor of 8 reduces vitamin D production in the skin by 95 per cent, while SPF15 reduces vitamin D production by 99 per cent. Most people do not apply enough sunscreen, however, and the development of a tan suggests that enough UVB radiation strikes the skin to stimulate production of both melanin (a natural sunscreen produced in response to UV damage) and some vitamin D regardless of sunscreen use.

Lack of vitamin D, due to poor diet and little sun exposure, reduces bone mineralization. This can lead to the deficiency diseases of rickets in children, and osteomalacia in adults. Bone thinning (osteoporosis) in menopausal women is partly regulated by the amount of vitamin D obtained in the diet or from supplements. When vitamin D is in short supply, less calcium is absorbed from the diet and blood levels therefore have to be maintained by leaching calcium from bones. Four out of five people with hip fracture have evidence of vitamin D deficiency. Other conditions that have been linked with a lack of vitamin D include constipation, muscle weakness, increased susceptibility to infections, poor growth, irritability, bone pain, bone deformities (in rickets) and deafness (in osteomalacia).

Benefits

There is renewed interest in the importance of vitamin D to health and the prevention of chronic disease. A meta-analysis of data from 18 clinical trials, involving over 57,000 people found that those taking vitamin D supplements (300–2000 IU daily, average 528 IU) were 7 per cent less likely to die *from any medical cause* during the average follow-up period of 5.7 years[1]. Researchers have also found that, among patients admitted to intensive care units, those who are most sick have the lowest vitamin D levels.

Osteoarthritis: Vitamin D appears to be important for people with osteoarthritis. Some studies have found a three- to four-fold increase in the risk of osteoarthritis progression in those with low vitamin D intakes, compared with people obtaining high intakes[2,3]. A study involving 82 women and 35 men undergoing total hip or knee replacement found that 85 per cent had a vitamin D deficiency[4]. This compares with a background level of around 15 per cent of men and women having a low vitamin D intake, as shown in the UK National Diet and Nutrition Survey of adults aged 19–64. Some evidence suggests that high vitamin D levels may protect against both the development and progression of hip OA, but other studies found no link between vitamin D levels and the risk of joint space narrowing or cartilage loss in people with osteoarthritis of the knee.

Osteoporosis: Vitamin D is important for calcium deposition in bone and for maintaining bone density. A meta-analysis of data from 29 clinical trials, involving almost 64,000 people aged 50 and over, suggests that taking calcium supplements can reduce the risk of bone fracture by 12 per cent, rising to 24 per cent where compliance was high. Treatment effects were best with calcium doses of 1200 mg or more, and with vitamin D doses of 20 mcg (800 IU) or more[5]. A meta-analysis of 12 studies, involving over 42,000 adults, found that taking vitamin D supplements alone reduced the risk of hip fractures by 9 per cent and other non-vertebral fractures by 14 per cent[6]. When they

1. Autier P, Gandini S. Arch Intern Med 2007;167(16):1730–7
2. McAlindon TE et al. Annals Int Med 1996;125:353–9
3. Felson DT et al. Annals Int Med 2000; 133:635–46
4. Breijawi N et al. Eur Surg Res 2009; 42(1):1–10
5. Tang BM et al. Lancet 2007; 370(9588):657–66
6. Bischoff-Ferrari HA et al. Arch Int Med 2009; 169(6):551–561

looked at studies using higher doses of over 10 mcg (400 IU) vitamin D per day the benefits increased, and they concluded that this higher dose could reduce non-vertebral fractures by at least 20 per cent. The lead author later commented that everyone aged 65 and older should take around 20 mcg (800 IU) vitamin D3 per day for bone health benefits.

Cancer: Is caused by uncontrolled growth of cells, which do not stick together properly, or respond to the usual signals from neighbouring cells telling them to self-destruct when they behave abnormally. Vitamin D is believed to bind to receptors in cancer cells and enter the nucleus to improve regulation of gene expression and reduce abnormal proliferation. By improving signalling responses between cells, it has the ability to halt cancer growth. Vitamin D has been shown to reduce growth and division of cancer cells in over 25,000 laboratory studies, and may play a role in reducing the risk of certain cancers, especially those affecting the prostate, colon and breast. Genetic differences in vitamin D receptors may be involved in cancer risk, and women taking 25 mcg (1000 IU) vitamin D daily have been shown to have a lower incidence of cancer over a four year follow-up period[1]. A meta-analysis of data from 17 studies suggests that people with the highest intakes of vitamin D are 11 per cent less likely to develop adenomas and therefore less likely to develop cancer of the colon/rectum than those with the lowest intakes[2]. A study involving more than 34,000 postmenopausal women also suggests that intakes of vitamin D above 20 mcg (800 IU) per day are associated with an 11 per cent lower risk of developing breast cancer compared with women whose intake is less than 10 mcg (400 IU) per day[3]. Other studies have shown no benefit, however, possibly because of the confounding effects of oestrogen hormone replacement therapy used by some women in these trials.

Heart disease: Vitamin D appears to be as important for a healthy heart and circulation as it is for healthy bones. It is involved in calcium metabolism and may help to reduce the amount of calcium laid down

1. Lappe JM et al. Am J Clin Nutr 2007; 85:1586–91
2. Wei MY et al. Cancer Epidemiol, Biomarkers Prev 2008;17:2958–69
3. Robien K et al. Cancer Causes Control 2007; 18:775–82

in artery walls as part of the hardening and furring up process. It may also have effects on blood pressure control through the renin-angiotensin-aldosterone hormone system, or through effects on parathyroid hormone. People with the lowest vitamin D levels were 30 per cent more likely to have high blood pressure and 98 per cent more likely to have diabetes in a study involving 15,000 US adults[1]. Other studies suggest that low vitamin D intakes are a risk factor for heart attack, heart failure and both Type 1 and Type 2 diabetes. Recent data from the Framingham Heart Study also suggest that people with low vitamin D levels are twice as likely to experience a heart attack, stroke or other cardiovascular event over a five year period than those with higher levels. This risk remained even when researchers adjusted for more usual cardiovascular risk factors.

Common cold: A recent study involving over 19,000 adults and adolescents found that those with the lowest vitamin D levels were 40 per cent more likely develop a common cold[2].

Asthma: Children with the lowest vitamin D levels appear to have a higher risk of developing asthma, and of being admitted to hospital with an asthma attack[3].

Brain: Scientists recently discovered that vitamin D receptors are widely distributed throughout the brain, and appear to be directly involved in learning, memory and mood. It may have a protective role in dementia, Parkinson's disease and multiple sclerosis. It has also been suggested that low levels of vitamin D may play a role in the development of long-term (chronic) pain, and those with low levels appear to need twice as much narcotic analgesia for pain-relief than those with lower vitamin D levels.

Teeth: Vitamin D may help to reduce mottling of teeth due to excess intake of fluoride (fluorosis). This was thought to be irreversible, but a study in which children with fluorosis were given vitamin C (500 mg), calcium (250 mg) and vitamin D (20 mcg or 800 IU) daily showed marked reversal of dental mottling.

1. Martins D et al. Arch Int Med 2007;167:1159–65
2. Ginde AA et al. Arch Int Med 2009; 169(4):384–390
3. Brehm JM. Am J Respir Crit Care Med 2009; 179(9):765–771

Skin: Vitamin D also has an important action on skin health and may be effective in treating some forms of psoriasis.

Bacterial vaginosis: Lack of vitamin D has recently been linked with an increased risk of bacterial vaginosis in pregnancy[1], a common bacterial imbalance that can cause increased vaginal discharge. It also increases the risk of miscarriage and premature labour. This finding may be linked to the effects of vitamin D on immune function.

Dose

The EU RDA is 5 mcg (200 IU) per day. No UK RNIs have been set for adults aged 19–50 years, but for adults confined indoors (no sunlight exposure) and for those aged 65 and over, the RNI for vitamin D is 10 (400 IU) mcg per day. Most experts believe that the current RNIs are inadequate, and that in the absence of exposure to sunlight, a minimum intake of 20 mcg (800 IU) is needed per day to maintain healthy blood levels of vitamin D during winter months. Others argue that intakes of 40 mcg per day are needed – irrespective of sun exposure[2].

The upper safe level for long-term use from supplements is suggested as 25 mcg per day. This is generally considered to be too low, however. An upper safe level of 50 mcg has been suggested by the European Food Safety Authority and in the US, while an upper safe level of 80 mcg per day has been set in Australia and New Zealand.

Toxic effects can occur at intakes exceeding 500 mcg per day, including headache, loss of appetite, nausea, vomiting, diarrhoea or constipation, palpitations and fatigue.

Look for supplements supplying vitamin D3 (cholecalciferol) as this appears to be 20–40 per cent more effective in maintaining blood vitamin D levels than the vitamin D2 (ergocalciferol) form.

200 IU vitamin D is equivalent to 5 mcg.

---

1. Bodnar LM et al. J Nutr 2009; 139(9):1157–61
2. Ruxton CHS, Derbyshire E. Nutrition Bulletin 2009;34:185–197

Vitamin E

Vitamin E consists of two groups of fat-soluble compounds, the tocopherols and tocotrienols. Until recently, eight fat-soluble substances were known to have vitamin E activity: four tocopherols (alpha, beta, gamma, delta) and four tocotrienols (alpha, beta, gamma, delta). In 2009, a ninth substance, delta-tocomonoenol, with vitamin E activity was identified in kiwifruit skin.

Alpha-tocopherol is the main source of vitamin E in the European diet, while gamma-tocopherol is the most common form in the American diet. Synthetic alpha-tocopherol (dl-alpha tocopherol) has less biological strength than natural source vitamin E (d-alpha tocopherol) due to the different symmetries of the molecules present. The main food sources of vitamin E include wheatgerm oil, avocado, butter, wholegrain cereals, nuts and seeds. Vitamin E is unstable when frozen – up to 80 per cent of the vitamin E content is destroyed. Heating also destroys around 30 per cent vitamin E content. Fresh raw foods and supplements are therefore the best sources.

Vitamin E is antioxidant protecting cell membranes, nerve sheaths, circulating cholesterol molecules, dietary fats and body fat stores from oxidation. It also has a mild anti-inflammatory action. In general, the more polyunsaturated fatty acids you eat, the more vitamin E you need. Vitamin E also has a strengthening effect on muscle fibres to relieve muscle cramps, and boosts immunity (by working together with selenium to increase antibody production).

Vitamin E activity is sometimes expressed in International Units (IU) rather than milligrams. 1 IU = 0.67 mg alpha-tocopherol equivalents or conversely: 1 mg = 1.5 IU.

Research

Glucose control: Vitamin E seems to improve glucose balance. Low dietary intakes have been linked with an increased risk of developing Type 2 diabetes[1]. Double-blind studies show that vitamin E improves glucose tolerance in people with Type 2 diabetes[2,3,4]

1. Salonen JT et al. BMJ 1995; 311(7013):1124–7
2. Bierenbaum ML et al. Nutr Rep Internat 1985;31:1171–80
3. Paolisso G et al. Am J Clin Nutr 1993;57:650–6
4. Paolisso G et al. Diabetes Care 1993;16:1433–7

although it may take three months or more for the benefits of supplementation to become apparent. Studies suggest that at least 800 IU vitamin E is needed for significant improvements in glucose control[1].

Coronary heart disease: Vitamin E protects circulating fats from oxidation, reduces platelet clumping, and has blood thinning and anti-inflammatory effects. It may therefore slow the progression of atherosclerosis. Large prospective trials show a 40 per cent reduction in coronary heart disease rates in both men and women taking vitamin E supplements – risk is lowest in those taking 100 IU (around 67 mg) vitamin E per day for at least two years[2,3]. Vitamin E gained widespread medical acceptance following results of the Cambridge Heart Antioxidant Study (CHAOS) in 1996[4]. Just over 2,000 patients with coronary heart disease were divided into two groups, with half taking vitamin E and half taking placebo for 18 months. Taking high dose vitamin E (at least 400 IU daily) was found to reduce the risk of a heart attack by 77 per cent. A recent meta-analysis of the results of 15 trials suggests that people with the highest intake of vitamin E, from both diet and supplements, have a 24 per cent lower risk of coronary heart disease than those with the lowest intakes[5].

Statins: Statin drugs lower blood levels of fat-soluble vitamin E by as much as 17 per cent[6]. As a result of reduced CoQ10 and reduced vitamin E levels, LDL-cholesterol is less able to withstand oxidative stress in people taking a statin[7]. If you are taking a statin, it's worth ensuring that your supplement regime includes vitamin E as well as co-enzyme Q10 (see page 104).

Brain function: By protecting brain cells from oxidation, high levels of vitamin E are also strongly associated with better cognitive scores

1. Duntas L et al. Curr Ther Res 1996;57:682–90
2. Stampfer MJ et al. N Engl J Med 1993;328:1444–1449
3. Rimm EB et al. N Eng J Med 1993;328:1450–1456
4. Stephens NG et al. Lancet 1996;347:781–785
5. Ye Z, Song H. Eur J Cardiovasc Prev Rehabil 2008; 15(1):26–34
6. Colquhoun DM et al. Eur J Clin Invest 2005;35(4):251–8
7. Palomaki A et al. FEBS Lett 1997; 410(2–3):254–8

compared with those having the lowest vitamin E intakes[1].

Osteoarthritis: A dietary analysis of 640 people with ostearthritis of the knee found reduced risk of OA progression with increasing vitamin E intakes in males[2]. Another study involving 56 people with OA found that taking 400 mg vitamin E (d-alpha-tocopherol) per day for six weeks reduced pain at rest, pain on movement and the need for painkillers, compared with those taking inactive placebo[3].

Cataracts: People with the highest dietary intake of vitamin E have a lower risk of developing cataracts severe enough to need extraction compared to those with the lowest intakes[4,5]. A study involving 1,380 people attending an ophthalmology outpatient clinic found that regular use of multivitamin and antioxidant supplements decreased the risk of developing cataracts by 37 per cent, with dietary intake of vitamin E, among other nutrients, decreasing the risk[6]. Other studies using high dose vitamin E have not shown a benefit, however, most likely because of the short duration of these trials.

Deficiency

Lack of vitamin E has a harmful effect on the nervous system and can produce symptoms such as lack of energy, lethargy, poor concentration, irritability, muscle weakness and poor co-ordination. In severe, long-term lack (such as that due to malabsorption) serious effects such as blindness, dementia and abnormal heart rhythms can occur.

Dose

There is no UK RNI for vitamin E, but intakes above 4 mg for men and above 3 mg for women are thought to be adequate. The old EU RDA for vitamin E was 10 mg per day. The newly set EU RDA has increased to 12 mg. The upper safe level for long-term use from supplements is suggested as 540 mg (800 IU).

Select supplements containing natural source vitamin E (d-alpha

1. Schmidt R et al. J Am Geriat Soc 1998;46:1407–1410
2. McAlindon TE et al. Arthritis Rheumatism 1996; 39(4), 648–56
3. McAlindon T & Felson DT. Annals Rheumatic Dis 1997;56,397–402
4. Tavani A et al. Ann Epidemiol 1996;6;1:41–6
5. Christen WG et al. Arch Ophthalmol 2008;126(1):102–9
6. Leske MC et al. Arch Ophthalmol 1991;109;2:244–51

tocopherol). High dose vitamin E is best taken together with other antioxidants, such as vitamin C, mixed carotenoids and selenium. Adequate supplies of vitamin C in particular are important as this regenerates vitamin E after it has acted as an antioxidant.

Side effects/Safety
High intakes of vitamin E can cause headache, fatigue, gastrointestinal distress, double vision, muscle weakness, but this only usually occurs above doses of 3000 mg daily.

Vitamin K

Vitamin K is a fat-soluble vitamin named after the initial from the German word *koagulation*. Three types of compound have vitamin K activity: phylloquinone (K1), menaquinones (vitamin K2) and menadione (vitamin K3). Ninety per cent of our dietary intake is in the form of vitamin K1, and just 10 per cent in the form of K2. Probiotic bacteria in the gut also produce some vitamin K2 which we can absorb and use.

Dietary sources include cauliflower, broccoli, and dark green leafy vegetables such as spinach and some lettuces which provide more than 100 mcg vitamin K1 per 100 g. Useful amounts are also found in yoghurt (produced by the bacteria present), egg yolk, alfalfa, safflower, rapeseed, soya and olive oils, fish liver oils, liver, tomatoes, meat, potatoes and pulses.

Vitamin K is essential for normal blood clotting. It acts as an essential co-factor for the production of clotting proteins II, VII, IX, X, protein C and protein S in the liver, and is used as an antidote for warfarin. Vitamin K is now also known to play important roles in bone metabolism and cardiovascular health.

Benefits
Neonatal health: A single dose of vitamin K (by injection or orally) is offered to babies after delivery to prevent a condition known as haemorrhagic disease of the newborn. This arises during the first few days of life and causes haemorrhage into the brain due to vitamin K deficiency.

Osteoporosis: Vitamin K is needed for the synthesis of osteocalcin – a calcium-binding protein found in bone matrix. Vitamin K is now recognized as being as important for bone health as the mineral, calcium. Lack of vitamin K has been linked to osteoporosis, and research suggests vitamin K supplements can reduce loss of bone calcium in post-menopausal women by up to 50 per cent and can also strengthen bones that are already weakened. In a meta-analysis of the results from 13 trials, all but one showed a significant protective effect of vitamin K supplements against bone loss. Seven trials showed that vitamin K2 could reduce the risk of vertebral fractures by 60 per cent, hip fractures by 77 per cent and all other non-vertebral fractures by 81 per cent[1]. Vitamin K2 is approved as a treatment for osteoporosis in Japan.

Vitamin K2 has also been shown to improve ostecalcin activity in children. This is important, as there is a growing awareness that maximizing bone strength during childhood can help to prevent osteoporosis in later life.

Atherosclerosis: Vitamin K2 (but not vitamin K1) may reduce the risk of coronary heart disease in older people, especially postmenopausal women. Researchers looking at dietary intakes of over 16,000 women aged 49–70 years found that every 10 mcg increase in dietary vitamin K2 intake is associated with a 9 per cent reduction in the risk of developing coronary heart disease[2].

Diabetes: Vitamin K1 supplements may reduce the development of insulin resistance in older men, and protect against Type 2 diabetes. In a recent study, 355 men and women aged 60–80, who did not have diabetes, received either 500 mcg vitamin K1 per day, or placebo for three years. All were also given calcium and vitamin D supplements. The men taking vitamin K showed significant improvements in insulin sensitivity, but the men receiving placebo, and all the women, continued to show progression of insulin resistance[3]. The mechanism is not clear, but may be linked with the vitamin-K dependent bone protein, osteocalcin, which is thought to

1. Cockayne S et al. Arch Intern Med 2006; 166(12):1256–61
2. Gast CG et al. Nutr Metab Cardiovasc Dis 2009;19(7):504–10
3. Yoshida M et al. Diabetes Care 2008; 31:2092–2096

play a role in glucose metabolism, or with an anti-inflammatory effect of vitamin K.

Deficiency

Symptoms that may be due to lack of vitamin K include prolonged bleeding time, easy bruising, recurrent nose bleeds, heavy periods and diarrhoea.

Dose

There is no UK RNI for vitamin K, but requirements are thought to be around 1 mcg per kilogram of body weight per day. The newly set EU RDA for vitamin K is 75 mcg. The upper safe level for long-term use from supplements is suggested as 1000 mcg (1 mg).

Supplements are usually taken at doses of 25–300 mcg. Higher doses may be suggested for treating osteoporosis. Where possible look for supplements containing vitamin K2 rather than vitamin K1 to also obtain the circulatory benefits.

Best taken with meals for optimum absorption.

Safety

Seek medical advice before taking supplements containing vitamin K if you are taking warfarin treatment (e.g. for a previous blood clotting disorder).

Significant changes to dietary intake of vegetables such as broccoli or cauliflower can also affect blood clotting control in patients on warfarin. You therefore need to maintain a fairly constant intake of these foods to ensure blood clotting control remains stable.

Wheatgrass

Wheatgrass is a green food supplement, similar in action to blue-green algae. Wheatgrass juice is prepared from three-to-four-day-old germinated wheat grain sprouts which are naturally rich in vitamins, minerals, trace elements and enzymes – including the important antioxidant superoxide dismutase. It is said to boost energy levels and immunity, help heal ulcers and to reduce body odours – including bad breath. It is mainly taken for its nutritional benefits, however. According to one estimate, 1 kg fresh wheatgrass juice is nutritionally equivalent to over 20 kg vegetables. Converts tend to grow their own in the kitchen and harvest the grass when it is 6–7 cm high for home-juicing. It needs to be drunk immediately before it oxidizes (e.g. 30 ml plus water to dilute at least 1:1) but it is an acquired taste.

Organically grown, vacuum-dried juice extracts are therefore popular, although purists say that this destroys some enzyme activity.

A dose of around 5 g dried wheatgrass juice is nutritionally equivalent to an average portion of dark-green leafy vegetables such as spinach or kale.

Wild yam
(Dioscorea villosa)

Wild yam is a Mexican vine whose root is rich in steroidal saponins such as diosgenin. Diosgenin was originally used to synthesize the synthetic form of progesterone (norethisterone) used in the first oral contraceptive pills. It is important to realize that wild yam does not contain progesterone, however, although it does seem to have progesterone-like actions and is widely used as a female remedy.

Wild yam acts as a general tonic that is traditionally used to improve mood and general feelings of well-being. It is also known as the colic root as it is used to help relieve painful spasms, including painful periods, uterine contractions during labour and pain due to gallstones. Wild yam is also used to help treat endometriosis.

It has anti-inflammatory actions and is used to treat rheumatoid arthritis and diverticulitis. Laboratory research suggests that it has an antioxidant action that prevents breakdown of fatty molecules in the body (lipid peroxidation) and increases beneficial levels of HDL-cholesterol.

Benefits
Menopause: In a trial 23 women with menopausal symptoms were asked to use a cream containing wild yam, or placebo, for three months. The results suggest that, although wild yam cream is free

from side effects, it appears to have little effect on menopausal symptoms[1].

Dose

Capsules: 250–500 mg once or twice a day.

Excess may cause nausea or diarrhoea.

Yerba maté
(Ilex paraguariensis)

Yerba maté is a tree that only grows in the rain forests of Paraguay. Its leaves are used to make a nutritional supplement rich in vitamins and minerals, especially vitamin C. Missionaries have been said to go for months at a time in the rain forests subsisting only on yerba maté tea made from the tree's leaves, with no ill effects other than some weight loss. The plant must be allowed to dry for at least 12 months before use.

The leaves of yerba maté contain xanthine alkaloids – related to those in coffee and guarana – which increase mental alertness and acuity without side effects of nervousness or sleep disturbance. They may even improve sleep architecture by normalizing the amount of time spent in REM (rapid eye movement) and deep, delta-wave sleep. Because yerba maté promotes a deeper, more relaxing sleep, some users find they actually need less sleep when taking it.

Yerba maté is classed as an adaptogen as it stimulates adrenal gland function to normalize the production of corticosteroids during times of stress. It is mainly used as a general energy boost, overcoming physical exhaustion and mental fatigue, especially when linked with stress. Yerba maté is a calming tonic for anxiety, poor concentration and nervousness, lifting a low mood and relieving headaches, migraine and neuralgia.

Dose

2–3 cups yerba maté tea a day.

---

1. Komesaroff PA et al. Climacteric 2001;4(2):144–50

Note: Yerba maté contains high levels of tannins, so it is best not taken with meals as it may impair the absorption of nutrients.

Yerba maté has been suggested to increase the risk of developing cancers of the mouth and throat[1].

Zinc

Zinc is an important mineral that acts as a co-factor for over 200 metabolic enzymes. It forms an integral part of the enzyme which switches on genes to produce specific proteins in response to hormone triggers. It plays a major role in the sensitivity of the tissues to circulating sex hormones and is vital for growth, sexual maturity and wound healing. Zinc also plays a central role in immunity and helps to protect against infections such as the common cold.

Dietary sources of zinc include red meat, seafood (especially oysters), offal, brewer's yeast, wholegrains (although processing removes most of their mineral zinc), pulses, eggs and cheese.

Low intakes of dietary zinc (less than 5 mg per day) are associated with low testosterone levels and, in some parts of the world, dietary zinc deficiency is common and results in delayed male puberty.

Zinc is so important for sperm health that it is actively concentrated in prostate tissues. Each ejaculate contains around 110 mg zinc per litre – equivalent to around 5 mg per ejaculation. This represents at least a third of a man's daily requirement. Men who are sexually active are therefore more at risk of zinc deficiency than women. Zinc is important for male fertility as it helps to keep mature sperm in a quiet state to prevent premature release of the acrosome enzymes that are needed to drill a hole through the egg during fertilization. Once in the female reproductive tract, where zinc levels are low, sperm become more active and start releasing the enzymes (acrosome reaction) so fertilization can occur. Zinc is also needed to keep the genetic material tightly packed within the sperm head. Men who are zinc deficient may be sub-fertile because their sperm have released their egg-boring enzymes too soon.

---

1. Goldenberg D. Oral Oncol 2002;38(7):646–9

The prostate gland has the highest concentration of zinc in any body tissue. Lack of zinc is associated with an increased risk of prostatitis (inflammation of the prostate gland). Measuring the zinc content of prostate biopsy samples can also help to determine whether or not prostate cancer is present, as prostate cancer cells lose their ability to concentrate zinc so levels are lower than normal if cancer is present.

Benefits

Colds: Zinc can inhibit viral replication. Sucking lozenges containing zinc gluconate stimulates immune cells in the throat to boost local immunity against throat infections. This was first shown in 1984 when sucking lozenges every two hours was shown to reduce the duration of cold symptoms by as much as seven days. Between then and 2004, ten further studies found benefits in some trials, but not in others. This appears to be due to the solubility and bioavailability of the zinc present in each preparation. A meta-analysis of these 11 trials, which assessed the amount of soluble zinc ions released, confirms that zinc lozenges with high zinc bioavailability are effective. The authors suggest using as much as 200 mg zinc on the first day of treatment, and 100–150 mg on following days to obtain seven day reductions in duration of a cold. Lozenges should contain 14.2 mg zinc and sucked at least every two hours while awake[1]. Daily doses of less than 75 mg were described as more like candy than medicine! It seems to be important to start treatment within 48 hours of the onset of symptoms.

Herpes simplex: Zinc has been shown to inhibit replication of Herpes simplex viruses by up to 90 per cent. Among 20 people with more than six episodes of recurrent herpes cold sores per year, taking zinc supplements (22.5 mg twice daily for four months) was shown to more than halve average recurrences to three per year, and to reduce the duration of each episode to an average of 5.7 days[2]. Applying a zinc oxide cream is also effective at shortening duration of sores[3].

1. Eby GA. Bioscience Reports 2004;24(1):23–39
2. Femiano F et al. J Oral Pathol Med 2005;34(7):423–5
3. Godfrey HR et al. Altern Ther Health Med 2001;7(3):49–56

Gastroenteritis: Zinc supplements have been used to treat acute gastroenteritis in children in the third world. A meta-analysis of 18 studies involving 11,180 children under the age of five years, investigated whether or not supplements were also beneficial in Europe where zinc deficiency is less common than in developing countries. Compared with placebo, zinc supplements significantly reduced diarrhoea duration and reduced the risk of diarrhoea lasting for longer than seven days by 30 per cent. There was no significant decrease in stool volume compared with placebo, but the incidence of vomiting was 20 per cent greater with zinc supplements[1]. How zinc reduces diarrhoea is not fully understood but probably relates to its ability to inhibit viral replication.

Respiratory infections: A meta-analysis of data from 17 studies found that children receiving zinc supplements are 20 per cent less likely to develop lower respiratory tract infections and pneumonia than those not taking them[2].

Osteoporosis: Some studies have found that men and women with osteoporosis have blood and bone levels of zinc that are up to 30 per cent lower than in those with healthy bones. However, no trials have investigated whether or not zinc can improve bone mineral mass.

Senses of smell and taste: Lack of zinc is one of the most common causes of loss of the sense of taste (ageusia) and sense of smell (anosmia). This can be tested for by obtaining a solution of zinc sulphate (e.g. 15 mg/5 ml) from a chemist. Swirl a teaspoonful in your mouth; if the solution seems tasteless, zinc deficiency is likely. If the solution tastes furry, of minerals or slightly sweet, zinc levels are borderline, and if it tastes strongly unpleasant, zinc levels are normal. Some people with pica – an odd craving for non-nutritive substances (e.g. coal, soil, paper) – have zinc deficiency, and this should always be checked for.

Anorexia nervosa: Loss of taste occurs in anorexia nervosa and may

1. Patro B et al. Aliment Pharmacol Ther 2008;28(6):713–23
2. Agarwal R et al. Pediatrics 2007;119(6):1120–30

be related to zinc deficiency. Taking zinc supplements has been shown to stimulate appetite and improve food intake in people with anorexia nervosa, and can double the rate of increase in body mass index compared with placebo[1].

Dose

The UK RNI for zinc is 9.5 mg a day for adult males (19–50 years) and 7 mg per day for women. The old EU RDA for zinc was 15 mg per day. The newly set EU RDA has decreased by one third to 10 mg. The upper safe level for long-term use from supplements is suggested as 25 mg per day.

Occasionally higher doses are recommended under medical advice – but need to be taken together with copper at a ratio of 10:1 (e.g. 15 mg zinc:1.5 mg copper).

1. Birmingham CL, Gritner S. Eat Weight Disord 2006;11(4):e109–11

PART 2

A–Z
OF
PROBLEMS AND
SOLUTIONS

Acne

Acne is an inflammatory skin disease associated with oversensitivity of sebaceous (oil) glands to the effects of a male hormone, dihydrotestosterone (DHT). This hormone is produced from the androgen, testosterone, within sebaceous glands that open into hair follicles. These are found on the face, back, chest, groin and outer ear canal. In severe cases, acne may spread down the arms, lower trunk, buttocks and even the upper legs. Sebaceous glands found on hairless skin such as the eyelids and foreskin are unaffected. Although most sufferers are in their teens, one in 20 is in their 30s or 40s.

Oily skin, blackheads and pimples that are characteristic of acne occur as a result of:

- Increased secretion of skin oil (sebum) under the influence of DHT
- Blockage of sebaceous gland ducts by skin cells (keratinocytes) that stick together rather than separating and being shed; this traps oil within the gland to form a blackhead (comedone) – the black colour is due to the skin pigment, melanin, rather than dirt
- Colonization of black heads with the skin bacterium, Propionibacterium acnes; this triggers an inflammatory immune reaction with the development of papules, pustules and nodules.

Acne is linked with nodules, cysts and scarring if not treated properly – always seek medical advice; up to 50 per cent of women with acne beyond their teens have increased circulating levels of testosterone which can usually be treated.

Treatment
Although it is widely claimed that acne is not linked with diet, researchers are now finding increasing evidence that good nutrition can improve symptoms. Diet can influence all three of the factors involved in acne: the production of DHT within oil glands, the

---

Do not take supplements if you are pregnant, breast-feeding, or taking prescribed drugs without first seeking advice from a pharmacist about possible interactions or adverse effects.

'stickiness' of keratinocytes, and the degree of inflammation that results. A healthy, wholefood diet full of fresh fruit and vegetables that supply antioxidant vitamins and minerals should be eaten, including nuts, seeds, oily fish and wholegrain cereals; these contain essential fatty acids (EFAs) that have an anti-inflammatory action.

The effects of DHT are stimulated by a substance called insulin-like growth factor (IGF-1). Levels of IGF-1 rise during puberty, typically around the age of 15 years in girls, and 18 years in boys. Acne is not just an adolescence problem, however, for as many as 54 per cent of women and 45 per cent of men over the age of 25 show some degree of facial acne. Acne symptoms in later life are often linked with being overweight, and increased production of insulin and IGF-1 as a result of following a high-glycaemic diet. The increased secretion of insulin and IGF-1 that is associated with a high-glycaemic diet stimulates proliferation of keratinocytes and also affects testosterone metabolism. Males with acne following a low GI diet for 12 weeks found that the number of acne lesions decreased more than in those on a high GI diet (an average of 25.5 fewer spots versus 12 fewer spots).

Milk contains sugars such as lactose, plus growth factors and hormones that can increase insulin and androgen levels. The effect of milk on the production of insulin and IGF-1 is three times greater than would be expected from its carbohydrate content alone. Research involving over 4,200 boys found that those consuming more than two servings of milk per day were more likely to have acne than those consuming dairy products less than once a week. Similar results were found in a group of over 6,000 adolescent girls. At least one dermatologist now recommends a 'no dairy, low glycaemic' dietary approach to help improve symptoms of acne. More information is available at www.acnemilk.com.

Red meat contains hormone-like substances that may affect DHT levels in body tissues. Cut back on intakes of red meat and eat more fish and vegetables in its place.

Omega-3 fish oils (especially DHA and EPA found in oily fish) are converted in the body into substances (series 3 prostaglandins

---

Do not take supplements if you are pregnant, breast-feeding, or taking prescribed drugs without first seeking advice from a pharmacist about possible interactions or adverse effects.

and series 5 leukotrienes) that reduce inflammation. In contrast, most omega-6 fatty acids (derived from vegetable oils such as sunflower, safflower and corn oils) are converted into substances that promote inflammation. GLA (gammalinolenic acid found in *evening primrose oil*, for example), is one of the few omega-6 fatty acids that has an anti-inflammatory action. An imbalance between intakes of omega-3s and omega-6s has been linked with worsening of symptoms in inflammatory diseases such as asthma and rheumatoid arthritis, and may also play a role in acne symptoms. Omega-3 fish oils (1–3 g daily) will not make your skin more oily.

Although it is often claimed that chocolate makes acne worse, there is actually no evidence that this is the case. In fact, dark chocolate containing at least 72 per cent cocoa solids might be expected to improve symptoms as it is one of the richest dietary sources of anti-inflammatory antioxidants. Dark chocolate provides an extraordinary 103,971 ORAC units per 100 g – over ten times more than is obtained from pomegranates (10,500 ORAC units). NB: Avoid white chocolate which contains few antioxidant and lots of fat and sugar.

Also eat more zinc-rich foods and consider testing for zinc deficiency (*see* **Zinc**). Where zinc deficiency is present, oral *zinc picolinate* supplements can be more effective than antibiotics. These are best taken under the supervision of a nutritional therapist, as extra copper and selenium will also be needed.

Vitamin A is required for healthy skin, and deficiency can lead to scaliness, raised pimply hair follicles and increased susceptibility to acne. Vitamin A supplements therefore sometimes help and, in fact, powerful drugs derived from vitamin A are used to treat severe acne. Antioxidants such as vitamins E (400 IU a day) and C (1000 g a day) help to damp down inflammation, as can grapeseed or pine bark extracts (Pycnogenol®).

Note: Vitamin A should be avoided by women who are pregnant or who are likely to become pregnant.

See also: **Agnus castus, Aloe vera, Biotin, Brewer's yeast, Myrrh, Sarsaparilla, Vitamin A, Vitamin B5, Vitamin B6.**

Adenomyosis

See **Endometriosis**.

Age spots

Age, or 'liver' spots, are the result of a lifetime's accumulation of sun damage. Every time skin is exposed to the sun, it is damaged by ultraviolet rays. This generates free radicals which set up an inflammatory reaction known as heliodermatitis. This inflammation damages skin structures and interferes with normal cell division. Enzymes released during the inflammatory process are also thought to dissolve elastin and collagen fibres leading to premature wrinkles and areas of pigmentation commonly known as age spots. These are most often seen on the backs of the hands, face and neck, and are related to damage from previous sunburn.

Dermatologists estimate that 30–40 per cent of the UK population who are fair-skinned have appreciable photo-damage caused by chronic exposure to sunlight. Studies by the American Academy of Dermatology reveal that by the age of 18 we have already received half of our lifetime's quota of sun damage – much of it while playing outdoors as a child. Always wear sunscreen outdoors with a protection factor of at least SPF16.

Treatment

As an antioxidant, *selenium* provides important skin protection against sun damage, and those with low intakes are most likely to develop age spots and certain types of skin cancer. Taking selenium supplements has been shown to decrease damage of skin cell membranes (lipid peroxidation) following UV exposure. Taking supplements containing selenium *and vitamins A, C and E* showed systemic protection against UV irradiation. The protection was greatest if taken before exposure to UV light.

Creams containing co-enzyme Q10 have been shown to reduce oxidation and wrinkle depth in human skin and to suppress produc-

---

Do not take supplements if you are pregnant, breast-feeding, or taking prescribed drugs without first seeking advice from a pharmacist about possible interactions or adverse effects.

tion of collagenase following UVA irradiation. Researchers suggest that oral *co-enzyme Q10* can also prevent many of the detrimental effects of photoageing.

Pine bark extracts (Pycnogenol®) can be taken both orally and applied to the skin in cosmetic creams for dual benefit. As well as reducing free radical damage, these bind to collagen and elastin in the skin, to protect them from degradation by collagenase and elastase enzymes. It therefore has the potential to improve skin smoothness and elasticity, and to discourage wrinkles. By increasing blood flow through small vessels in the skin it also brightens the complexion, and reduces red blotches.

Over-the-counter fade creams will also help. *See also:* **Vitamin B5**.

Note: Photo-ageing significantly increases the risk of developing skin cancer. Always seek medical advice if any skin lesion starts to get bigger, turns darker, becomes scaly, itchy, weepy, crusts over or scabs without healing, develops a raised, rolled edge or ulcerates.

Alcohol intake – excessive

Current recommendations suggest that men should drink no more than three to four units of alcohol per day, and women no more than two to three units per day. You should also have several alcohol-free days per week so that, overall, men consume no more than 21 units per week, and women no more than 14 units.

The form of alcohol that seems most beneficial to health, in moderation, is red wine, which is a rich source of antioxidant, procyanidin polyphenols. According to experts, the red wines with the highest antioxidant ratings are those made from the Sangiovese grape in Umbria, Italy, from the Tannat grape in the Madiran region of Gascony, France, or from the Cabernet Sauvignan grape in Chile (Vina MontGras).

Wine should ideally be drunk with food rather than on its own, however, as this protects dietary fats from oxidation when levels are at their highest, after a meal.

Do not take supplements if you are pregnant, breast-feeding, or taking prescribed drugs without first seeking advice from a pharmacist about possible interactions or adverse effects.

While a low to moderate intake is beneficial in reducing stress and possible coronary heart disease, excess is harmful to health. Alcohol is metabolized in the liver to acetaldehyde – a poison that can damage liver, brain and heart muscle cells. If alcohol intake remains excessive, fatty degeneration occurs as liver cells drop their normal housekeeping metabolic reactions and work overtime to eliminate alcohol from the body. Because liver enzymes are diverted from their normal tasks to metabolize alcohol, fewer dietary fatty acids are processed and liver cells start to swell from the accumulation of unprocessed globules of fat.

The impaired metabolic reactions inside liver cells generate large numbers of damaging free radicals. This increases the damaging effects of a continued excessive alcohol intake and liver cells accumulate more and more fatty globules so that the liver enlarges and takes on a yellow appearance. If high alcohol intake continues, cirrhosis eventually develops. If you are worried about your alcohol intake, it is important to have a blood test to check liver function.

Treatment
Extracts of *milk thistle* (*Silybum marianum*) – known as silymarin – protect liver cells from the poisonous effects of excess alcohol. They can even improve liver function when cirrhosis is present. By supporting liver function, silymarin helps to maintain levels of one of the liver's own antioxidant enzymes, glutathione, boosting its level by over a third. Silymarin also appears to alter the outer structure of liver cell walls so poisons do not enter so quickly and liver cells are not overwhelmed. Silymarin has also been shown to stimulate liver cell regeneration by increasing the rate at which new proteins are made and by reducing the formation of scar tissue.

The other main remedy for liver health is *globe artichoke* (*Cynara scolymus*). Globe artichoke is related to the milk thistle and has similar liver regenerating and protective properties. Its fleshy leaves contain several unique substances (e.g. cynarin, cynaropicrin, cynaroside) that help to increase bile secretion by over 150 per cent within one hour. Globe artichoke also protects liver cells from toxins

---

Do not take supplements if you are pregnant, breast-feeding, or taking prescribed drugs without first seeking advice from a pharmacist about possible interactions or adverse effects.

such as alcohol, and has a beneficial effect on cholesterol levels. Where milk thistle is used to protect the liver before a heavy night out, globe artichoke is an excellent remedy to take afterwards, helping to reduce hangover effects the morning after. Both can be taken together.

Lactic-acid producing, *probiotic* bacteria (e.g. Lactobacilli, Bifidobacteria) play an important role in liver health. They digest dietary fibre to produce short-chain fatty acids such as propionate, which is absorbed into the circulation and used as an energy source in the liver. Propionate is chemically related to non-steroidal anti-inflammatory painkillers such as ibuprofen, and research suggests it also has an anti-inflammatory effect in the liver. Probiotic bacteria also support the liver by helping to digest a number of dietary and intestinal toxins so the liver is not overwhelmed by them. When people with alcoholic liver disease are given probiotics to improve the balance of healthy intestinal bacteria, their liver function has improved. This is believed to result from reduced gut 'leakiness' and the absorption of fewer bacterial endotoxins into the circulation.

B group vitamins are needed for energy production in liver cells, and for the metabolism of alcohol. A vitamin B complex supplement is therefore a good idea for anyone who drinks alcohol regularly, and is often given by injection to people with alcoholic liver disease who are admitted to hospital.

For those who find it difficult to go without alcohol, the herb kudzu can dramatically decrease alcohol cravings. *Kudzu* (*Pueraria lobata*) is a traditional Chinese food whose starchy root is used in soups and stews as a thickening agent similar to cornstarch. It contains beneficial plant hormones (betasitosterol and isoflavones such as daidzein and formononetin) similar to those found in soya. Extracts have been used to treat those under the influence of alcohol – both to sober them up, and to reduce their alcohol intake.

Yerba maté tea is an energizing tonic that is also used as a substitute for alcohol, and to help liver regeneration, especially when trying to reduce alcohol intake.

NB: If you have liver disease or gallstones do not take supplements except under the advice of a medical doctor or qualified medical herbalist.

Women who are pregnant or planning to be should ideally avoid alcohol altogether, certainly for at least the first 12 weeks. Thereafter, they will probably not experience serious problems from drinking one or two units of alcohol, once or twice a week. This is controversial, however.

See also: **Artichoke, Isoflavones, Kudzu, Milk thistle, St John's Wort, Vitamin B1**.

Alopecia

Alopecia areata is a non-scarring, inflammatory condition in which the hair follicles switch off and lie dormant. The exact cause is unknown, although an imbalance of enzymes responsible for the production of hair fibre and an abnormal T-lymphocyte immune response are implicated. Occasionally alopecia is linked with iron-deficiency anaemia, or with an underactive thyroid gland. Stress plays a major role as it reduces blood supply to the scalp, and also seems to increase production of oily secretions by the sebaceous glands connected to each hair follicle.

There are four main types:

- *Alopecia areata* in which hair is lost in patches, usually on the scalp
- *Alopecia totalis*, in which there is total loss of scalp hair
- *Alopecia universalis* – loss of hair over the entire body, including eyebrows and eyelashes
- Diffuse alopecia, a condition sometimes known as *alopecia androgenetica* in which widespread hair loss affects the whole scalp, causing a 'moth-eaten' appearance.

In half of all cases, the hair follicles start to recover within a year so that the hair grows back, and altogether four out of five people

---

Do not take supplements if you are pregnant, breast-feeding, or taking prescribed drugs without first seeking advice from a pharmacist about possible interactions or adverse effects.

regrow their hair within five years, although some people always retain a small bald area. In around one in ten people affected, the condition progressively worsens.

Treatment

Nutrient deficiencies – especially of *iron* – can play a role in hair loss, and several supplements designed to counter this problem are now widely available in healthfood shops or chemists. These usually include vitamins such as *B5* and *biotin*, minerals such as *iron* and *silica*, and may also include herbs such as *ginkgo* (which increase peripheral blood circulation) and seaweed extracts as a source of *iodine. Evening primrose oil* is also useful for hair problems as it supplies essential fatty acids needed for healthy cell membranes within hair follicles. Massage your scalp regularly with your fingers, at least once a week, and preferably every day to stimulate circulation – this increases the flow of nutrients to hair follicles.

See also: **Kelp**.

Alzheimer's disease

Alzheimer's disease is the most common form of dementia. It is associated with the formation of abnormal clumps of protein (beta-amyloid plaques) that accumulate outside brain cells, and bundles of altered proteins (neurofibrillary tangles) that form inside brain cells. Symptoms vary from person to person. The first inkling that something is wrong is usually forgetfulness and loss of memory. Long-ago occurrences from childhood are often recalled while more recent events such as a television programme just the previous evening are not. It then becomes increasingly difficult to concentrate, add numbers and to find the right words when describing something. Although mild versions of these symptoms are perfectly normal with increasing age, overwork and stress, it soon becomes apparent that problems are more severe in someone suffering from this condition. Mood swings and personality changes occur and,

---

Do not take supplements if you are pregnant, breast-feeding, or taking prescribed drugs without first seeking advice from a pharmacist about possible interactions or adverse effects.

eventually, a person with Alzheimer's becomes disorientated and confused.

Treatment

Some people with Alzheimer's disease are helped by taking supplements of *choline* or *lecithin*, which boost brain levels of a neurotransmitter, acetylcholine. Volunteers taking a 10 g dose of choline were found to remember a list of words more rapidly than before. Lecithin is one of the most important dietary sources of choline. Foods rich in lecithin include soya beans, sunflower oil, maize, egg yolk and liver.

Faulty memory is occasionally due to *thiamin* (vitamin B1) deficiency, especially in people who drink a lot of alcohol. This is treated with high doses of around 50 mg vitamin B1 a day. Foods rich in thiamin include: brewer's yeast, brown rice, wheat germ, wholegrain bread and cereals.

Garlic tablets improve blood flow in the brain and may help to improve memory.

Ginkgo supplements also boost blood supply to the brain and have been shown to improve memory and concentration in some studies, but not in others.

Antioxidants such *as vitamins C, E, grapeseed* or *Pycnogenol®* (pine bark extracts) will also help to reduce free radical damage that may be linked with brain cell damage.

See also: **Alpha-lipoic acid, Antioxidants, Choline, Folic acid, Phosphatidylcholine, Reishi, Sage, Selenium, Zinc**.

Anaemia

Anaemia due to low concentrations of the red blood pigment, haemoglobin, is associated with weakness and profound exhaustion. Haemoglobin is needed to transport oxygen to body tissues, without which muscle and brain cells in particular cannot function properly.

There are three main causes of anaemia:

Do not take supplements if you are pregnant, breast-feeding, or taking prescribed drugs without first seeking advice from a pharmacist about possible interactions or adverse effects.

- Reduced or defective production of red blood cells in the marrow (due to lack of iron, vitamin B12, folic acid, or to bone marrow disease, for example)
- Excessive destruction of red blood cells (haemolytic anaemia due to malaria, for example, and immune or genetic conditions such as sickle cell anaemia)
- Excessive blood loss (such as that associated with heavy, frequent periods, peptic ulceration or occasionally a bowel tumour).

Treatment

It is vital to determine the underlying cause of anaemia before beginning any sort of treatment. *Iron* supplementation may be recommended once the cause is established, but not before, as it may mask deficiency. Those most at risk of iron-deficiency anaemia are outlined on page 193 (under Iron).

If you have iron-deficiency anaemia, you may be advised to select iron-rich foods such as shellfish, red meats, sardines, wheatgerm, wholemeal bread, egg yolk, green vegetables and dried fruit. The form of iron found in red meat (heme iron) is up to ten times more easily absorbed than non-haem iron in vegetables, and over boiling vegetables decreases their iron availability by a further 20 per cent. Vitamin C (found in citrus and berry fruits, blackcurrants, kiwi fruit and green leafy vegetables) increases the absorption of inorganic (non-haem) iron by keeping it in the more easily absorbed ferrous form. Phytate fibre, calcium, tea and coffee decrease iron absorption so iron supplements are best taken on an empty stomach unless this causes irritation. Ferrous fumarate or ferrous gluconate are usually better tolerated and less constipating than ferrous sulphate. Wash down iron tablets with *vitamin C*-rich juice to increase absorption. Naturopaths recommend beetroot and beetroot juice to help increase haemoglobin concentration. *Coenzyme Q10* supplements help to increase oxygen uptake in cells and are also beneficial.

Lack of *vitamin B12* (pernicious anaemia) is treated with B12 injections although high-dose oral supplements are becoming more

---

Do not take supplements if you are pregnant, breast-feeding, or taking prescribed drugs without first seeking advice from a pharmacist about possible interactions or adverse effects.

available – select those that are absorbed under the tongue (sub-lingual).

Echinacea is also believed to promote formation of red blood cells.

See also: **Astragalus, Copper, Folic acid, Gymnema, Iron, Molybdenum, Nickel, Phosphorus, Pumpkin seed, Vitamin B2, Vitamin B6, Vitamin B12, Vitamin C**.

Angina

Coronary heart disease (CHD) is due to hardening and furring up of the coronary arteries so heart muscle is starved of oxygen-rich blood. This triggers pain (angina) which is usually:

* Felt behind the chest bone
* Tight and crushing – like a bear hug
* Described as spreading through the chest and may radiate up into the neck, jaw or down the left arm
* Brought on by exertion and relieved by rest.

If heart muscle cells die due to prolonged oxygen starvation, a heart attack occurs. Heart attack pain is similar to angina but:

* Lasts longer
* Is more intense
* Is usually accompanied by sweating, breathlessness and paleness
* Can come on at any time and is unrelieved by rest.

Sudden chest pain should always be taken seriously and medical assistance sought without delay.

Treatment
The number of deaths attributed to CHD is slowly falling as more people are taking stock of their diet and lifestyle. Making changes

such as stopping smoking, losing at least some excess weight, and taking regular exercise (ideally 60 minutes' brisk walking per day) can, together with improving diet, significantly lower your risk of a heart attack. One in three heart attacks is linked with an unhealthy diet with too much fat of the wrong sort, not enough fat of the right sort, and too few wholegrains, fruit and vegetables.

Eat at least five portions of fresh fruit, vegetables and salads per day: fruit and vegetables contain important vitamins, minerals, antioxidants and beneficial plant hormones that protect against CHD. Eating at least five servings (and preferably 8–10) per day reduces the risk of premature death from any cause (but especially from coronary heart disease) compared with those who eat fewer. Vegetables may be more important than fruit so if having five portions in a day, make three vegetables and two fruits. Potatoes do not count towards your five-a-day as they are classed as a starchy food. Variety is important – a serving of berries, a kiwi and an orange is better than, for example, three oranges, as different types provide different phytonutrients.

Watch the fats in your diet: The average adult needs to reduce their total fat intake by at least a quarter. Concentrate on obtaining beneficial fats such as fish, olive, rapeseed, walnut, almond, macadamia and evening primrose oils rather than hydrogenated fats and excess saturated fats found in doughnuts, chips and cream. Choose reduced fat foods where possible. Grill rather than fry. Eat red meat only once or twice a week and have more vegetarian meals instead. The effects of a high-fat diet can partly be offset by taking antioxidant supplements (see below) that protect circulating fats from oxidation and reduce the risk of hardening and furring up of the arteries (*see* **Atherosclerosis**).

Eat more fish: fish oils have a blood thinning action, lower blood pressure, reduce triglyceride levels, may reduce abnormal heart rhythms and reduce the risk of a heart attack. If you already suffer from heart disease, they can reduce your risk of a fatal heart attack by a third (see *Omega-3 fish oils*, page 139). Aim to eat fish – especially oily fish (salmon, herrings, sardines, mackerel) two or

Do not take supplements if you are pregnant, breast-feeding, or taking prescribed drugs without first seeking advice from a pharmacist about possible interactions or adverse effects.

four times per week (if pregnant or planning to be, restrict intakes to twice a week). If you don't like fish, consider taking an omega-3 fish oil supplement instead (1–3 g daily). Emulsified products are available that improve absorption from the gut so you get fewer 'fishy' burps.

Eat more fibre: dietary fibre absorbs fats and slows their absorption so your body can handle them more easily. Eating 3 g or more of soluble oat fibre (roughly equal to two large bowls of porridge) every day has been shown to lower harmful blood cholesterol levels by a small but significant amount. *Fibre* supplements are also available, and usually contain inulin or psyllium.

Cut back on salt: if everyone reduced the amount of salt in their diet, at least one in seven heart attacks would be prevented. Although only an estimated one in two people are sensitive to the effects of sodium chloride, it is worth avoiding obviously salty foods (such as products tinned in brine) and to stop adding salt during cooking or at the table. Obtain flavour from herbs, spices and black pepper instead. Adding lime juice reduces the need for salt flavour.

In addition to the above, it is sensible to keep alcohol intake within safe limits, avoid excess stress, have regular blood pressure, blood fat level, and urine checks.

As well as the omega-3 fish oils supplements recommended above, the following are worth considering.

Garlic tablets: Taking garlic tablets can lower high blood pressure, reduce high blood fat levels and thin the blood (see page 154).

Antioxidants: People with high blood levels of the antioxidant vitamins C and E (usually through taking supplements) are three times less likely to have a heart attack than those with low levels. (*See* **Vitamins C, E**). Antioxidant supplements are especially important for smokers and people with diabetes.

Folic acid: Around one in ten people has inherited high blood levels of the amino acid homocysteine. This damages artery linings and more than triples the risk of a heart attack. High levels of

Do not take supplements if you are pregnant, breast-feeding, or taking prescribed drugs without first seeking advice from a pharmacist about possible interactions or adverse effects.

homocysteine can be reduced by taking supplements of folic acid (400–800 mcg per day). Vitamins B6 and B12 also have a beneficial effect. Foods rich in folic acid include green leafy vegetables (spinach, broccoli, Brussel sprouts) and wholegrains.

Drink more tea: Drinking four cups of tea per day may halve your risk of a heart attack. Both green and black tea are rich sources of antioxidants known as flavonoids. Other important sources of flavonoids include garlic, onions and apples.

See also: **Arginine, Astragalus, Bromelain, Carnitine, Iron, Magnesium, Tribulus terrestris, Vitamin C**.

Anosmia

Every day, we breathe over 23,000 times, bringing up to 10,000 different aromas into our noses. Smell receptors are located at the top of the nasal cavity and depend on tiny, hair-like nerve endings detecting aromatic substances dissolved in overlying mucus. Complete lack of smell (anosmia) is commonly related to chronic rhinitis in which inflammation and increased production of mucus block smell receptors. Two types – perennial allergic rhinitis and vasomotor rhinitis – are both associated with nasal polyps and loss of smell. It is worth undergoing investigations into either of these conditions to pinpoint dietary or environmental allergies.

Treatment

Curcumin (extracted from the spice turmeric) has powerful anti-inflammatory actions equivalent to those of some steroids. High-dose *vitamin C* also helps to reduce inflammation (this should be taken in the form of ester-C by sufferers of indigestion). The amino acid, *N-actylcysteine* makes mucus less viscous and may improve symptoms.

Taking a daily multi-nutrient supplement containing 10–15 mg zinc may be helpful as poor sense of smell is often linked to zinc deficiency (*see* **Zinc** for information on a zinc deficiency test). *Zinc* is best taken in a supplement that also provides potassium, magnesium, calcium and vitamin B12 which are important for smell/taste sensation.

Anxiety

Anxiety is a common symptom of stress and is associated with feelings of apprehension, dread, panic and impending doom. While short-lived anxiety is appropriate in some situations (such as when going for an interview) those who worry excessively about trivial matters frequently experience other typical stress symptoms such as restlessness, palpitations, tremor, flushing, dizziness, hyperventilation, loose bowels, sweating, muscle tension and insomnia. This is often related to over breathing, and can lead to panic attacks (see page 548).

Treatment

Valerian is one of the most calming herbs available and can help to relieve anxiety, muscle tension and promote tranquillity. It is often used together with other herbs with similar effects such as lemon balm and hops to ease nervous anxiety, insomnia and to help avoid panic attacks.

Rhodiola is also helpful to combat mild anxiety and associated symptoms such as fatigue and exhaustion. It acts on the adrenal glands to reduce levels of stress hormones, has an energizing effect and improves sleep quality.

Chamomile has a gentle anxiety-reducing action and also promotes sleep.

Where anxiety is associated with depression, *St John's Wort* will help to lift a low mood, but medical advice should be sought by anyone taking prescribed medications or antidepressants to check for potential drug interactions.

Supplements containing *calcium, magnesium* and *B group vitamins* are also important for healthy function of the nervous system.

See also: **Agnus castus, Ashwagandha, Black cohosh, Chamomile, Damiana, Ginkgo, Ginseng, Gotu kola, Hawthorn,**

Holy basil, 5-HTP, Lemon balm, Maca, Magnesium, Muira puama, Oatstraw, Rhodiola, Sage, St John's Wort, Siberian ginseng, Valerian, Vitamin B6, Yerba maté.

Asthma

Asthma is a long-term, inflammatory disease of the lungs. Inflammation is thought to result from abnormal immune responses that cause the lining of the airways to become red, swollen and produce increased amounts of mucus. This triggers airway spasm producing symptoms of cough, wheezing and shortness of breath. Once irritation has set in, the airways become increasingly sensitive to a wide range of triggers such as viral infections, exercise, emotion and exposure to the cold. Even between attacks, when you are symptom-free, the airways are still red and inflamed. This inflammation produces irritation and spasm of the airways that triggers wheeze and difficulty breathing. It also increases production of secretions that block the airways and interfere with breathing – even if the tubes are fully dilated. For more information about my book on Overcoming Asthma, visit my website www.naturalhealthguru.co.uk.

Treatment
Medical treatment involves the use of drugs that dilate the bronchioles usually together with anti-inflammatory corticosteroids. General measures include avoiding cigarette smoke, and keeping the home as dust free as possible by dusting with a damp cloth and using a vacuum cleaner fitted with a HEPA filter. Special covers over mattresses, pillows and duvets are recommended to overcome bed mites. Identify any triggers that seem to set off your asthma symptoms, including certain foods (e.g. those containing sulphite or benzoate preservatives).

Eat a Mediterranean-style wholefood diet providing plenty of fruit, vegetables, garlic, olive oil and fish. Coffee, dark chocolate and unsweetened cocoa are beneficial as they contain methyl-

---

xanthines such as caffeine and theobromine which open up the airways and reduce cough. Regular coffee intake reduces the chance of current asthma symptoms by 30 per cent compared with non-coffee drinkers. Drinking three to six cups of coffee per day can reduce the number of asthma attacks and improve exercise induced asthma. Ground coffee provides more benefit than instant coffee. Excess can cause tremor, sleep problems and withdrawal symptoms, however.

The increased incidence of chronic inflammatory diseases such as asthma is strongly linked with an imbalance of dietary fats. Ideally, we need a balanced intake of omega-3s and omega-6s, but the average British diet currently contains seven times more omega-6s which promote inflammation, than omega-3s which reduce inflammation in the airways by limiting the production of leukotrienes (chemicals involved in asthma symptoms). People who eat oily fish at least twice a week are half as likely to experience asthma, wheezing or chest tightness on waking compared to those who eat little oily fish – even when other factors such as smoking are taken into account. Fish oils can also reduce the severity of exercise-induced asthma. Aim to eat 150 g oily fish (salmon, herrings, fresh but not tinned tuna, mackerel, sardines, pilchards, kippers, sprats) two to four times a week, or take an omega-3 fish oil supplement supplying a total of 1–3 g *omega-3 essential fatty acids* (EPA and DHA, see page 120). Eat fish as fresh as possible, and preferably raw (sushi, sashimi), steamed, grilled or baked. NB: Girls and women who may become pregnant at some time in the future should limit their intake to two portions a week to limit their exposure to sea pollutants such as mercury.

Chamomile tea contains chamazulene and alpha-bisabolol which have anti-allergic, anti-inflammatory and antispasmodic actions. Drinking camomile tea can reduce histamine release and reduce nocturnal cough. It may also protect against viral colds which can trigger asthma symptoms.

Garlic is a source of allicin (diallyl thiosulphinate) and its sulphur degradation products which have a powerful antioxidant action. It

---

Do not take supplements if you are pregnant, breast-feeding, or taking prescribed drugs without first seeking advice from a pharmacist about possible interactions or adverse effects.

also has antibacterial and anti-viral properties, and stimulates an immune response known as T-cell proliferation.

Ginger contains volatile oils that can improve asthma symptoms by reducing the effect of platelet-activating factor (PAF) which initiates inflammatory processes. It also reduces the production of inflammatory leukotrienes, loosens phlegm and acts as an expectorant.

White, green, oolong and black teas contain high levels (up to 30 per cent by weight) of flavonoid catechins such as epigallocatechin-3-gallate (EGCG) and gallic acid, plus methylxanthines such as caffeine, theobromine, and small quantities of theophylline (an anti-asthma drug first extracted from tea leaves). EGCG has anti-allergy properties. Gallic acid has antioxidant, anti-inflammatory and antimicrobial actions. Theophylline is a powerful bronchodilator. Theanine, an amino acid in tea, reduces stress and promotes relaxation. Drinking tea two to three times a day can reduce the risk of asthma by 28 per cent. Green tea supplements are also available.

Tomatoes are a rich source of the red carotenoid, lycopene. Women with the highest intake of tomatoes are 15 per cent less likely to have asthma than those with the lowest intakes. Lycopene can protect against exercise-induced asthma. Cooking releases more lycopene for absorption. *Lycopene* supplements are also available.

Turmeric contains curcumin which has a powerful anti-inflammatory action equivalent to that of some prescribed corticosteroids. It also relaxes smooth muscles to reduce bronchospasm. Turmeric is used as a traditional asthma treatment in Ayurvedic and Chinese medicine to relieve cough and reduce mucus production.

Vitamin C is a powerful antioxidant in the fluid parts of the body, and is the main antioxidant protecting lung airways. It reduces inflammation triggered by inhaled antigens so that less histamine is released. It also protects against colds by blocking viral replication in cells. Blood levels are lower in people with asthma, and several studies suggest that those taking vitamin C supplements are less likely to experience an asthma attack than those taking placebo. It may also reduce the dose of corticosteroids needed to control asthma

Do not take supplements if you are pregnant, breast-feeding, or taking prescribed drugs without first seeking advice from a pharmacist about possible interactions or adverse effects.

symptoms, and helps to protect against exercise-induced asthma when taken 30 minutes beforehand.

Vitamin E is a powerful antioxidant in the lipid parts of the body, protecting cell membranes from oxidation. It improves immune function of T lymphocytes in people with asthma, increases the number of mature B lymphocytes and reduces circulating levels of immature B cells. Increased dietary intake of vitamin E is associated with a reduced incidence of asthma.

Vitamin B6 is needed for protein and energy production in cells. It also corrects abnormalities of tryptophan metabolism which occur in some people with severe asthma, as a result of B6 deficiency. Supplements may help to reduce the frequency and severity of wheezing in some people with asthma, and is especially important for those taking the anti-asthma drug, theophylline, which depletes B6 levels even further.

Magnesium inhibits constriction of airways, reduces bronchial reactivity and improves symptom control. It may also reduce dose of corticosteroids needed to control symptoms.

Selenium is needed for the formation of powerful antioxidant enzymes called glutathione peroxidases. Lowered activity of these enzymes is linked with aspirin induced asthma. Interestingly, blood levels of selenium appear to be lower in people with asthma than in those without.

Green-lipped mussel extracts have an anti-inflammatory action. They reduce production of leukotrienes and can significantly reduce day-time wheeze.

Quercetin is a flavonoid antioxidant that inhibits the release of histamine. It has a relaxant effect on smooth muscle cells in the airways, stabilizes airway mast cells (which produce histamine) and promotes bronchial relaxation. Apples are an important dietary source of quercetins, which may explain why people who eat five or more apples per week have significantly better lung function than non-apple eaters, and are 38 per cent less likely to have asthma.

N-acetyl cysteine (NAC) is an antioxidant amino acid which thins excess mucus by breaking it down into smaller, less viscous units. It also inhibits the activity of eosinophils – white blood cells involved in allergic inflammatory responses. It can improve asthma symptoms by reducing release of inflammatory chemicals and helping to clear excess mucus.

Co-enzyme Q10 (CoQ10) is a vitamin-like substance needed for oxygen utilization and energy production in cells. Blood levels are lower in people with asthma and, when combined with vitamins C and E, has reduced the dose of corticosteroids needed to control asthma symptoms.

Probiotics prime the immune system with 'friendly' bacteria to reduce development of allergic diseases. They appear to reduce airway hypersensitivity and allergic airway responses. When taken during pregnancy, and in infancy, for example, they offer some protection against childhood asthma.

Pycnogenol® (extracts from the bark of the French maritime pine) contains a powerful array of antioxidants. Research suggests it is as effective in preventing release of histamine as the anti-asthma drug, sodium cromoglicate, and can block 70 per cent of histamine release from mast cells when they are exposed to airborne allergens such as pollen. It reduces leukotriene synthesis, improves asthma frequency, reduces the severity of asthma symptoms and the frequency of inhaler use.

Reishi mushroom has antioxidant, anti-inflammatory, anti-viral and antibacterial actions. It also has an immune modulating effect to reduce production of inflammatory cytokines in the airways, to improve bronchial hypersensitivity.

Boswellia is used to treat chronic inflammatory conditions such as asthma, and has been shown to have anti-inflammatory properties, while *red clover*, known mainly for its oestrogenic actions, also has anti-spasmodic properties and is used to treat asthma.

Other supplements that can be helpful include *bromelain, magnesium, oregano* and the anti-inflammatory action of *liquorice*.

See also: **Boswellia, Brewer's Yeast, Bromelain, Butterbur, Chamomile, Essential Fatty Acids, Fish oils, Folic acid, Ginkgo,**

Do not take supplements if you are pregnant, breast-feeding, or taking prescribed drugs without first seeking advice from a pharmacist about possible interactions or adverse effects.

Green-lipped mussel, Holy basil, Magnesium, Oregano oil, Perilla, Pine bark, Selenium, Vitamin B6, Vitamin C, Vitamin D.

Atherosclerosis

Healthy arteries are elastic to even out the peaks and troughs in blood pressure that occur as the heart pumps blood around the circulation. Atherosclerosis, or hardening and furring up of the arteries, starts early in life, usually in the teens, and is triggered by normal wear-and-tear damage to the artery walls. Once the damage occurs, small cell fragments in the bloodstream – known as platelets – stick to the damaged area and form a tiny clot. These platelets release chemical signals to stimulate healing of the damaged area. Under normal circumstances, this would lead to healing, but if excessive damage continues (e.g. as a result of high blood pressure, raised cholesterol and/or homocysteine levels or lack of antioxidants in the diet) the damage continues and the area becomes inflamed and infiltrated with a porridge-like substance that builds up to form a fatty plaque (atheroma).

At the same time as the fatty plaques are developing, inflammation causes the underlying middle layer of the artery wall to degenerate, become fibrous and less compliant. Whereas the walls of healthy arteries are elastic and help to even out the surges of blood pressure produced every time the heart beats, the walls of arteries that have started to harden become more rigid. As a result, blood pressure surges caused by the heart beat are not evened out, and systolic blood pressure (when the heart contracts) shoots up higher. A vicious cycle then sets up, for just as atherosclerosis leads to high blood pressure, untreated hypertension can also lead to atherosclerosis by progressively damaging artery linings and hastening the hardening and furring up process.

If atherosclerosis is widespread throughout the body, it narrows the circulation so the diastolic BP – the pressure in the system when the heart is resting between beats – also becomes raised.

Do not take supplements if you are pregnant, breast-feeding, or taking prescribed drugs without first seeking advice from a pharmacist about possible interactions or adverse effects.

Atherosclerosis can therefore raise both diastolic and systolic blood pressure. If left untreated, the raised BP in turn causes damage to the arterial system which hastens the development of atherosclerotic plaques and blood pressure rises even further.

As a result, the heart has to pump blood out into a circulation whose vessels are narrowed and have lost their elasticity. This increases the workload of the heart – which has to pump blood out into the high pressure system – and its need for oxygen increases, at a time when its blood supply is often already compromised due to atherosclerosis of the coronary arteries. This may eventually lead to angina and a heart attack. In some people, two-thirds or more of a coronary artery may be furred up and blocked with atheroma without causing symptoms. In others, angina may be triggered even though only a small atheromatous plaque is present and the coronary artery is only narrowed slightly. It all depends on:

- The exact site where the atheroma and narrowing have developed – the most common site is within 3 cm of where a coronary artery originates from the aorta, so that the effects of ischaemia are likely to be more widespread and serious
- How well the two main coronary arteries join up to share the load of supplying blood
- How good the blood supply from the other coronary artery is
- The type of coronary arteries you have inherited – whether they are the vascular equivalent of motorways or winding country lanes.

Antioxidants protect dietary fats in the circulation from oxidation. It is only oxidized fats that are taken up by scavenger cells and transported into the blood vessel lining where they become 'stuck' to produce atheroma. Although the main culprits were thought to be saturated (animal) fats, increasing evidence suggests that these are less important than previously thought (though they do provide calories and are best avoided in excess). Excessive intakes of omega-6 fatty acids and trans-fatty acids (also known as partially

---

Do not take supplements if you are pregnant, breast-feeding, or taking prescribed drugs without first seeking advice from a pharmacist about possible interactions or adverse effects.

hydrogenated fats) are more harmful. Unlike saturated fats, omega-6 and trans fatty acids have a molecular structure that contains spare double bonds. This makes them highly reactive and more susceptible to chemical changes such as oxidation, especially if levels of circulating antioxidants are low. This chemical change produces toxic substances known as lipid peroxides that are linked with atherosclerosis. Omega-6s also promote inflammation.

Treatment
All the usual health guidelines apply. These include:

- Stopping smoking, which is a powerful trigger for atherosclerosis
- Following a healthy, low-salt, low-fat, high-fibre diet
- Maintaining a healthy weight
- Taking regular brisk exercise – at least 30 minutes per day and preferably 60.

Follow a relatively low-fat diet and concentrate on obtaining 'healthy' dietary fats: monounsaturates (e.g. found in olive, rapeseed, almond, avocado and macadamia nut oils) and omega-3s (from oily fish, see page 138). *Omega-3 fish oils* (at least 1 g per day) can protect against both a first heart attack (primary prevention) and subsequent heart attacks (secondary prevention) from occurring (see page 139).

Eat plenty of fruit and vegetables (at least five and preferably 8–10 servings per day). They are a rich source of antioxidants which can protect circulating fats from oxidation and help to protect against atherosclerosis. The evidence about whether or not anti-oxidant supplements can protect against atherosclerosis and coronary heart disease is conflicting. Some studies show benefit while others do not (but often involved older people who took antioxidants for relatively short periods of time). Overall, the evidence is promising for *vitamin C* (see page 327), *vitamin E* and some *carotenoids* (see page 86). High doses of single antioxidants are not a good idea, however, as they work together helping to

---

Do not take supplements if you are pregnant, breast-feeding, or taking prescribed drugs without first seeking advice from a pharmacist about possible interactions or adverse effects.

regenerate each other's activity. They are best taken in combination.

A raised level of the amino acid, homocysteine, damages artery walls to trigger atherosclerosis and is now recognized as an important risk factor for coronary heart disease and stroke. Taking *folic acid, B12* and *B6* supplements can lower homocysteine levels and may protect against atherosclerosis (see page 148).

Garlic tablets have been shown in some trials to reduce harmfully raised cholesterol levels, lower a raised blood pressure and increase the elasticity of the aorta. Some studies have also found that garlic could reduce and even partially reverse atherosclerosis, and reduce calcification of arterial walls.

Ginkgo biloba extracts can improve peripheral circulation due to atherosclerosis by up to 50 per cent. Ginkgo is particularly useful for atherosclerosis that causes poor blood flow to the legs so that calf pain develops on exercise (intermittent claudication).

The flowering tops and berries of the *hawthorn* (*Crataegus oxycantha* and *C. monogyna*) contain chemicals that normalize the cardiovascular system, and can:

- Relax peripheral blood vessels
- Dilate the coronary arteries, improving blood circulation to heart muscle
- Discourage fluid retention
- Slow and possibly even reverse the build-up of atheromatous plaques.

Hawthorn also increases the strength and efficiency of the heart's pumping action.

See also: **Antioxidants, Arginine, Astaxanthin, Carnitine, Choline, Co-enzyme Q10, Copper, Fish oils, Folic acid, Garlic, Grapeseed, Hawthorn, Iron, Lycopene, Pomegranate, Silicon, Sodium, Vitamin B6, Vitamin E, Vitamin K**.

Related entry: **Cholesterol – raised**.

Attention deficit hyperactivity disorder

Attention deficit hyperactivity disorder (ADHD) is an abnormality affecting psychological development in which a child is continually inattentive, restless, impulsive and often defiant, so he or she is unable to sit down quietly even when overly tired or exhausted. Any stimulation leads to feverish excitement and attempts to calm the child frequently result in screaming fits and hysteria.

ADHD comes on in early childhood with symptoms often appearing before the age of two, usually before five, and necessarily by the age of seven for diagnosis. Four times as many boys are affected as girls, and it is estimated to affect just over 1 per cent of boys of primary school age. Some children improve at puberty, and around 40 per cent seem to 'outgrow' ADHD. Behavioural problems often persist into adolescence and adulthood, however, with insomnia, abnormal thirst and difficulty in concentrating.

The exact cause of ADHD is poorly understood, but many researchers believe that diet plays a significant part – both during foetal development and in childhood.

Treatment

Children's behaviour and mental performance may be improved by following a wholefood diet containing plenty of fresh fruit and vegetables – preferably organic – and reducing intakes of white flour, white sugar, artificial colourings, flavourings, chocolate, monosodium glutamate, benzoate preservatives, caffeine and food additives. Food may be sweetened when necessary with raw Barbados sugar, muscovado sugar, honey or molasses used sparingly. This simple dietary approach is often effective but has proven unusually controversial. *Probiotic supplements* may help to improve associated intestinal problems, correct dysbiosis and improve immune function.

Mounting evidence suggests that *omega-3 fish oils* (DHA and EPA) are beneficial for children with learning and behavioural disorders including dyslexia, dyspraxia, ADHD and autistic

Do not take supplements if you are pregnant, breast-feeding, or taking prescribed drugs without first seeking advice from a pharmacist about possible interactions or adverse effects.

spectrum disorder (ASD) – conditions which are increasing in prevalence and which show considerable clinical overlap.

Some researchers in the USA have found that the behaviour of children and adults with attention deficit hyperactivity disorder improved when taking *glutamine* supplements.

See also: **Fish oils, Phosphatidylserine**.

Back pain

Back pain is common, and those most likely to suffer include those whose work involves heavy lifting or carrying, or people who spend long periods of time sitting in one position or bending awkwardly. Almost any day-to-day activity can bring it on, however, including housework, gardening and over-vigorous exercise. If you are overweight and unfit, with poor muscle tone, you are also at increased risk as apart from having to support a heavier load, your back will not receive the support it needs from your abdominal muscles.

Back pain most commonly affects the lower, lumbar region of the spine. Most cases are due to excessive strain on muscles, ligaments and small joints. As well as discomfort from the damaged tissues, the surrounding muscles may go into spasm so that pain and tenderness spread over a larger area. More severe symptoms will occur if the soft, jelly-like centre of an intervertebral disc ruptures through the outer fibrous coating under pressure – a condition popularly known as a slipped disc. The prolapsed centre of the disc may press on the root of a spinal nerve to cause muscle weakness, pins and needles, spasm and pain in the back. If the sciatic nerve is irritated, pain will shoot down the leg. This is known as sciatica.

Non-specific back pain is usually treated with simple painkillers such as aspirin, paracetamol and codeine. If necessary, muscle-relaxant drugs can be taken to reduce painful spasms and applying hot or cold compresses will also help. Prolonged bed rest is no longer recommended routinely as early mobilization is essential to

---

Do not take supplements if you are pregnant, breast-feeding, or taking prescribed drugs without first seeking advice from a pharmacist about possible interactions or adverse effects.

prevent the back from 'seizing up'. Manipulation from a chiropractor or osteopath is often helpful.

Treatment

To help strengthen bones, it is important to take a supplement containing bone-building nutrients such as *calcium, magnesium, manganese, boron, vitamin C, vitamin D* and *vitamin K. Evening primrose oil* helps to increase calcium absorption and deposition in bone.

Omega-3 fish oils contain essential fatty acids that help to reduce inflammation. Taking omega-3 fish oils, or extra-high-strength cod liver oil supplements, can improve back stiffness and pain. *MSM-sulphur* also has an anti-inflammatory action.

Glucosamine sulphate can improve symptoms related to a prolapsed intervertebral disc by strengthening the central nucleus pulposus of the disc.

Back pain is often helped by supplements containing raw extracts of *New Zealand green-lipped mussel*. Research suggests that these contain substances (glycoproteins) that prevent immune cells from entering inflamed joints and releasing powerful inflammatory chemicals that would make pain worse.

Devil's claw and *bromelain* are also helpful in relieving back pain.

See also: **Devil's claw, Fibre, Fish oils, Vitamin A, Vitamin D**.

Bacterial vaginosis

Anaerobic or bacterial vaginosis (BV) is due to an imbalance in the bacteria normally found in the vagina. Healthy *Lactobacilli* are reduced, or lost, and other bacteria that do not need oxygen to survive (anaerobes) start to flourish.

BV often seems to arise spontaneously around the time of menstruation and then resolves mid-cycle. Because of their strange metabolism, anaerobic bacteria produce chemicals that can cause irritation, an unpleasant fish odour – especially after sex – soreness,

---

Do not take supplements if you are pregnant, breast-feeding, or taking prescribed drugs without first seeking advice from a pharmacist about possible interactions or adverse effects.

and a heavy discharge, although 50 per cent of women do not notice any appreciable symptoms. BV can also irritate male sexual partners if condoms are not used.

While it is not classed as a sexually transmissible disease, it is more common in sexually active women. Medical treatment is with antibiotics (metronidazole tablets/gel or clindamycin cream) but, unfortunately, it often seems to recur.

BV has been linked with increased risk of miscarriage during the first three months of pregnancy, and with pre-term labour.

Treatment

Replenishing levels of healthy *Lactobacillus acidophilus* bacteria by taking a *probiotic* oral medication may help to prevent recurrences.

If general immunity is low, a multivitamin and mineral supplement providing around 100 per cent of as many micro-nutrients (including iron) as possible is beneficial.

It is also worth considering taking an immune-supporting supplement such as *Echinacea* to boost white cell function.

Bacterial vaginosis was recently found to be associated with lowered levels of *vitamin D*, and supplements may be worth trying.

See also: **Probiotics, Vitamin D**.

Bell's palsy

Bell's palsy is a weakness of muscles on one side of the face due to temporary paralysis of the facial nerve. The exact cause is unknown, but it is believed to be due to a viral infection which causes inflammation and swelling of the facial nerve as it passes through a narrow channel in the temporal bone. Pain behind the ear is common at the onset and there may be loss of taste on the front two-thirds of the tongue.

Left untreated, Bell's palsy usually starts to improve within two weeks but may take up to 12 months to resolve fully. Around one in seven sufferers retain some residual, permanent weakness. To

---

Do not take supplements if you are pregnant, breast-feeding, or taking prescribed drugs without first seeking advice from a pharmacist about possible interactions or adverse effects.

encourage full recovery, early treatment with prednisolone or adreno-corticotrophic hormone (ACTH) may be recommended at the onset of symptoms. Anti-viral drugs are sometimes tried but their efficacy is unknown. The eyelids may need to be temporarily closed (either with a pad or by stitching) to prevent drying and ulceration of the cornea. Electrical stimulation of muscle fibres is often helpful, and can also predict which patients are unlikely to recover. In these cases, cosmetic surgery may be suggested to improve the appearance of severe, permanent paralysis. It may also be possible to rejoin some of the remaining nerves to the facial nerve to help it to start working again.

Treatment
Taking *a vitamin B complex*, including high-dose vitamin B12 may help to improve nerve function. B vitamins are needed for the formation of healthy myelin nerve sheaths and the conduction of messages along nerves. Alpha lipoic acid is also worth considering.

Garlic, ginkgo and *ginger*, which stimulate circulation, are also used.

Bereavement

Bereavement is one of the worst emotional experiences anyone has to bear. Everyone copes differently with bereavement and, in time, it usually becomes easier to accept what has happened.

Treatment
Rhodiola helps to overcome anxiety and may help the bereaved get through the early days. For difficulty in sleeping, *valerian* and *lemon balm* are a good combination. Sometimes, people who have suffered a bereavement slowly sink into depression until they are overwhelmed with feelings of sadness, loneliness and despair. When this happens, anti-depressant drugs are the most effective route to recovery, by correcting imbalances of certain chemicals in the brain.

Do not take supplements if you are pregnant, breast-feeding, or taking prescribed drugs without first seeking advice from a pharmacist about possible interactions or adverse effects.

Natural alternatives for treating mild to moderate depression include *5-HTP* and *St John's Wort*. Do not take antidepressant remedies without first talking to your doctor. Check with a pharmacist for interactions with any prescribed medications you are taking.

Blepharitis

Blepharitis is an inflammation of the eyelids whose symptoms include redness, soreness, itching and scaling. It can be a difficult condition to treat as it often recurs, especially during times of stress.

Allergic reactions may play a role, so it is worth stopping the use of all creams, cosmetics, perfume/colognes and shampoos, then gradually re-introducing them, one at a time, to see if any retrigger the problem. Contact lenses should not be worn until the problem has resolved as some lens solutions and saline preservatives may be involved.

Hypoallergenic toiletries should be used wherever possible – the gentlest shampoos, soaps and moisturizers are those formulated for newborn babies.

Treatment

Sometimes all that is needed is gentle removal of the scales around the lashes using gauze or cotton buds and warm saline solution or a very dilute solution containing baby shampoo. Herbal practitioners suggest bathing the eye with a compress soaked in dilute infusions of chamomile. Use separate compresses and eyebaths for each eye. Aloe vera gel may be applied to damp down inflammation. If eyes also feel dry, artificial tears (available over the counter) will help.

Supplements that may be suggested include *vitamin C* and *omega-3 fish oils* as these are helpful in reducing inflammatory skin conditions. *Echinacea* by mouth helps to boost general immunity.

Do not take supplements if you are pregnant, breast-feeding, or taking prescribed drugs without first seeking advice from a pharmacist about possible interactions or adverse effects.

Bloating

Although bloating is commonly linked with overindulgence or eating a rich diet, it can also occur after eating relatively little in those with functional disorders of the gut such as irritable bowel syndrome (IBS). If symptoms have been present for a while, it is important to seek medical advice to find out the cause, but assuming a clean bill of health is given, symptoms may be related to insufficient bile production in the liver which is needed to emulsify dietary fats before they can be absorbed.

Treatment
Extracts of *globe artichoke* leaves (*Cynara scolymus*) stimulate bile production and can quickly relieve bloating without side effects. It is also helpful when bloating and indigestion are due to overly spicy food or drinking alcohol.

Other natural treatments that can help to reduce bloating include drinking *peppermint*, *ginger* or *fennel* tea, taking *probiotic supplements* containing digestive bacteria (e.g. *Lactobacilli*), and *aloe vera*.

See also: **Artichoke, Brewer's yeast, Dandelion, Digestive enzymes, Evening primrose oil, Fibre, Liquorice, Magnesium, Turmeric, Vitamin B6**.

Bronchitis

There are two types of bronchitis: acute and chronic. Acute bronchitis is a relatively mild inflammation of the larger lung airways – the bronchi – and can be due to a viral or bacterial infection. Symptoms are more common in winter and often follow on from a cold. They are due to inflammation of mucous membranes lining the bronchi, which swell and secrete increased amounts of yellow-green mucus. Airway narrowing can cause shortness of breath, cough and wheeze and you may notice a hoarse voice.

Do not take supplements if you are pregnant, breast-feeding, or taking prescribed drugs without first seeking advice from a pharmacist about possible interactions or adverse effects.

Feelings of soreness or rawness are often felt behind the breast bone (sternum) and a low-grade fever may occur. In most cases, symptoms come on suddenly and clear up quickly within a few days. Those most at risk include smokers, people who are exposed to atmospheric pollution, babies, the elderly and people with a pre-existing lung disease such as chronic bronchitis or asthma.

In contrast to acute bronchitis, chronic bronchitis is a long-term lung problem which is diagnosed when phlegm is coughed up:

• On most days
• During at least three consecutive months
• For at least two years.

The commonest causes of chronic bronchitis are smoking cigarettes and exposure to industrial pollution. Long-term inflammation of the bronchi results in widespread stiffening, narrowing and obstruction of the airways which, together with increased secretions, makes a secondary bacterial infection (i.e. acute bronchitis) more likely. Other symptoms of chronic bronchitis include cough, breathlessness, wheezing and sometimes chest pain or coughing up blood. The last two symptoms should always be investigated to rule out other causes.

Smoking can also cause widespread emphysema (overstretching and rupturing of air sacs). When emphysema and chronic bronchitis develop together, the condition is often referred to as Chronic Obstructive Airways Disease or COAD.

Treatment
Symptoms may be relieved by steam inhalations (plain, or with added essential oils of menthol or eucalyptus) and by drinking plenty of fluids – this helps to loosen the phlegm so you can cough it up more easily.

Zinc and vitamin C lozenges will help to boost immunity so that sore throat is less likely. Supplements containing *Echinacea, astragalus, lapacho, reishi, shiitake* or *maitake* are effective in boosting

Do not take supplements if you are pregnant, breast-feeding, or taking prescribed drugs without first seeking advice from a pharmacist about possible interactions or adverse effects.

immunity including the activity of white blood cells needed to fight infections. *Garlic* and *olive leaf* extracts have natural anti-viral and antibacterial actions.

Mucus dispersion can be improved by supplements containing *N-acetyl cysteine* (NAC) – an amino acid that boosts levels of a powerful antioxidant (glutathione) in the respiratory tract. NAC has a pronounced mucus-dissolving action and studies show it can significantly reduce mucus production and associated cough in chronic respiratory conditions such as bronchitis, emphysema and sinusitis.

In general, to help maintain a healthy respiratory system, regular exercise throughout the year is important to improve general fitness. Smoky or polluted atmospheres which can damage airways making infection more likely should be avoided, and smokers should make every effort to stop.

Antibiotics are needed when acute-on-chronic bronchitis develops, as it frequently does. Regular sufferers from bronchitis should speak to a doctor about being immunized against influenza and pneumococcal pneumonia.

Note: A doctor should be consulted especially by anyone who is susceptible to chest infections (due, for example, to a lung problem such as chronic bronchitis, asthma or emphysema) if:

- Their temperature goes above 38°C
- Severe breathlessness develops
- Thick, green-coloured phlegm is produced
- Symptoms last longer than three days
- There is a pre-existing lung problem
- There is chest pain.

See also: **Astragalus, Bromelain, Eucalyptus, Holy basil, Liquorice, N-acetyl cysteine, Pelargonium sidoides, Pomegranate, Reishi, Vitamin A**.

 Related entry: **Catarrh – excess**.

Do not take supplements if you are pregnant, breast-feeding, or taking prescribed drugs without first seeking advice from a pharmacist about possible interactions or adverse effects.

Bruising

Easy bruising is common in older people, partly due to increased fragility of skin and blood vessels (known as Easy Bruising Syndrome). If this is excessive, it is important to consult a doctor as a blood test may be needed to investigate the possibility of a bleeding tendency.

Treatment

Occasionally, lack of *vitamin K* can be a cause of easy bruising in older people, and a doctor should be asked about taking supplements containing this. General skin quality can be improved by taking *evening primrose oil* capsules (at least 1 g a day). *Horsechestnut, red vine leaf, pine bark extracts (Pycnogenol®)* or *gotu kola* extracts which help to strengthen the connective tissues supporting blood vessels may help.

Burns

The skin is designed to protect the body from a variety of environmental insults, including excessive heat. If the skin is heated above 49°C, its cells are damaged to cause a burn. If only the top layer of skin is injured, reddening and pain occur to form a first-degree burn. This will heal quickly and the dead cells often peel after a few days (the classic example is sunburn). If the damage is more severe, cells in the deeper layers of the skin are destroyed and a blister forms. This is known as a second-degree burn. Enough live cells remain for regeneration, so the burn usually heals without scarring. If the full thickness of the skin is affected, a third-degree burn results. Extensive treatment, including skin grafts, may be needed and there is a risk of scarring. If second- or third-degree burns cover more than 10 per cent of the body, the effects often trigger clinical shock, where the pulse speeds up and blood pressure falls.

Do not take supplements if you are pregnant, breast-feeding, or taking prescribed drugs without first seeking advice from a pharmacist about possible interactions or adverse effects.

Treatment

Immerse the burned area in cold, running water as soon as possible, for at least 10 minutes. If this isn't possible, soak a clean towel or pillow case in cold water and hold against the burn until pain disappears. Take off any jewellery before the area swells, then dress with a clean, non-stick, non-fluffy material such as sterile gauze. In an emergency, cling film will help to prevent fluid loss and infection until you can obtain urgent medical attention, but ensure it is not applied too tightly – keep checking for swelling.

Do not:

- Try to remove any clothing that is stuck to the wound
- Use adhesive plasters
- Apply butter, oil or grease
- Try to burst any blisters
- Use fluffy dressings (e.g. cotton wool).

Burns easily become infected. Seek medical advice for anything more than a mild burn, or if burns result from contact with chemicals and electricity.

Natural approaches that can help include applying burn gel, *aloe vera gel* or neat *lavender essential oil* to the burns to relieve pain and inflammation. *Calendula* (marigold) or *goldenseal* cream may be used for their antibacterial actions. High dose *vitamin C* supplements are useful for reducing inflammation, and promoting formation of collagen fibres during healing. *Vitamin E, zinc, selenium* and *co-enzyme Q10* can also help the healing process.

Cancer

Cancer will affect an estimated one in three people at some time in their life. If you are diagnosed with cancer, you should ideally seek individual advice from both a nutritionist and a herbalist to tailor a plan to your individual needs. This should only be done with the permission of your oncologist.

Do not take supplements if you are pregnant, breast-feeding, or taking prescribed drugs without first seeking advice from a pharmacist about possible interactions or adverse effects.

It is usually advisable to follow a low-fat, salt-free, mainly vegetarian diet which is as organic as possible, and to avoid junk food, alcohol and caffeine. Most practitioners advise high-dose *vitamin C* (the form known as ester-C is least likely to produce side effects such as indigestion, as it is acid free) plus other powerful antioxidants such as *vitamin E, selenium, green tea, grapeseed* and/or *pine bark extracts (Pycnogenol®)*. Other vitamins and minerals such as *folic acid* and other *B group vitamins* may also be suggested. Iron is thought to suppress immunity so it may be advisable to avoid supplements containing iron except in cases of anaemia. An immune-boosting supplement such as *Echinacea, maitake, lapacho* (*pau d'arco*) or *cat's claw* (*Uncaria tomentosa*) may be recommended to improve the destruction of abnormal body cells. Some researchers recommend that cat's claw is stopped two days before and until two days after receiving chemotherapy.

Milk thistle is often used to protect the liver when receiving chemotherapy. *Glutamine* has been used to enhance the effectiveness of chemotherapy and radiation treatments while reducing toxicity, decreasing infections and weight loss, and to improve healing of radiated intestines.

See also: **Antioxidants, Astralagus, Blue-green algae, Cat's claw, Echinacea, Fish oils, Glutamine, Lapacho, Maitake, Reishi, Selenium, Shiitake, Vitamin D.**

Cancer prevention

There are close links between cancer, diet and lifestyle. Fruit and vegetables are a rich source of protective antioxidants such as *carotenoids, vitamins C, E*, and mineral *selenium*. These neutralize harmful chemicals (free radicals) that form as a by-product of normal metabolism. Free radicals can damage genetic material to trigger cancer unless mopped up quickly by high circulating levels of antioxidants. Those people with high intakes of vitamin C (found in citrus and berry fruits), carotenoid pigments (e.g betacarotene,

---

lycopene found in yellow, orange, green and red fruit and vegetables) and selenium (found in Brazil nuts and fruit and vegetables grown in selenium-rich soils) seem to have a lower risk of developing some cancers.

Unfortunately, dietary antioxidant intakes are often low in the UK, especially for selenium (see page 283). In parts of the world where soil selenium levels are low, the incidence of cancer increases six-fold. In a study looking at the effects of 200 mcg selenium supplementation in 974 men, the incidence of a number of cancers – including colon and rectum – was reduced by over 50 per cent. As a result, the blinded phase of the trial was stopped early as it was considered unethical to withhold treatment from the placebo group.

Vitamin E may help to decrease the risk of colon cancer, and works synergistically with selenium to improve general immunity. It has also been found that those with highest intakes of *folic acid* are less likely to develop colorectal polyps (a risk factor for colonic cancer). Eating a diet high in *fibre* and low in sugar and fat (especially a vegetarian diet) also reduces the risk of colonic cancer.

Omega-3 fish oils have an anti-inflammatory effect and can inhibit the growth of colonic polyps and may have an anti-cancer action although this is still under investigation.

A variety of nutritional strategies will help to reduce the risk of hormonal cancers such as breast or prostate cancer. At least seven to ten servings of fruit and vegetables per day should be eaten – preferably those that are organic. Cruciferous vegetables such as broccoli are especially important as, along with soya, they are rich sources of protective plant hormones known as phyto-oestrogens. Although it is hard to include soy in a Western diet, soya/linseed bread and muesli-style bars are available (or pulses such as chickpeas, kidney, black eye or mung beans are just as good). It is important to ensure a good intake of fibre, and it is also a good idea to take a tablespoon of flax (linseed) per day. It is recommended to eat oily fish two to four times a week and olive oil should be used in cooking and salad dressings. Cut back on omega-6 polyunsaturated fats such as those

---

Do not take supplements if you are pregnant, breast-feeding, or taking prescribed drugs without first seeking advice from a pharmacist about possible interactions or adverse effects.

found in margarines and avoid excess sugar. Alcohol consumption should be limited to no more than three units per week – especially for pre-menopausal women or those who are taking HRT.

Eating red meat (beef, pork, lamb, sausages, hamburgers, ham, bacon) – especially if fried or barbecued – increases the risk of certain cancers. This is thought to be as a result of chemicals produced during these methods of cooking. The World Cancer Research Fund suggests eating no more than 500 g red meat per week, and to avoid processed meats such as ham, hot dogs, burgers, salami and some sausages. In addition, the World Cancer Research Fund also recommends the following general guidelines to help lower the risk of cancer:

- Be as lean as possible without becoming underweight
- Be active for at least 30 minutes per day
- Avoid exposure to cigarette smoke (responsible for an estimated 30 per cent of all cancer deaths)
- Limit consumption of energy-dense foods (foods that are high in fats and/or added sugars, and/or low in fibre, and avoid sugary drinks
- Follow a healthy, low-fat, high-fibre diet
- If consumed, limit alcoholic drinks to two a day for men and one a day for women
- Limit consumption of salty foods and foods processed with salt (sodium).

Always seek medical advice about any recurring symptoms, and accept invitations for health screening such as mammography and cervical screening.

See also: **Selenium, Vitamin D**.

Do not take supplements if you are pregnant, breast-feeding, or taking prescribed drugs without first seeking advice from a pharmacist about possible interactions or adverse effects.

Candidiasis

Candidiasis – a vaginal yeast infection also known as thrush – is common, affecting three out of four women at some time during their lives. It is caused by an overgrowth of a yeast, *Candida albicans*, that is normally present in the vagina of many women without causing symptoms. Candida spores are in the air and thrive in warm, moist places such as the groin and vagina. Infection can sometimes also be passed on during sexual intercourse.

Candidiasis is more likely to occur around the time of a period due to changes in the acidity of vaginal discharge. It is also more common in women who are pregnant, have uncontrolled diabetes mellitus, or who use oral contraceptives. Candida often occurs after taking antibiotics which kill off the healthy bacteria (e.g. *Lactobacillus acidophilus*) naturally found in the vagina which help to keep disease-causing organisms such as candida yeasts at bay.

Some women suffer repeated bouts, which may be due to slightly reduced levels of *iron* needed by white blood cells to make the chemicals used to destroy opportunistic infections such as these. This can be diagnosed by a blood test that measures serum levels of ferritin – an iron-binding protein. An inborn error of *biotin* metabolism may also be involved.

Symptoms of thrush vary and can include itching, soreness or burning, a yeasty smell, vaginal discharge, which is sometimes white and cottage-cheese-like, and discomfort during urination and/or intercourse.

Diagnosing candida from symptoms and examination alone is not always accurate as other conditions such as bacterial vaginosis and sensitivity reactions cause similar problems and need different treatment. For any genital symptoms, it is best to visit a genito-urinary medicine clinic for full screening and proper diagnosis.

Treatment

To help keep thrush at bay, avoid getting hot and sweaty. Use panty-liners and change them as necessary throughout the day, and avoid

---

Do not take supplements if you are pregnant, breast-feeding, or taking prescribed drugs without first seeking advice from a pharmacist about possible interactions or adverse effects.

wearing tight underwear, especially nylon tights or tight-fitting trousers. Stockings and cotton underwear are recommended. Boil cotton underwear or hot-iron underwear gussets after washing, as modern low-temperature washing machine cycles do not kill candida spores and re-infection may occur via underclothes. Avoid bath additives, vaginal deodorants or douches which can upset the naturally acidic vaginal environment.

Eat an *iron*-rich diet and take a *multivitamin and mineral supplement* containing iron – a *vitamin C* source such as orange juice will also increase iron absorption from the gut. It can help if male partners use an anti-fungal cream, as men can harbour yeast spores under the foreskin and pass infection back without developing symptoms themselves.

Some women find it helpful to smear the affected area with natural yoghurt containing a live Bio culture of *Lactobacillus acidophilus* or use acidophilus pessaries. This colonizes the vagina and may help to prevent overgrowth of candida. Taking *probiotic supplements* will replenish intestinal levels of friendly digestive bacteria that suppress candida overgrowth in the gut, reducing the reservoir for recurrent vaginal candida infections. *Biotin* supplements may also help.

Herbal remedies for candida include lapacho bark extracts (also known as *pau d'arco*), grapefruit seed extracts and olive leaf extracts. Siberian ginseng (*Eleutherococcus senticosus*) is useful for boosting immunity when under excess stress.

Although there is no scientific evidence to support dietary changes, some women have found it helpful to follow a yeast-free diet. Others avoid alcohol, mushrooms, sugary foods, tea, coffee and chocolate. A wholefood diet of salads, fruit, vegetables, pulses and wholegrain cereals is usually recommended instead.

See also: **Brewer's yeast, Digestive enzymes, Grapefruit seed, Lapacho, Olive leaf, Oregano oil, Probiotics, Vitamin A**.

Carpal tunnel syndrome

The carpal tunnel is a narrow space formed between bones in the wrist that are covered by a strong band of tissue, the transverse carpal ligament. The median nerve passes through this space, together with nine flexor tendons that bend the fingers and thumb. Because of this overcrowding in an anatomically narrow area, the median nerve can become pinched to cause painful tingling and sensations that resemble an electric shock. Symptoms classically involve the thumb, index and middle fingers plus the inner side of the ring finger, as these areas are supplied by the median nerve. In severe cases, numbness, weakness and muscle wasting may also occur.

Carpal tunnel syndrome (CTS) most commonly affects women. Heredity is another important factor, as having a tight carpal tunnel can run in some families. It is also associated with obesity, in which fatty tissue can cause further restriction, and with a number of other conditions associated with weight gain or tissue swelling such as pregnancy, diabetes, hypothyroidism, wrist fracture and kidney problems. Often, however, no obvious underlying risk factors are identified.

Treatment
Some people with CTS have a low level of *vitamin B6*, which is needed for optimum nerve functioning. Although supplements are not effective in everyone, the pioneer of B6 treatment for CTS claims that at least 85 per cent of people respond to doses of between 50–200 mg daily, with improvement starting in a few weeks, and complete resolution of symptoms occurring within eight to twelve weeks. It is generally recommended that high-dose vitamin B6 (e.g. 200 mg daily) is only taken under medical supervision, short term, as excess may, in itself, lead to nerve conduction problems.

Vitamin B3 also seems to be important, as are essential fatty acids found, for example in *omega-3 fish oils*, which are important for optimal nerve sheath function.

Do not take supplements if you are pregnant, breast-feeding, or taking prescribed drugs without first seeking advice from a pharmacist about possible interactions or adverse effects.

Diuretic herbs such as *dandelion* may relieve symptoms where these are linked with fluid retention, while *bromelain* may help to reduce inflammation and pain especially when combined with vitamin B6 supplements.

Alpha lipoic acid is also important for nerve health.

See also: **Vitamin B6**.

Cataracts

A cataract is an opacity in the normally crystal clear eye lens, caused by changes in lens proteins similar to those that turn cooked egg white cloudy. This results in blurring, sensitivity to sun glare, changes in colour perception, and seeing haloes around light.

Most cataracts are due to degenerative changes with increasing age, worsened by exposure to ultraviolet light. Most people over the age of 65 have some degree of cataract, which progresses with age and – like macular degeneration – is linked with damaging oxidative reactions. In order to transmit light without scatter, the lens does not contain any blood vessels, and is made of cells that lack a nucleus. Cells within the lens must therefore obtain their oxygen and nutrients by diffusion from the eye fluids in which the lens is suspended. This leaves the lens increasingly vulnerable to free radical attack when levels of antioxidant nutrients are poor. Smokers and anyone who is diabetic or overweight are more prone to cataracts than others as they generate more free radicals than usual.

Treatment

Cataract extraction and replacement of the eye lens with an artificial prosthesis is now a common and routine surgery.

People with the highest dietary intakes of antioxidants (*vitamins C, E, selenium* and carotenoids such as *lutein, zeaxanthin* and *lycopene*) are less likely to develop cataracts than those with low intakes. Research involving over 50,000 nurses aged 45–67 found that those whose diet was rich in spinach and carrots, or who had been taking

---

Do not take supplements if you are pregnant, breast-feeding, or taking prescribed drugs without first seeking advice from a pharmacist about possible interactions or adverse effects.

vitamin C supplements for ten or more years, had up to a 45 per cent lower risk of cataracts than women whose antioxidant intake was poor (i.e. they ate little fruit and vegetables and/or took no supplements). Antioxidant vitamins prevent damaging oxidative chemical reactions in the body by mopping up free radicals (oxidizing molecular fragments produced by the metabolism and by smoking).

Bilberry extracts are rich in antioxidants and carotenoids and can help to protect against cataracts and macular degeneration of the eye, as well as reducing the progression of cataracts once they have started to appear.

See also: **Anthocyanins, Antioxidants, Bilberry, Chromium, Folic acid, Ginkgo, Lutein, Selenium, Vitamin A, Vitamin B2, Vitamin B3, Vitamin C, Vitamin E.**

Catarrh – excess

Catarrh is excess phlegm, or mucus, produced by the respiratory tract, and is a very common problem.

Treatment
Excess catarrh can sometimes be helped by cutting out dairy products, red meat, wheat and excess refined carbohydrates. Try following a restricted diet for a few weeks, then reintroducing products one at a time to see if any seem to trigger your symptoms. If a particular group of foods is omitted long term, it is important to seek nutritional advice so that important micro-nutrients such as calcium or iron are not lost.

Excess mucus can be dissolved by supplements containing *N-acetyl cysteine* (NAC), an amino acid that makes phlegm less viscid (do not take if you have peptic ulcers). Steam inhalations with essential oils of lavender, eucalyptus or tea tree oil can also help. Avoid exposure to cigarette smoke and other pollutants.

See also: **Aloe vera, Bromelain, Cayenne, Iodine, Liquorice, N-acetyl cysteine, Sarsaparilla.**

Do not take supplements if you are pregnant, breast-feeding, or taking prescribed drugs without first seeking advice from a pharmacist about possible interactions or adverse effects.

Chapped lips

Chapped lips are due to repeated wetting and drying of the skin around the mouth (e.g. due to nervous licking) which removes natural, protective skin oils. Exposure to cold winds is another common cause.

Treatment
A protective lip salve is essential but choose one that is non-flavoured as toffee or fruit flavours just encourage more licking. Piercing a capsule containing evening primrose oil and gently rubbing the oil into the sore area and surrounding skin will also soothe and protect. When going out in the cold, apply a protective layer of marigold ointment (or petroleum jelly) on the skin around the lips, and cover your lower face with a scarf.

Cracking and soreness at the corners of the mouth where the lips meet may indicate a fungal infection which will respond to an oral anti-fungal gel – ask a pharmacist for advice. Cracked corners can also be a sign of low levels of *iron* or *B group vitamins*. If you feel tired, have heavy periods or suspect you are anaemic, seek medical advice.

See also: **Vitamins B2, B6**.

Chemotherapy

It is important to seek individual advice from a nutritionist and/or herbal practitioner for support during and after receiving chemotherapy. Checking levels of *iron, folic acid* and *B12* may be recommended as anaemia can cause weakness and lack of stamina after cancer treatment.

Supplements such as *milk thistle, globe artichoke* and high-dose *antioxidants* may be suggested to help support liver function.

Siberian ginseng (Eleutherococcus senticosus) has been extensively investigated in Russia, and found to improve energy levels

---

Do not take supplements if you are pregnant, breast-feeding, or taking prescribed drugs without first seeking advice from a pharmacist about possible interactions or adverse effects.

and increase sense of well-being during and following both chemo- and radiotherapy. It also had beneficial effects on immunity during convalescence.

Co-enzyme Q10 can boost general energy levels by encouraging oxygen uptake in cells, but it usually takes three weeks – and occasionally up to three months – for energy levels to be noticeably improved.

B group vitamins and *evening primrose oil* may be helpful, while *5-HTP* or *St John's Wort* can relieve fatigue associated with low mood. Honey produced by bees fed on immune-boosting herbs can help to maintain white blood cell count during chemotherapy (see www.during-chemotherapy.org.uk).

See also: **Astralagus, Bee products – honey, Cat's claw, Glutamine, Maitake, Milk thistle, Reishi, Shiitake**.

Chickenpox

Chickenpox is a highly infectious illness, to which the majority of adults are immune as a result of exposure during childhood. Unfortunately, when chickenpox does occur in adults, it can be severe and may lead to complications including viral pneumonia. If an adult develops typical vesicles, it is important to consult a doctor as soon as possible, as an anti-viral drug, acyclovir, helps to reduce the duration and severity of adult chickenpox. Treatment must be started early for best results however – preferably within 72 hours of the onset of symptoms.

Treatment
Herbal extracts that boost immunity against viral infections include *Echinacea, cat's claw (una de gāto), reishi, shiitake* or *maitake*.

Antioxidants such as high-dose *vitamin C* and *vitamin E* or *olive leaf extract* can help to reduce inflammation. *Aloe vera gel* may be applied to the rash to help soothe and heal.

Related entry: **Shingles**.

Do not take supplements if you are pregnant, breast-feeding, or taking prescribed drugs without first seeking advice from a pharmacist about possible interactions or adverse effects.

Chilblains

Chilblains – known medically as *Erythema pernio* – are itchy, purple areas of inflammation that occur on parts of the body exposed to the cold for a prolonged period of time. They usually appear a day or two later on fingers, toes and even ears. They occur when small blood vessels in the skin go into spasm, which reduces blood supply to the affected area and causes local cell damage. In severe cases, they can develop into painful blisters. After they first occur, the area tends to be more sensitive to the effects of cold in the future so chilblains often recur each year. For some reason, chilblains are six times more common in women than men, and are more likely to affect the very young and the elderly. Chilblains may also be triggered by wearing tight clothing that constricts the circulation during cold weather.

Treatment

Hands and feet should be massaged daily with a good moisturizing skin cream containing omega-3s, evening primrose oil and/or aloe vera.

Eat plenty of oily fish (e.g. salmon, sardines, herrings, mackerel) which help to damp down inflammation as well as having a useful thinning effect on blood. *Omega-3 fish oil* supplements may also be taken.

Garlic tablets reduce the risk of chilblains by improving circulation through a thinning effect on blood, and by dilating small arteries in the skin. *Ginkgo biloba* also increases circulation to the extremities and may be taken together with garlic for additional benefit. *Ginger* also has a beneficial warming effect and some supplements combine all three extracts.

In addition, avoid tight, restrictive clothing, exercise regularly and, when going out in cold weather, wear several layers of thin, loose clothing to trap body heat, plus gloves, thick socks, scarf and hat.

Related entry: **Splits in Fingers**.

Do not take supplements if you are pregnant, breast-feeding, or taking prescribed drugs without first seeking advice from a pharmacist about possible interactions or adverse effects.

Childbirth

Many midwives recommend raspberry leaf tea or tablets to reduce both the duration and pain of childbirth. Raspberry leaf is thought to strengthen the contraction of longitudinal uterine muscles and should only be taken during the last eight weeks of pregnancy.

The homoeopathic remedy, Caulophyllum 30c, is recommended to strengthen uterine contractions, soften the cervix and reduce the need for interventions such as episiotomy, Caesarian or forceps delivery. Take twice a week (but not on consecutive days) from the 37th week of pregnancy, until labour starts. Two other homoeopathic remedies, Arnica 30c and Hypericum 30c, can be taken as soon as labour is established to reduce blood loss, bruising and hasten healing.

See also: **Agnus castus, Black cohosh, Bromelain, Raspberry leaf**.

Cholesterol – raised

Cholesterol is a fatty substance that is made in your liver from certain fats in your diet. A small amount is also obtained ready-made from animal-based foods such as meat, egg yolks and prawns.

Cholesterol acts as an important building block used to make:

- Healthy cell membranes
- Steroid hormones (e.g. cortisol, oestrogen, testosterone, progesterone)
- Vitamin D
- Bile acids
- Co-enzyme Q10 – a vitamin-like substance essential for processing oxygen and generating energy within cells (see page 103).

A certain amount of cholesterol is therefore vital for health. If you

---

Do not take supplements if you are pregnant, breast-feeding, or taking prescribed drugs without first seeking advice from a pharmacist about possible interactions or adverse effects.

make or consume too much, however, the amount circulating in your blood stream increases. If you lack antioxidants (from eating vegetables and fruit) to protect this circulating fat, it undergoes a chemical reaction called oxidation. Oxidized cholesterol is recognized as 'foreign' by scavenger cells (macrophages), which engulf it to form bloated 'foam' cells. As these foam cells try to leave your circulation by squeezing through the lining of your artery walls, they become trapped. As they accumulate, they cause hardening and furring up of the arteries – a process known as atherosclerosis (see page 378).

There are two main types of cholesterol in the circulation. The main difference between them is in their relative size and weight. High-density lipoprotein (HDL) cholesterol forms large, heavy particles that are too big to be engulfed by scavenger cells, or to seep into artery walls. HDL-cholesterol is referred to as 'good' cholesterol, as it stays in your blood stream and carries LDL-cholesterol back to the liver for processing. This is known as reversed cholesterol transport. The higher your level of HDL-cholesterol, the lower your risk of cardiovascular disease. In fact, for every 1 per cent rise in your blood level of HDL cholesterol, your risk of a heart attack falls by as much as 2 per cent.

Low-density lipoprotein (LDL) cholesterol, on the other hand, is referred to as 'bad cholesterol'. These tiny, light particles are readily oxidized and engulfed by scavenger cells. They can also seep into gaps between cells lining your artery walls, to hasten atherosclerosis. Some people make very small, dense LDL-cholesterol particles and have an unusually high risk of developing coronary heart disease. Others make LDL-particles that are closer in size to the gaps between artery lining cells and have an intermediate risk of heart disease. If you are lucky, you make relatively large, less dense LDL-cholesterol particles and have a lower risk of heart disease. The size of LDL-particle you make depends partly on the genes you inherit, and partly on your diet and lifestyle.

Blood fat levels are measured first thing in the morning before you have had anything to eat or drink (fasting level). In general, you want your cholesterol levels to be as follows:

- Total cholesterol less than 5 mmol/l
- LDL-cholesterol less than 3 mmol/l
- HDL greater than 1 mmol/l for men, or 1.2 mmol/l for women.

If you have other coronary heart disease factors such as high blood pressure, diabetes or smoke cigarettes, then your recommended total cholesterol level is even lower – below 4 mmol/l – with your LDL-cholesterol ideally less than 2 mmol/l. This usually means having to take a cholesterol-lowering drug such as a statin.

If you are told you have a raised cholesterol it is important to know the ratio between beneficial HDL cholesterol and harmful LDL cholesterol:

- If your cholesterol is mostly in the form of HDL-cholesterol, your risk of CHD is significantly reduced
- If your cholesterol is mostly in the form of LDL-cholesterol, your risk of CHD is significantly increased.

Divide the number for your total cholesterol (e.g. 5.8 mmol) by the number for your HDL-cholesterol (e.g. 1.4 mmol) to get your total cholesterol/HDL ratio (in this case, 5.8/1.4 = 4.1).

It is only a total cholesterol/HDL ratio of above 4.5 that is thought to be associated with a significantly increased risk of coronary heart disease.

Another type of fat, triglyceride, also increases the risk of circulatory problems if it is raised. The levels of these blood fats are related to diet (especially increased carbohydrate intake) and exercise levels, but heredity also has a significant role. Luckily, triglycerides are readily lowered by taking omega-3 fish oil supplements (see page 139).

Treatment
Statin drugs (atorvastatin, fluvastatin, pravastatin, rosuvastatin and simvastatin) reduce cholesterol production in your liver by inhibiting an enzyme, HMG-CoA reductase, which is involved in

---

Do not take supplements if you are pregnant, breast-feeding, or taking prescribed drugs without first seeking advice from a pharmacist about possible interactions or adverse effects.

the synthesis of both cholesterol and co-enzyme Q10. Statins are excellent at reducing cholesterol levels, but as well as lowering levels of LDL-cholesterol, statins also lower production of co-enzyme Q10 in the body. In fact, taking a statin can halve your circulating blood levels of co-enzyme Q10 within just two weeks. This is thought to account for the fact that around 1 in 10 people taking a statin develop tiredness and muscle aches and pains. These side effects can usually be overcome by taking *co-enzyme Q10* supplements. Importantly, taking a co-enzyme Q10 supplement does not affect the cholesterol-lowering action of statin drugs.

A good intake of dietary *antioxidants* is essential to protect circulating fats from oxidation (only oxidized fats are thought to enter vessel walls to cause atherosclerosis). Consume plenty of fresh fruit and vegetables. Antioxidant supplements may also help. *Pycnogenol®*, for example, extracted from the bark of the French maritime pine, contains a variety of potent antioxidants that can significantly reduce LDL-cholesterol and increase HDL-cholesterol as well as having other beneficial effects on the circulation.

Garlic tablets may prove beneficial. Some trials have shown that these could reduce cholesterol levels by an average of 11 per cent (and up to 25 per cent), but others have shown no benefit. Interestingly, however, some studies have found that garlic tablets could reduce and even reverse hardening and furring up of the arteries compared with those not taking them.

Omega-3 fish oils lower triglycerides but mostly have a neutral effect on total cholesterol levels. They can, however, increase good HDL-cholesterol and lower harmful LDL-cholesterol to improve your total cholesterol/HDL ratio.

Vitamin B3 (niacin) is needed to process fatty acids and is prescribed to lower stubbornly high triglycerides and LDL-cholesterol levels, while increasing levels of good HDL-cholesterol. At high doses (under medical supervision) it reduces the risk of both fatal and non-fatal heart attacks. Higher prescription doses can produce facial flushing, but this effect is now reduced by combining niacin with another drug (laropiprant) that helps to stop this. Low

Do not take supplements if you are pregnant, breast-feeding, or taking prescribed drugs without first seeking advice from a pharmacist about possible interactions or adverse effects.

dose aspirin taken half an hour beforehand can also reduce this effect.

Lecithin (phosphatidyl choline) is a type of fat that inhibits intestinal absorption of cholesterol, and increases its excretion into bile. Taking 10.5 g lecithin for 30 days can reduce average total cholesterol, LDL-cholesterol and triglycerides by over one third, while increasing beneficial HDL-cholesterol by 46 per cent.

Isoflavones are especially helpful for post-menopausal women for their oestrogen-like action. Regular intake can lower total cholesterol and LDL-cholesterol by 4 per cent or more. Research consistently shows an association between diets rich in phytoestrogens, and a reduced risk of cardiovascular disease.

Psyllium seed and husks are a natural fibre source that binds dietary cholesterol and other fats to slow their absorption. Taking 10 g psyllium seed daily for at least six weeks can reduce LDL-cholesterol levels by between 5–20 per cent. Drink plenty of water.

Probiotics are live, friendly digestive bacteria that produce short-chain fatty acids. These act on the liver to reduce blood stickiness and lower a raised cholesterol level.

Plant sterols such as campesterol, sitosterol and stigmasterol closely resemble cholesterol. They block absorption of dietary cholesterol to reduce LDL-cholesterol levels by up to 15 per cent. In those with Type 2 diabetes, this effect is almost doubled (26.8 per cent reduction). Adding plant sterols to statin medication is more effective than doubling the statin dose.

Red yeast rice is made by fermenting a type of yeast, *Monascus purpureus*, over rice, and is often used as a food colouring in foods such as Peking duck. Red yeast rice is the Chinese medicine equivalent of a statin, lowering cholesterol in the same way by inhibiting the enzyme (HMG-CoA reductase) needed to synthesize cholesterol in the liver. It can reduce total cholesterol by 23 per cent, LDL-cholesterol by 31 per cent and triglycerides by 34 per cent while increasing beneficial HDL-cholesterol by 20 per cent. Some muscle side effects similar to those seen with statin drugs have been reported, however, so this supplement should also be combined with co-Q10.

Do not take supplements if you are pregnant, breast-feeding, or taking prescribed drugs without first seeking advice from a pharmacist about possible interactions or adverse effects.

Cholesterol: Increasing evidence suggests that, by improving bile flow, artichoke extracts can lower 'bad' LDL-cholesterol levels and triglyceride levels while raising 'good' HDL-cholesterol. This effect is due to cynaroside and luteolin blocking synthesis of excess cholesterol in the liver. Studies suggest that taking artichoke extract for six to 12 weeks can lower total cholesterol levels by between 4.2 per cent and 18.5 per cent.

In addition to the above, the following supplements have all been used to help people with raised cholesterol levels.

See also: **Antioxidants, Arginine, Artichoke, Ashwaganda, Astaxanthin, Blue-green algae, Carnitine, Choline, Chromium, Conjugated linoleic acid, Copper, Devil's claw, Evening primrose oil, Fenugreek, Fibre, Flaxseed oil, Folic acid, Fo-ti, Garlic, Ginger, Ginseng, Grapeseed, Green tea, Hempseed oil, Holy basil, Iron, Isoflavones, Kelp, Krill oil, Lycopene, Magnesium, Myrrh, Oatstraw, Olive oil, Pfaffia, Pine bark, Probiotics, Rapeseed oil, Red vine leaf, Reishi, Shiitake, Turmeric, Vitamin B3, Vitamin C, Vitamin E.**

Chondromalacia patellae

Chondromalacia patellae is a common but painful condition of adolescence in which cartilage behind the patella becomes roughened rather than smooth. The exact cause is unknown, but it usually resolves after a few years. Orthodox treatment is with rest, painkillers, avoiding high heels and warmth.

Treatment
Supplements containing *glucosamine sulphate* will ensure optimum production of synovial fluid and cartilage, and in one study it was found helpful for athletes with chondromalacia patellae.

MSM-Sulphur is also helpful in reducing joint pain. Some evidence suggests that *isoflavones, vitamin C* and *vitamin D* are also

---

Do not take supplements if you are pregnant, breast-feeding, or taking prescribed drugs without first seeking advice from a pharmacist about possible interactions or adverse effects.

helpful. Other supplements such as *devil's claw* and *omega-3 fish oils* that are beneficial in treating arthritis are also worth trying.

Chronic fatigue syndrome

Chronic fatigue syndrome – also known as post-viral fatigue syndrome and myalgic encephalomyelitis (ME) – are linked with persistent feelings of extreme weakness, tiredness and loss of energy. The diagnosis of chronic fatigue syndrome is made when fatigue has been present for four months in an adult, or three months in a child where symptoms are:

- New or had a specific time of onset (i.e. not life long)
- Persistent and/or recurrent
- Not explained by other conditions
- Have resulted in a substantial reduction in activity level
- Are accompanied by post-exercise fatigue which is typically delayed usually by at least 24 hours, with slow recovery over several days
- And where one or more of the following are present:
  ▷ Difficulty in sleeping
  ▷ Muscle and/or joint pain at multiple sites without evidence of inflammation
  ▷ Headaches
  ▷ Painful lymph nodes that are not enlarged
  ▷ Sore throat
  ▷ Difficulty in thinking straight or concentrating
  ▷ Symptoms worsen with physical or mental exertion
  ▷ General malaise or flu-like symptoms
  ▷ Dizziness and/or nausea
  ▷ Palpitations with no obvious heart problem.

The exact cause is unknown and many different factors are thought to be involved, including abnormal immune responses. Most people

---

Do not take supplements if you are pregnant, breast-feeding, or taking prescribed drugs without first seeking advice from a pharmacist about possible interactions or adverse effects.

with chronic fatigue improve over time and some recover enough to resume normal work and activities. Some, however, experience relapses.

Treatment
Cognitive behavioural therapy (CBT) and graded exercise therapy (GET) can help. Avoid day-time sleeping and naps, which can further disrupt the sleep-wake cycle without improving physical or mental symptoms.

Many people with CFS benefit from a wholefood, balanced diet that is low in animal fat and high in fibre, and provides plenty of fresh fruits, vegetables and low-glycaemic foods such as wholegrains and pulses/beans.

Antioxidants such as *vitamin C* and mixed *carotenoids* may be recommended. Some evidence suggests that *B vitamin* status, especially *pyridoxine (vitamin B6)* is low in people with chronic fatigue syndrome and it is therefore worth trying an oral B complex supplement to see if this helps. A few physicians use a modified 'Myers cocktail' of vitamins and minerals (magnesium, calcium, B vitamins, vitamin C) injected into a vein.

Levels of *co-enzyme Q10* naturally start to decline from the age of 20 and taking supplements can improve fatigue – it usually takes three weeks and occasionally up to three months for energy levels to become noticeably increased, however.

L-carnitine is needed to transport fatty acids into the parts of the cell (mitochondria) that are responsible for burning them as a fuel. Some people have benefited from taking L-carnitine supplements (often taken together with *alpha-lipoic acid*).

Up to 80 per cent of people with chronic fatigue have benefited from taking high doses of *evening primrose oil* and *omega-3 fish oil* which are rich in essential fatty acids.

Immune-stimulating herbs are often tried, such as *Echinacea, astragalus, reishi* and *lapacho*, which also have anti-viral actions. *Olive leaf extracts* also have an anti-viral action and are often helpful for people with chronic fatigue syndrome.

Do not take supplements if you are pregnant, breast-feeding, or taking prescribed drugs without first seeking advice from a pharmacist about possible interactions or adverse effects.

St John's Wort may be helpful if mild to moderate depression is present, but *5-HTP* is the better option as it also improves sleep quality.

Liquorice root extracts are often recommended for chronic fatigue syndrome but are not appropriate for everyone and, in some cases, can make symptoms worse. Liquorice contains substances that reduce the breakdown of some steroid hormones made in the adrenal glands, and so increases levels of the body's natural steroids which can give you a temporary boost. This effect can wear off, however, as the adrenal glands produce fewer steroid hormones to compensate. Some practitioners suggest trying liquorice root extracts for a few weeks then switching to another form of adaptogen such as Korean or Siberian ginseng.

Note: Liquorice root extracts should only be taken under supervision of a doctor or medical herbalist, as they can cause side effects of high blood pressure and water retention in some people when used in high doses long term. *See under* **Liquorice**.

See also: **Aloe vera, Alpha-lipoic acid, Carnitine, Goldenseal, 5-HTP, Liquorice, Magnesium, Maitake, Olive leaf, Oregano oil, Pfaffia, Rhodiola, Shiitake, Vitamin B2, Vitamin B5, Vitamin B6, Vitamin D**.

Related entry: **Tiredness All the Time**.

Colds

As many as 200 different viruses can infect the upper respiratory tract to cause symptoms of the common cold. Cold viruses attack the lining of the nose, throat and sinuses which swell and produce increased amounts of mucus and fluids. At first, nasal secretions are clear, but they often turn yellow due to pus cells (white blood cells) rushing in to fight the infection. Other symptoms include sore throat, runny nose, watering eyes, coughing and sneezing. Often senses of smell and taste are also affected and a slight fever, headache and muscle pains may be experienced. Symptoms usually last from three

---

Do not take supplements if you are pregnant, breast-feeding, or taking prescribed drugs without first seeking advice from a pharmacist about possible interactions or adverse effects.

to seven days unless complications such as chronic rhinitis, sinusitis or chest infection set in.

Cold viruses are highly infectious and spread through nasal droplets passed on from person to person through coughing and sneezing. If one member of a family becomes infected, it is likely that three-quarters of those in the same house will suffer too. Young adults get an average of two to three colds per year while children may suffer as many as eight to 12 colds annually. Once infected with a cold, the body makes specific antibodies against that virus which are secreted into the nasal fluids for at least two years. These will protect against closely related viruses, but will not protect against the many other viruses that can also produce cold symptoms. To make matters worse, cold viruses frequently change their surface markers, so that as soon as the immune system gets to grips with one, it could mutate enough to cause problems again next time it is encountered.

Prevention

If you are fit, healthy and eat a nutritious diet, you can often shrug off a cold with few, if any, symptoms. To help prevent a cold, try to avoid excess stress which increases your chance of developing symptoms on exposure to a cold virus. If you are under stress, taking an adaptogen such as *Siberian ginseng, Korean ginseng*, *Rhodiola* or *astragalus* may help to reduce infections. *Valerian* (and Rhodiola) have a calming effect and can reduce anxiety as well as improving sleep.

Avoid cigarette smoke as both active and passive smoking damage the nasal lining and suppress your natural defences against cold viruses.

Ensure you get a regular good night's sleep. People who sleep for less than seven hours at night are more likely to develop a cold than those who regularly sleep for eight hours or more. People exposed to a common cold virus are five times more likely to develop symptoms if they have a low sleep efficiency score (time asleep divided by total time in bed) of 85 per cent, or less, than those with a higher sleep efficiency.

Do not take supplements if you are pregnant, breast-feeding, or taking prescribed drugs without first seeking advice from a pharmacist about possible interactions or adverse effects.

Take regular exercise which has a beneficial effect on immunity. Don't over do things, however, as over training lowers immunity and increases your chance of developing cold symptoms.

Avoid getting too cold. Researchers at the Common Cold Centre, Cardiff University, asked 90 people to sit with their feet in bowls of iced water for 20 minutes. Another 90 people sat with their feet in empty bowls. Three times more people who were chilled went on to develop cold symptoms than those who kept warm (29 per cent versus 9 per cent). Constriction of blood flow to the nose is thought to reduce the presence of disease-fighting white blood cells. So, a mild infection you would normally fight off without symptoms is able to take hold.

Good hygiene is vital to limit the transmission of respiratory infections, especially if you have children at home, who tend to harbour cold viruses outside the usual peak winter season. Encourage them to wash their hands regularly, including after blowing their nose and before eating. Using antibacterial hand wipes or sprays will provide extra protection. If possible, avoid people with obvious cold symptoms and try not to shake their hand! Wipe down door handles regularly as micro-organisms can survive on plastics and stainless steel for many hours. Another good strategy is to use anti-viral tissues that are impregnated with substances such as vitamin C, which kills 99 per cent of cold and flu viruses within 15 minutes. In contrast, viruses can survive for at least 24 hours in normal tissues.

Many vitamins and minerals play an important role in immunity. Diet should always come first, so aim to eat a healthy, wholefood diet providing plenty of fresh fruit, vegetables and nuts. Omega-3 oils found in oily fish, nuts and seeds boost immune function and can reduce susceptibility to respiratory allergies, as well as reducing the inflammation associated with cold infections. Several studies have found that people who take a *multivitamin and mineral supplement* are less likely to develop cold symptoms than those not taking supplements.

Try drinking *green tea*. Green tea contains antioxidant polyphe-

Do not take supplements if you are pregnant, breast-feeding, or taking prescribed drugs without first seeking advice from a pharmacist about possible interactions or adverse effects.

nols which help to protect against infection. Taking green tea supplements for three months has been shown to reduce the frequency and severity of cold symptoms by around a third compared to those taking inactive placebo.

Probiotic bacteria appear to stimulate immunity against both bacterial and viral infections. Taking supplements containing probiotics (plus vitamins and minerals) has been shown to significantly reduce the severity of cold symptoms, and to shorten the duration of a cold by almost two days compared with inactive placebo. These effects appear to be due to increased activity of immune cells called T lymphocytes, which regulate immune responses.

Obtain a good intake of *vitamin D* (from fortified foods, oily fish, supplements, sensible sun exposure) which has an important role in immunity and the prevention of upper respiratory tract infections. People with the highest vitamin D levels are less likely to have experienced a recent cold than those with low levels.

Echinacea increases the number and activity of white blood cells involved in fighting infections, and can reduce the susceptibility to colds. An analysis of data from 14 different trials confirms that Echinacea can reduce the chance of developing a cold by 58 per cent and shorten the duration of those that do occur by 1.4 days. It may be taken in low dose, long term, to reduce infections, or in a higher dose just when you feel an infection coming on. Follow instructions on packs as different products vary.

Vitamin C is one of the most popular supplements for preventing the common cold. Research suggests that viruses cannot multiply and survive in cells containing high levels of vitamin C so taking supplements regularly helps to lessen the chance of a respiratory infection taking hold. Studies involving school children and students, for example, found that taking vitamin C reduced the risk of catching a cold by as much as 30 per cent. When 168 people took ester-C (a non-acidic form that is readily absorbed) or placebo for two months, those taking ester-C experienced significantly fewer colds than those on placebo (37 versus 50), had shorter duration of symptoms (1.8 versus 3.1 days) and, overall, experienced fewer

Do not take supplements if you are pregnant, breast-feeding, or taking prescribed drugs without first seeking advice from a pharmacist about possible interactions or adverse effects.

days affected by cold symptoms (85 versus 178 days).

Taking *garlic* powder tablets may help to protect against viral infections.

Treatment

Saturate your circulation with vitamin C as soon as you feel symptoms coming on to help boost your resistance and reduce the severity and duration of a cold. Take 1 g of vitamin C (e.g. non-acidic ester-C) every hour until symptoms start to improve up to a total dose of 6 g. Vitamin C suppresses viral replication and also has an antioxidant action that reduces inflammation.

Sucking lozenges containing *zinc gluconate* may shorten the duration of a sore throat.

A systematic review of eight trials involving a Zulu herbal remedy, *Pelargonium sidoides,* confirms that it successfully treats symptoms of acute rhinosinusitis and common cold, such as sore throat, cough, runny and blocked nose. It can also relieve acute bronchitis.

Elderberry extracts contain anti-viral compounds that have been shown in double-blind, placebo-controlled trials to reduce the severity and duration of common cold and influenza infections. In one trial involving 40 patients (children and adults) with viral respiratory infections, 93 per cent receiving elderberry extracts showed significant clinical improvement within two days versus six days with a placebo.

Olive leaf extracts have a powerful anti-viral action against the common cold and influenza. Other supplements used to treat respiratory infections include *propolis* (a natural antiseptic produced by honey bees) and *Siberian ginseng* (*Eleutherococcus senticosus*) which is a powerful immune stimulant and, according to Russian research, reduces the incidence of colds, flu and other respiratory infections by 40 per cent in those taking it regularly.

Echinacea may be taken as soon as symptoms start, to boost general immunity. Most studies show that this reduces susceptibility to colds by around a third. In one study of just over 100 people with

---

Do not take supplements if you are pregnant, breast-feeding, or taking prescribed drugs without first seeking advice from a pharmacist about possible interactions or adverse effects.

a common cold, some were given Echinacea and others a placebo. After eight weeks, those taking Echinacea had longer intervals between recurrent infections, less severe symptoms and a quicker recovery if infection did occur than those taking the placebo. On average, it seems to lengthen the time between infections by around 60 per cent.

Nasal congestion can be relieved by plain steam inhalation, but adding essential oils such as menthol, eucalyptus, cinnamon, or pine will bring immediate relief.

See also: **Astragalus, Bee products – Propolis, Garlic, Ginger, Lapacho, Liquorice, Olive Leaf, Peppermint, Probiotics, Reishi, Shiitake, Siberian ginseng, Vitamin C, Zinc**.

Related entry: **Catarrh – excess**.

Conception

One of the most important times in a baby's development is the first four weeks after conception – often before an expectant mother is even aware she is pregnant. If a baby is undernourished at this critical time, it is more likely that he or she will develop certain illnesses such as coronary heart disease, high blood pressure, stroke or diabetes in later life, possibly because of the way the circulatory system is laid down.

Studies have shown a significant relationship between size of a baby at birth and maternal diet at or around the time of conception. These first few weeks of gestation are a time of rapid division of cells and a baby's brain and spinal cord are often fully developed before the pregnancy has even been recognized.

A woman needs twice as much folic acid during pregnancy as at any other time. Folic acid is essential for copying genetic material correctly during cell division, and deficiency during the first few weeks of pregnancy can cause faulty development of the brain or spinal cord – a condition known as a neural tube defect (e.g. spina bifida). Lack of folic acid is also associated with chromosome

---

Do not take supplements if you are pregnant, breast-feeding, or taking prescribed drugs without first seeking advice from a pharmacist about possible interactions or adverse effects.

abnormalities. Taking 400 mcg folic acid a day from the time of first trying to conceive (and preferably earlier) can reduce the risk of conceiving a child with a neural tube defect by as much as 70 per cent. Women with a family history of this condition are advised to take around ten times as much (4–5 mg a day) – a doctor should be consulted for advice. Foods naturally rich in folic acid should be eaten (e.g. dark green leafy vegetables) and fortified foods (such as cereals).

Vitamin B12 works together with folic acid and deficiency seems to be an independent risk factor for neural tube defects. These are five times more common in babies whose mothers have low blood levels of vitamin B12. Some researchers now suggest that B12 supplements should be included in programmes designed to reduce the risk of neural tube defects.

To guard against other vitamin and mineral deficiencies, a varied, healthy diet should be followed, and a multivitamin and mineral supplement is also worth considering. It is important to take one especially designed for pregnancy as megadoses of some micro-nutrients (such as vitamin A) can be just as harmful as not enough. A supplement containing an essential fatty acid (DHA) derived from oily fish or algae which is important for development of your baby's eyes and brain is also helpful (only select one specifically designed for use during pregnancy).

Supplements containing evening primrose oil help to keep skin in good condition during pregnancy and may reduce the risk of stretch marks.

See also: **Agnus castus, Folic acid, Vitamin C**.

Advice for future dads

Men who are planning to father a child should stop smoking – smokers have damaged sperm and are only half as fertile as non-smokers. If they don't stop, at the very least they should take anti-oxidant supplements – including *vitamin C, vitamin E, selenium and carotenoids*; these are essential to help protect sperm from the damaging effects of cigarette smoke. Folic acid and zinc are also

---

Do not take supplements if you are pregnant, breast-feeding, or taking prescribed drugs without first seeking advice from a pharmacist about possible interactions or adverse effects.

important for sperm health. Alcohol intake should be lowered, and preferably cut out altogether as 40 per cent of male infertility is linked with just a moderate intake of alcohol.

See also: **Antioxidants, Arginine, Astralagus, Carnitine, Chromium, Co-enzyme Q10, Maca, Selenium, Vitamin C, Zinc.**
Related entry: **Sperm count – low.**

Constipation

Most doctors define constipation as passing bowel motions less than twice a week, or straining more than 25 per cent of the time. A number of factors can contribute to constipation, including poor fibre intake, poor fluid intake, lack of exercise and poor muscle tone, poor toilet habit (putting off going due to being busy), pregnancy, an underactive thyroid gland and depression. Old age, the side effects of some drugs (e.g. codeine phosphate) or supplements (such as iron), bowel obstruction (a bowel tumour or scar tissue) and abnormal masses (e.g. large fibroid or ovarian cyst) can also be a cause. Chronic constipation and straining at stools can lead to a number of other problems including haemorrhoids, diverticular disease, anal fissures and even rectal prolapse which will in turn make constipation worse.

Treatment
To help overcome constipation, a wholefood diet is recommended, containing more brown bread, brown rice, wholegrain cereals, salads, fresh fruit and vegetables for fibre. Apples, bananas, pears, grapes, dried apricots or figs are good snacks, rather than crisps, cakes or biscuits. Five to six prunes soaked in water or cold tea overnight may be eaten for breakfast with natural bio yoghurt, and seeds (such as sunflower, pumpkin, fenugreek, fennel and linseed) should be added to salads and yoghurt for extra roughage.

Natural bulking agents (e.g. bran, wheat husks, psyllium/ispaghula taken with plenty of water) can increase the

---

Do not take supplements if you are pregnant, breast-feeding, or taking prescribed drugs without first seeking advice from a pharmacist about possible interactions or adverse effects.

volume of bowel motions and soften them by absorbing fluid. The seed and husks of psyllium are a safe and effective remedy for constipation, increasing the frequency of bowel movements and making stools softer and easier to pass. When taking fibre supplements, it is vital to drink plenty of fluid: at least six glasses of mineral water per day to swell up the dietary fibre and get things moving.

Other supplements that will help include *probiotic bacteria, dandelion root, dong quai* and *aloe vera* juice. *Goldenseal* may be recommended to help to normalize muscular action in the bowel.

See also: **African prune, Aloe vera, Arginine, Artichoke, Calcium, Dandelion, Fibre, Flaxseed, Iron, Magnesium, MSM, Oatstraw, Potassium, Vitamin D**.

Coronary heart disease

See: **Angina**.

Corticosteroids – taking oral treatment

Oral corticosteroids are powerful drugs that damp down inflammation and abnormal immune reactions. Those taking oral corticosteroids may benefit from taking herbs that support liver function. These include *dandelion* extracts which are also diuretic and help to reduce fluid retention) and *milk thistle* extracts (silymarin). *Curcumin,* which is extracted from turmeric, is also used to support liver function and has been shown to have a strong anti-inflammatory action similar to that of the corticosteroid, hydrocortisone, in its own right. Herbal preparations that enhance immunity such as *Echinacea* or *cat's claw* may also be beneficial.

Note: It is important for each individual to consult a medically qualified herbal practitioner for specific treatments tailored to suit him or her.

Do not take supplements if you are pregnant, breast-feeding, or taking prescribed drugs without first seeking advice from a pharmacist about possible interactions or adverse effects.

Coughs

A cough is the most common symptom of respiratory disease, and is designed as a protective reflex that helps to bring up excess phlegm or irritant substances from the lungs, or which prevents foreign particles from being inhaled. If mucus is brought up, the cough is described as productive. If there is no phlegm, the cough is said to be dry. An irritating, repetitive cough with annoying sensations at the back of the throat is called a tickly cough, while whooping cough is due to a bacterial infection (pertussis) in which long paroxysms of coughing are followed by a desperate whoop as air is drawn back into the lungs. A smoker's cough contains mucky grey discoloured phlegm.

Coughs are usually due to irritation of the airways from dust and smoke, from mucus constantly dripping down from the back of the nose or to infection and inflammation of your upper airways. When somebody with a cold coughs or sneezes over people near by, they will be showered with droplets teeming with millions of infectious viral particles and will then be at risk of catching the infection themselves.

Treatment

In general, a dry, irritating, tickly cough that interferes with sleep may be damped down with a cough suppressant, but a productive cough should not usually be damped down with anti-cough medicines as the excess mucus needs to be brought up. An expectorant can help to bring up infected phlegm from the lungs.

Infective coughs benefit from drinking plenty of fluids (especially hot drinks) to loosen secretions, and from steam inhalations.

Liquorice or *slippery elm* lozenges may be used to soothe an irritating cough and sore throat, while *zinc* lozenges can also reduce tickling coughs.

Olive leaf extracts and *Pelargonium sidoides* extracts have a natural antibiotic effect and can help cough linked with bronchitis or other infection. Tinctures or teas containing *thyme* can help to

---

Do not take supplements if you are pregnant, breast-feeding, or taking prescribed drugs without first seeking advice from a pharmacist about possible interactions or adverse effects.

reduce cough and have traditionally been used to help children with whooping cough infection.

See also: **Eucalyptus, Liquorice, N-acetyl cysteine**.

Note: Always seek medical advice about a cough that is troublesome, recurrent or associated with coughing up blood, as it may be an important sign of chronic lung infection (e.g bronchitis), inflammation (e.g. asthma) or irritation (e.g. lung cancer).

Cradle cap

Cradle cap (*Crusta lutea*) is a form of seborrhoeic dermatitis that commonly affects newborn infants. In severe cases, a thick circle of yellow, waxy crusts build up on the scalp to resemble a cap. The face, neck, behind the ears and nappy area can be affected, too. The cause is unknown but sensitivity to a common skin yeast, *Pityrosporum ovale*, overactivity of sebaceous glands, lack of essential fatty acids and failure of immature skin cells to shed properly have all been suggested as possibilities.

Treatment

Scales are traditionally loosened by gently massaging in a little warm olive oil, leaving overnight, then washing off next morning using a simple shampoo designed for use on newborns. This should be repeated until all the scales have been loosened and washed off. Brushing the hair with a clean soft-bristled brush will also help, but care should be taken not to scratch the skin.

Improvements have also been seen in many babies who are given *evening primrose oil* drops – whether these are added into their feeds, or rubbed directly on to the affected skin. Nursing mothers can also take evening primrose oil supplements to enrich the essential fatty acid content of their milk.

Do not take supplements if you are pregnant, breast-feeding, or taking prescribed drugs without first seeking advice from a pharmacist about possible interactions or adverse effects.

Cramp

Cramp is the popular name for the painful, excessive contraction of a muscle. It is most commonly felt in the leg, but any muscle can be affected. Cramps are linked with a build-up of lactic acid and other waste products of muscle metabolism – usually during or after physical exercise. They can also be triggered by repetitive movements (as in writer's cramp) and or by sitting or lying in an awkward position. Poor circulation decreases the oxygen supply to muscles and interferes with the flushing away of lactic acids and other chemicals. This can happen at night in elderly people with hardening and furring up of their leg arteries. Night cramps are also common during pregnancy, possibly because of changes in blood circulation. After eating a heavy meal, blood is diverted away from peripheral muscles to aid digestion; this is why swimming immediately after eating is not advised. Excessive sweating, a fever, and hot weather can also cause cramps due to dehydration.

Treatment

Increasing dietary intakes of calcium (low-fat milk, cheese, yoghurt and other dairy products, dark green leafy vegetables) and magnesium (nuts, seafood, dairy products, wholegrains, dark green, leafy vegetables) can help to prevent cramps, and plenty of fluids should be drunk during the day, especially mineral water.

Supplements containing *calcium, magnesium* and *vitamin E* are also beneficial. Poor circulation may be improved by taking *garlic tablets, omega-3 fish oil* supplements or *ginkgo biloba* extracts. Many sufferers also find *co-enzyme Q10* – which increases oxygen uptake in muscle cells – effective, especially where circulation is poor.

Cramps can usually be relieved by vigorous massage, applying a hot or cold compress, or by gently stretching the affected muscle. Applying a warm compress will increase circulation and help to bring relief.

Do not take supplements if you are pregnant, breast-feeding, or taking prescribed drugs without first seeking advice from a pharmacist about possible interactions or adverse effects.

Note: Seek medical advice if cramps last longer than an hour.
See also: **Pine bark**.

Crawling sensations

A prickling sensation that resembles ants crawling over the skin is known as formication. It is a form of pins and needles (paraesthesiae) which may be due to irritation or compression of part of the nervous system. It can also occur in diabetes, liver or thyroid disease, as a side effect of some drugs (e.g. alcohol, cocaine), and from taking excessively high amounts of some supplements (e.g. *agnus castus* or *vitamin B6*). Confusingly, however, it can also occur due to severe lack of certain micronutrients such as *B12* or *phosphorus*. If sensations persist, it is best to seek medical advice.

Crohn's disease

Crohn's disease is a chronic inflammatory disease of the bowel whose origin is unknown. Some researchers believe it to be an abnormal allergic reaction – possibly due to dietary components or an as-yet unidentified bacterial, viral or parasitic infection. Particular foods often exacerbate symptoms, and should be avoided to help reduce symptoms or maintain clinical remission. Unfortunately, it is not always easy to identify the culprits. In one study, the foods most commonly implicated were corn, wheat, milk, yeast, egg, potato, rye, tea, coffee, apples, mushrooms, oats and chocolate. A 19-year study in Japan found that the strongest independent dietary risk factor for Crohn's was an increased intake of animal protein.

Treatment
The so-called LOFFLEX (low-fibre, fat-limited exclusion) diet is designed for people with Crohn's disease. It suggests not eating

---

Do not take supplements if you are pregnant, breast-feeding, or taking prescribed drugs without first seeking advice from a pharmacist about possible interactions or adverse effects.

foods identified by bowel specialists as most likely to worsen symptoms in their patients. The list of foods you are advised to exclude, and those that you are allowed to eat, is as follows:

Foods that are NOT allowed	Foods that ARE allowed
Pork	Other lean meat and poultry
Fish in batter/oil/tomato	All other fish and shellfish
Milk (cow's, goat, sheep) and dairy products	Soy products
Wheat, rye, barley, millet, buckwheat, corn, oats	Rice, rice cakes, rice milk and rice cereals
Yeast	Tapioca, sago
Pulses, onion, tomatoes, sweetcorn	All other vegetables, including potatoes (2 portions per day, no skins)
Citrus fruit, apples, bananas, dried fruits	All other fruits (2 portions a day, no skins)
Vegetable, corn and nut oils	Sugar, honey, jam
Nuts and seeds	Fruit and herbal teas
Tea, coffee, alcohol, squashes, cola	Water

After following the LOFFLEX diet for two weeks, you start re-introducing new foods as long as you are symptom free. It is not recommended that you follow the full restriction part of this diet for more than four weeks.

New 'test' foods are then introduced, one at a time, over the course of four days, to see if you can tolerate them. The exception is wheat products, which you must test for seven days, as the onset of symptoms is often delayed after re-introducing this cereal into your diet. If a test food causes side effects, you continue to avoid it and wait until all symptoms have improved before testing another food. If no reactions occur, you start testing a new food after four days.

Do not take supplements if you are pregnant, breast-feeding, or taking prescribed drugs without first seeking advice from a pharmacist about possible interactions or adverse effects.

You are advised to introduce new foods in the following order, starting with those that are less likely to cause problems: pork, oats, tea, rye, eggs, onions, coffee, yeast, banana, apple, milk, butter/margarine, white wine, peas, chocolate, tomato, cheese, corn, citrus fruit, wheat, bread, yoghurt, nuts, sweetcorn. Keeping a food and symptom diary will help identify foods that you need to avoid long term.

In one study, over half of people who followed the LOFFLEX diet were still free from symptoms after two years.

This diet can be nutritionally balanced if you eat a variety of allowed foods, and you start introducing new 'test' foods within two to four weeks. If you find you need to avoid lots of foods because they worsen your symptoms, it is important to seek dietary advice. When avoiding dairy products, for example, you can obtain calcium from a calcium-enriched soy milk and from green vegetables such as kale and broccoli.

People with inflammatory bowel disease are at risk of a number of vitamin and mineral deficiencies. This is partly because they may follow a restricted diet, and partly because bowel inflammation can reduce absorption of some nutrients. As a result, even people with newly diagnosed Crohn's disease may have low levels of riboflavin (B2), folate, betacarotene, vitamin B12, calcium, phosphorus, magnesium, selenium, zinc and vitamin D. People with long-standing Crohn's are also likely to have low levels of iron and of fat-soluble vitamins, including vitamin K.

As well as regulating calcium absorption, vitamin D may also regulate immune responses linked with inflammatory bowel disease, making it important to avoid deficiency of this nutrient. You should therefore strongly consider taking a *multivitamin and mineral* supplement.

Probiotics are friendly, digestive bacteria that produce beneficial substances such as butyrate. Butyrate is a short fatty acid that acts as a 'food' for bowel lining cells (colonocytes). Abnormal metabolism of butyrate has been suggested as a possible cause of ulcerative inflammatory bowel disease. Butyrate levels are reduced by the

Do not take supplements if you are pregnant, breast-feeding, or taking prescribed drugs without first seeking advice from a pharmacist about possible interactions or adverse effects.

action of sulphur compounds in the bowel and, by helping to maintain butyrate levels, probiotic bacteria may have a beneficial role to play in inflammatory bowel disease.

The number of probiotic bacteria in the bowel can be improved by eating resistant fibre, such as that found in oat bran. This type of fibre (sometimes referred to as prebiotics) is not digested by humans, but can be used by probiotic bacteria to fuel their growth in the colon.

As oat bran may offer other health benefits, such as helping to lower cholesterol levels, it is worth increasing your intake of this fibre source if you have an inflammatory bowel disease.

Omega-3 fish oils help to reduce inflammation in the body. Eating oily fish has been shown to help people with other inflammatory conditions, such as rheumatoid arthritis, and might also have a beneficial effect on inflammatory bowel diseases. Unfortunately, the evidence does not currently support this theory. Research looking at whether fish oils might help to maintain remission in Crohn's disease has not found significant benefit. Of those studies that are available, those using enteric coated capsules may provide more positive benefits in Crohn's disease than ordinary gelatin capsules. For example, in one study involving enteric-coated fish oil capsules (supplying 1.8 g of EPA and 0.9 g DHA taken for one year), only 28 per cent of the 39 patients taking fish oils relapsed to active disease versus 69 per cent of 39 patients receiving a placebo. As fish oils have other beneficial effects in the body on heart, circulatory and joint health, it is worth increasing your intake of oily fish (e.g. salmon, herring, mackerel, sardines) to see if this helps you as an individual.

Aloe vera gel, and herbal supplements with a natural anti-microbial action such as grapefruit seed extract, goldenseal or garlic are sometimes helpful.

People with Crohn's disease tend to be smokers, and giving up smoking can help to improve symptoms.

See also: **Aloe vera, Boswellia, Copper, Glutamine, Liquorice, Mastic gum, Vitamin B12**.

Do not take supplements if you are pregnant, breast-feeding, or taking prescribed drugs without first seeking advice from a pharmacist about possible interactions or adverse effects.

Cystitis

Cystitis is an inflammation or infection of the bladder. It is more common in women than men as the passage from the bladder to the outside world (urethra) is much shorter in females than males (2 cm as compared with around 20 cm), making it easier for infection to pass up the urinary tract. As many as one in two women experiences symptoms at some time during her life.

Symptoms depend on the severity of the infection. In mild cases, only one or two symptoms may occur. In severe cases, a sufferer may develop every symptom. These include:

- Burning, stinging or discomfort on passing urine (dysuria)
- A need to rush to the toilet (urgency)
- Passing frequent, small amounts of urine
- Low abdominal pain or backache
- Unpleasant smelling urine which may appear cloudy or blood-stained.

Infection is usually due to bacteria from the vagina or bowel. Seventy per cent of cases are due to *Escherichia coli* which normally lives in the large intestines. Sexual intercourse is one of the commonest triggers of cystitis as it can push bacteria up into the urethra. This is sometimes referred to as honeymoon cystitis. Research suggests that sexual activity can multiply a woman's risk of a UTI by fourteen times. Some attacks of cystitis are thought to be caused by wearing tight trousers or nylon tights as these can increase warmth and humidity which encourage bacterial growth.

Sufferers of recurrent cystitis should be investigated for conditions such as diabetes, anaemia and anatomical abnormalities of the urinary system.

Treatment
Supplements containing a combination of extracts from the herbs *dandelion, bearberry* and *peppermint* can help to prevent the

---

Do not take supplements if you are pregnant, breast-feeding, or taking prescribed drugs without first seeking advice from a pharmacist about possible interactions or adverse effects.

symptoms of cystitis. In one study, 57 women who had suffered at least three episodes of cystitis during the previous year were given either a preparation containing dandelion, bearberry and peppermint or inactive placebo tablets. After 12 months, none of the women taking the herbal product had developed cystitis during treatment, while around one in four of those receiving the placebo suffered at least one bout of cystitis.

Drinking 300 ml *cranberry* juice daily can almost halve the risk of developing cystitis. Studies also suggest that cranberries contain an anti-adhesin that prevents bacteria from sticking to the urinary tract wall. Concentrated cranberry extracts are also beneficial.

Olive leaf extracts have an antibacterial action and are often helpful for treating cystitis.

Note: Medical advice should be sought in any of the following circumstances:

- Symptoms that last longer than a day or keep recurring
- Pregnancy
- Urine is cloudy or stained with blood
- A fever or uncontrollable shakes develop.

See also: **Bilberry, Cranberry, Grapefruit seed, Oregano oil, Peppermint, Sarsaparilla.**

Dandruff

Dandruff is the shedding of tiny flakes of skin from the scalp which does not usually cause any discomfort. Severe cases, known as seborrhoeic dermatitis, can produce an itchy, scaly rash on the scalp, and affected skin may look red and inflamed. Dry or greasy scales form around the hairline and, in severe cases, a yellow-red crust appears.

Seborrhoeic dermatitis is thought to be triggered by a hypersensitivity to the skin yeast, *Pityrosporum ovale*. On the face, the red, scaly rash commonly affects the eyebrows and forehead, with greasy scaling of skin folds running between the nose and lips. A wide range of shampoos/lotions is available containing anti-fungal agents (such as pyrithione zinc, selenium sulphide, ketoconazole) which reduce flaking and help to control the number of yeast cells present. Corticosteroids (hydrocortisone, betametasone) may be prescribed to damp down inflammation, while products containing salicylic acid may be used to help loosen scales.

Treatment
Dry, scaly skin is sometimes linked with a lack of certain vitamins and minerals, especially vitamins A, B2, B3, C, biotin and the minerals iodine, manganese, selenium and zinc. A good *multi-vitamin and mineral* supplement containing around 100 per cent of the recommended daily amount (RDA) for as many vitamins and minerals as possible might be beneficial.

Kelp supplements contain 13 vitamins, 20 essential amino acids and 60 minerals and trace elements, and are a particularly rich source of calcium, magnesium, potassium, iron and iodine so are often recommended to improve any associated hair problems.

Inflammation can be reduced by increasing intakes of omega-3 fatty acids, and cutting back on omega-6s (*see* **Essential Fatty Acids**). Eat more oily fish, nuts, seeds and take *evening primrose oil* and/or *omega-3 fish oil* supplements.

A solution of seven drops of rosemary or tea tree essential oil diluted with 1 tablespoon (15 ml) carrier oil should be rubbed into the scalp before washing the hair with a tea tree shampoo.

See also: **Brewer's yeast, Essential Fatty Acids**.

Deep vein thrombosis

A deep vein thrombosis (DVT) is the formation of a blood clot within a deep lying vein, most commonly in the lower leg. DVT may occur when blood flow is sluggish (e.g. due to varicose veins, or

---

Do not take supplements if you are pregnant, breast-feeding, or taking prescribed drugs without first seeking advice from a pharmacist about possible interactions or adverse effects.

prolonged inactivity such as bed rest or long-haul air flights) and when an increased level of blood clotting factors are produced (e.g. some blood diseases, in pregnancy, when taking the oral contraceptive pill or following extensive injury, infection or surgery). Increasing age and being overweight also makes deep vein thrombosis more likely.

Symptoms of a DVT can include pain, tenderness, discoloration and swelling of the affected area. This is most easily detected when the DVT forms in veins running through the calf, but it is not always easy to diagnose especially if an unusual site is affected.

DVT is potentially serious as a clot interferes with blood flow to the affected area. Part of a clot may break off and travel in the blood stream to the heart or lungs as an embolus which can cause pulmonary embolism (a clot on the lung), stroke or heart attack, and, in severe cases, may be fatal.

Treatment

Treatment of DVT is with anticoagulant drugs (e.g. heparin, warfarin) and sometimes fibrinolytic drugs which dissolve dangerous clots. Where thrombosis is life-threatening, surgery may be needed to remove the clot.

Regular exercise, especially when confined to cramped space (e.g. on a long-haul flight) can reduce the risk of DVT. Wearing elasticated support socks/tights can also help by reducing blood pooling in the lower limbs. It is important to have them fitted for the correct size – too tight will restrict blood flow.

Research suggests 125 mg *Pycnogenol®* is as effective in preventing increased susceptibility to blood clotting as 500 mg aspirin in smokers. As a bonus, it does not irritate the stomach, and does not increase bleeding time so will not lead to easy bruising.

Omega-3 fish oils have a blood thinning action which helps to increase bleeding time and reduce formation of unwanted blood clots.

Guarana lowers levels of fibrinogen (a blood coagulation factor) to reduce risk of DVT.

Do not take supplements if you are pregnant, breast-feeding, or taking prescribed drugs without first seeking advice from a pharmacist about possible interactions or adverse effects.

Ginkgo biloba, garlic and *ginger* improve general circulation to the peripheries.

During a long-haul flight, drink plenty of fluids, avoid excess alcohol, walk around frequently, and wear support socks. An in-flight blow-up exerciser cushion that simulates the action of walking is also very effective in boosting blood flow through veins in the lower leg to minimize the risk of DVT.

Note: Because of the risk of over-thinning the blood, it is inadvisable to combine different supplements without seeking advice from a qualified nutritionist/herbalist. Also, they should not be combined with heparin, or warfarin, unless under specialist advice.

See also: **Pine bark**.

Depression

Depression is common and affects as many as one in eight men and one in five women at some time during their life. It is caused by an imbalance of chemical messengers in the brain that are responsible for passing signals from one brain cell to another. If levels of one or more fall too low, the brain does not function properly and a variety of psychological and physical symptoms can occur including:

- Low mood with crying and sadness
- Tiredness or exhaustion
- Nervousness, anxiety and agitation
- Headache, difficulty in concentrating
- Loss of self-esteem and lack of confidence
- Low sex drive
- Loss of interest in everyday life.

Women are more susceptible to depressive illness than men and are up to three times more likely to suffer due to hormone changes linked with menstruation, childbirth and the menopause.

At least half of all people with depression do not seek help, yet it

---

is important to address low mood quickly before more serious symptoms set in. It is one of the commonest reasons why people consult their doctor yet it is estimated that only half of all cases are diagnosed, as sufferers either do not realize they have a depressive illness or are unwilling to seek help. Once a diagnosis or assessment has been made, a doctor should advise on whether an antidepressant drug or referral for a psychiatric assessment is needed.

Treatment

One of the most effective natural treatments is *5-HTP* which provides building blocks for making several brain neurotransmitters, including serotonin. It should not be taken together with other antidepressant medications.

Treatment with standardized preparations of the herb *St John's Wort* (*Hypericum perforatum*) are often effective in treating mild to moderate depression. St John's Wort extracts providing 900 mcg hypericin a day are at least as effective as prescribed anti-depressants in treating moderate depression, but with less risk of side effects.

St John's Wort does interact with numerous prescribed drugs, however, so anyone who is on other medication should check with a doctor or pharmacist before taking it.

The fish oil consumption of populations worldwide is strongly inversely correlated with the prevalence of depression – those who eat fish infrequently are more likely to become depressed than those who eat fish regularly. Several studies show that the omega-3 fish oil, EPA, can improve depression. It is thought to work by affecting serotonin metabolism or to have an action similar to that of the prescribed anti-depressant drugs, lithium and valproate. A dose of 1 g EPA daily appears to be most effective. The other main omega-3 essential fatty acid found in fish oils (DHA) does not appear to offer significant benefit in treating depression.

See also: **Agnus castus, Biotin, Black cohosh, Choline, Chromium, Damiana, Essential Fatty Acids, Fish oils, Folic acid, Ginkgo, Gotu kola, Holy basil, 5-HTP, Lemon balm, Maca,**

Do not take supplements if you are pregnant, breast-feeding, or taking prescribed drugs without first seeking advice from a pharmacist about possible interactions or adverse effects.

Magnesium, Muira puama, Oatstraw, Rhodiola, St John's Wort, Valerian, Vitamin B1, Vitamin B3, Vitamin B5, Vitamin B6, Vitamin B12.

Diabetes

Diabetes mellitus occurs when the body is unable to make enough insulin hormone in the pancreas gland (Type 1) or when the body does not respond properly to the insulin that is made (Type 2). Insulin controls blood sugar levels by helping to transport glucose into muscle and fat cells, where it is used as a fuel. Without insulin, glucose builds up in the bloodstream, and the way in which cells process carbohydrate, protein and fat becomes abnormal.

Symptoms of untreated Type 1 diabetes include thirst, producing excess urine, blurred vision, raging hunger and weight loss. In Type 2 diabetes, symptoms are often less specific and can include lack of energy, tiredness, listlessness and easy fatigue. Raised glucose levels also encourage recurrent infections such as cystitis, thrush and boils.

Type 2 diabetes accounts for 95 per cent of cases and is linked with obesity – especially where excess fat accumulates around the internal organs to increase waist size. This type of centrally deposited fat is metabolically active. It releases chemicals that increase insulin resistance, blood pressure, blood stickiness and triglycerides and reduces production of 'good' HDL-cholesterol. The aim of diabetes treatment, which usually involves drugs (e.g. insulin, metformin) is to maintain blood glucose levels within the normal range (4–6 mmol/l) before breakfast (fasting) and below 7mmol/l two hours after a meal. The tighter your glucose control, the lower your risk of developing long-term complications linked to damage to the circulation and internal organs such as diabetic retinopathy, kidney disease, heart attack and leg ulcers. For more information about my book on Overcoming Diabetes, visit my website www.naturalhealthguru.co.uk.

When glucose levels are raised, glucose molecules become

irreversibly bound to proteins in the circulation, causing damage to blood vessel walls that hastens hardening and furring up of the arteries. At the same time, some excess glucose is converted to a sugar alcohol, sorbitol, inside cells. Sorbitol causes the cell to swell and disrupts the normal flow of salts and amino acids across the cell membrane – especially in the eyes, kidneys and nerve sheaths. This hastens the onset of complications. NB: Sorbitol used as an artificial sweetener is not linked to this damage as it does not accumulate inside cells.

Treatment
People with diabetes are advised to follow the same healthy eating guidelines as everyone else. This involves:

- Reducing energy intake to help you lose excess weight (adjusting your dose of glucose-lowering drugs to compensate for reduced energy intake)
- Reducing your intake of excess, rapidly-digested (high-glycaemic load) carbohydrates to lower triglyceride levels and improve insulin sensitivity
- Increasing your intake of healthy monounsaturated and omega-3 fats to improve cholesterol balance and to protect against coronary heart disease and stroke
- Cutting down on salt to reduce the sodium and fluid retention that can trigger high blood pressure
- Increasing your fibre intake to slow absorption of dietary carbohydrates and fats, thereby improving your glucose control and blood cholesterol balance
- Eating more fresh fruit and vegetables to provide antioxidants and isoflavones that protect against the circulatory damage linked with diabetic complications
- Eating more wholegrains for the trace elements such as chromium, manganese and magnesium which can improve glucose control
- Following a diet rich in vitamins B6, B12 and folic acid to reduce elevated levels of homocysteine

---

Do not take supplements if you are pregnant, breast-feeding, or taking prescribed drugs without first seeking advice from a pharmacist about possible interactions or adverse effects.

• Cutting back on partially-hydrogenated trans-fatty acids to lower your risk of heart disease.

Exercising for 30 minutes (and preferably 60 minutes) every day can significantly improve glucose control and help with weight maintenance. Exercise has been shown to increase the tissue levels of chromium, which improves glucose control and cholesterol levels. Exercise helps some people with Type 2 diabetes regain normal glucose tolerance.

If you smoke, do your utmost to stop.

Antioxidants help to neutralize excess harmful free radicals produced during diabetes and can improve glucose metabolism and reduce the risk of complications.

Vitamin C has a similar structure to glucose and plays a role in glucose tolerance. Vitamin C significantly reduces the harmful glycosylation of proteins, including haemoglobin (1 g daily reduces HbA1c by 18 per cent within 12 weeks). It also reduces sorbitol formation within cells which may reduce long-term complications including cataracts. NB: Vitamin C will affect HbA1c blood tests and urinary glucose tests, so always tell your doctor if taking supplements.

Vitamin E protects body fats from oxidation and strengthens capillaries and muscle fibres. Vitamin E can significantly lower levels of glycosylated haemoglobin and fasting glucose. As it becomes a free radical itself as a result of its antioxidant action, it is best taken together with vitamin C and/or alpha-lipoic acid that help to regenerate it.

Alpha lipoic acid speeds energy production in cells, and regenerates vitamins C and E to enhance their effectiveness. Monitor blood glucose levels carefully as ALA stimulates glucose uptake into muscle cells to significantly improve glucose tolerance in people with Type 2 diabetes. ALA protects nerve sheaths from oxidative damage, improves nerve conduction and is used in the treatment of diabetic neuropathy, to improve pain, burning sensations, numbness and pins and needles. ALA also reduces the amount of albumin

Do not take supplements if you are pregnant, breast-feeding, or taking prescribed drugs without first seeking advice from a pharmacist about possible interactions or adverse effects.

protein that leaks into the urine, suggesting that it helps to preserve kidney function in people with diabetes.

Co-enzyme Q10 is needed to process oxygen in cells, and to generate energy-rich molecules. It can improve glucose control in people with Type 2 diabetes by increasing energy levels within pancreatic beta-cells and increasing insulin secretion. It can also reduce abnormal blood clotting. Lack of co-enzyme Q10 is linked with coronary heart disease, congestive heart failure and diabetic cardiomyopathy. Supplements are important for people taking statin drugs to lower cholesterol levels, as statins block production of co-enzyme Q10 in the body.

Pine bark extracts (Pycnogenol®) contain a rich blend of anti-oxidant proanthocyanidins. These reduce hardening and furring up of the arteries, reduce abnormal blood clots and reduce the risk of coronary heart disease and stroke. Pycnogenol improves fasting blood glucose levels and improves poor circulation. It can reduce the progression of retinopathy and preserve vision. A growing body of evidence suggests it helps to prevent macular degeneration, peripheral vascular disease, intermittent claudication and leg cramps.

Carotenoids can improve glucose tolerance and protect against diabetes complications. Lutein and zeaxanthin can reduce the risk of macular degeneration and cataracts, while lycopene lowers LDL-cholesterol and can reduce the risk of heart attack.

Selenium has an insulin-like action that stimulates uptake of glucose and improves glucose control. It is thought to activate proteins that tell the cells when insulin is present. Selenium reduces platelet clumping in the circulation to protect against coronary heart disease and stroke.

Bilberry fruit contains an antioxidant anthocyanidin called myrtillin, which has an insulin-like action. Other components strengthen blood vessels and improve circulation, especially in the retina of the eye. Bilberry extracts can improve visible retinal abnormalities associated with diabetic retinopathy and slow the progression of cataracts.

Folic acid is needed to process an amino acid, homocysteine which, if allowed to rise, damages artery walls and can trigger coronary heart disease, stroke, peripheral vascular disease and other conditions associated with abnormal blood clotting. People with diabetes appear to be more susceptible to the harmful effects of homocysteine on the circulation than those without diabetes, developing more pronounced thickening of arterial walls than those without diabetes. Folic acid can also improve dilation of small blood vessels in people with Type 1 diabetes. Folic acid supplements are especially important for people with Type 2 diabetes who take metformin (a drug used to treat insulin resistance). Metformin lowers folic acid and vitamin B12 levels enough to produce a 4 per cent increase in homocysteine levels after four months' treatment.

Vitamin B6 may reduce diabetic retinopathy. In a study involving 18 people with diabetes, none went on to develop diabetic retinopathy after their carpal tunnel syndrome was treated with vitamin B6 supplements for between eight months and 28 years. This may partly be due to lowered homocysteine levels. Lack of vitamin B6 has been linked with nerve damage and one study found that vitamin B6 levels were significantly lower in people with diabetic neuropathy compared with a similar group of people who had diabetes but were free from neuropathy.

Chromium, together with *vitamin B3*, is needed to make chromium dinicotinic acid glutathione, also known as Glucose Tolerance Factor (GTF). GTF boosts insulin sensitivity by increasing the number of insulin receptors present on muscle and fat cell membranes, improves insulin binding to cells and activates receptors to increase insulin sensitivity. It promotes uptake of glucose into cells, the breakdown of glucose for energy (glycolysis) and lowers LDL-cholesterol levels. Chromium deficiency is common, especially in people with diabetes who have significantly lower levels of chromium inside their cells compared with people without diabetes and tend to lose twice as much chromium through their urine. Taking chromium supplements can improve blood glucose levels, insulin levels, and reduce glycosylated haemoglobin A1c indicating better long-term glucose control. Chromium is also

Do not take supplements if you are pregnant, breast-feeding, or taking prescribed drugs without first seeking advice from a pharmacist about possible interactions or adverse effects.

beneficial in people with Type 1 diabetes who are receiving insulin injections if they have a degree of insulin resistance. Some studies have found that taking 200 mcg chromium per day can lower the amount of hypoglycaemic medication needed. Other studies have shown little improvement, possibly because they used low doses, used a poorly absorbed inorganic form (chromium chloride), or because the people taking part did not have a chromium deficiency.

Select supplements containing chromium already incorporated into GTF from chromium-enriched yeast cultures, or combined with vitamin B3 (niacin) as chromium nicotinate or polynicotinate. Niacin-bound chromium is absorbed and retained 600 per cent better than chromium chloride, and 300 per cent better than chromium picolinate.

Cinnamon bark contains polyphenols that enhance insulin sensitivity by activating insulin receptors. Taking cinnamon extracts has been shown to reduce fasting glucose levels, triglycerides and LDL-cholesterol.

Echinacea contains several unique polysaccharides (echinacins) that increase the number and activity of white blood cells. It can reduce susceptibility to infection that is associated with diabetes – especially against the yeast, *Candida albicans*. Combining oral Echinacea with a topical anti-fungal cream (e.g. econazole nitrate) can reduce the rate of recurrence of vaginal candidiasis compared with those using the anti-fungal cream alone.

Magnesium is important for glucose intolerance and blood pressure control. People with diabetes are three times more likely to have low magnesium levels than those without diabetes. Taking magnesium supplements improves insulin-stimulated uptake of glucose into cells to produce significant improvements in glucose levels, insulin sensitivity and HbA1c levels compared with placebo. Insulin requirements appear to be lower in people with Type 1 diabetes who take magnesium supplements. Low magnesium levels are associated with an increased risk of developing diabetic foot ulcers. No trials appear to have investigated whether or not magnesium supplements can produce clinical improvement of foot ulcers, however.

Do not take supplements if you are pregnant, breast-feeding, or taking prescribed drugs without first seeking advice from a pharmacist about possible interactions or adverse effects.

Zinc is important for the synthesis, storage and secretion of insulin, and the zinc content of pancreatic beta cells is one of the highest in the body. Zinc improves insulin production from pancreatic beta cells, and taking zinc supplements has helped to lower glucose levels in people with Type 1 diabetes. In those with Type 2 diabetes, zinc supplements have not been shown to significantly improve glucose control – perhaps because of an inability to transport zinc into the beta cells where it is needed.

Conjugated linoleic acid (CLA) transports fatty acids away from fatty tissues to muscle cells where they are burned for fuel. It helps to reduce central obesity, improves insulin sensitivity, glucose tolerance and triglyceride levels.

Ginkgo biloba contains a variety of unique substances (ginkgolides, bilobalides) that relax blood vessels and improve circulation to the peripheries. Research suggests that ginkgo biloba extracts can improve insulin resistance, and lower insulin levels in people with impaired glucose tolerance. In people with Type 2 diabetes, who need oral hypoglycaemic drugs, Ginkgo biloba significantly increases insulin production in response to a glucose load. It improves blood flow to the eye and has been shown to improve visual impairment in people with diabetes, producing significant improvements in blue-yellow colour differentiation. A study involving 99 people with macular degeneration, found marked improvements in visual acuity after four weeks' treatment.

Garlic is a source of allicin (diallyl thiosulphinate) which reduces cholesterol production in the liver and hastens excretion of fatty acids. Antioxidant compounds formed from the degradation of allicin also protect circulating LDL-cholesterol from oxidation and promote blood vessel dilation to lower a raised blood pressure and reduce atherosclerosis. Garlic also contains ajoene, which reduces both glucose and triglyceride levels.

Korean ginseng contains five glycans (panaxans A to E) that lower blood glucose levels by stimulating the release of insulin from the pancreas. They also reduce insulin resistance by increasing the number of insulin receptors on cell membranes. Ginseng can reduce

Do not take supplements if you are pregnant, breast-feeding, or taking prescribed drugs without first seeking advice from a pharmacist about possible interactions or adverse effects.

fasting blood glucose levels and, in one study, a third of those taking ginseng achieved normal blood glucose control with no change in blood insulin levels. Taking ginseng just before or with a meal can significantly reduce the post-prandial rise in glucose levels that occurs in people with Type 2 diabetes. Ginseng also has a beneficial effect on erectile dysfunction, and works in a similar way to anti-impotence drugs such as sildenafil.

Aloe vera gel extracted from aloe leaves appears to have blood glucose lowering properties but the mechanism remains unknown. Taking aloe vera gel has been shown to reduce fasting glucose levels by around 45 per cent in people with Type 2 diabetes. Analysis of ten controlled clinical trials suggests aloe vera may have beneficial effects on both glucose tolerance and cholesterol levels.

Bitter melon (Momordica charantia) is the unripened fruit of an Asian vine. It is often referred to as 'plant insulin' as it contains a small protein chain (polypeptide-p) that has structural similarities to insulin. Studies suggest it improves glucose tolerance by slowing glucose absorption from the intestines, and reducing production of new glucose in the liver.

Coccinia indica is a wild, Indian creeper that also appears to have an insulin-like action to improve glucose tolerance. In a controlled trial involving 32 people with Type 2 diabetes, 62 per cent of those taking Coccinia showed marked improvement in glucose tolerance compared with no improvements in those taking inactive placebo.

Fenugreek (Trigonella foenum-graecum) is an Ayurvedic herb that can reduce insulin resistance by increasing the number of insulin receptors present in cell membranes. It also decreases triglyceride and LDL-cholesterol levels. In people with Type 2 diabetes, it helps to reduce fasting blood glucose levels, improves glucose tolerance, lowers raised insulin levels and halves the amount of glucose excreted in the urine.

Gymnema sylvestre is an Ayurvedic herb that reduces the ability to detect sweet flavours for up to 90 minutes. This reduces the amount of sugary foods eaten and may help to control food intake. It improves insulin production and normalizes blood sugar levels in diabetes. Some evidence suggests it may also help regeneration or improve the function of residual insulin-producing beta-cells in the pancreas. It can reduce fasting blood glucose levels in both Type 1 and Type 2 diabetes, lowering the requirement for insulin or other hypoglycaemic drugs. It also reduces LDL-cholesterol and triglyceride levels.

Holy basil (*Ocimum sanctum* and *Ocimum album*) is an Ayurvedic herb used to lower blood glucose levels, reduce high blood pressure and for its anti-inflammatory actions. It increases uptake of glucose into cells by improving insulin secretion from residual pancreatic beta cells. In people with Type 2 diabetes it can reduce average fasting blood glucose levels by between 17 per cent and 20 per cent compared with placebo, as well as reducing LDL-cholesterol and triglycerides.

A Tibetan preparation, *Padma 28*, contains a complex mix of 19 Tibetan medicinal herbs (including Iceland moss, red sandalwood, cardamom, allspice, liquorice, cloves, gingerlily and marigold). It promotes blood vessel dilation and is used to treat intermittent claudication – calf pain on exercise due to poor circulation through peripheral arteries.

NB: Blood glucose levels must be carefully monitored if using supplements or herbal remedies. Supplements are best used under the supervision of a medical nutritionist if prescribed drugs are already being taken to lower blood glucose levels – it is important to avoid hypoglycaemic attacks.

See also: **African prune, Aloe vera, Alpha-lipoic acid, Anthocyanins, Antioxidants, Arginine, Artichoke, Astralagus, Bilberry, Biotin, Bitter melon, Blue-green algae, Brewer's yeast, Carnitine, Carotenoids, Chamomile, Chromium, Cinnamon, Coccinia indica, Evening primrose oil, Fenugreek, Fish oils, Flaxseed, Folic acid, Ginkgo, Ginseng, Grapeseed, Gymnema, Hawthorn, Holy basil, Iron, Magnesium, Maitake, Olive oil, Plant sterols, Shiitake, Vitamin B1, Vitamin B2, Vitamin B3, Vitamin B6, Vitamin B12, Vitamin C, Vitamin D, Vitamin E, Vitamin K.**

Diarrhoea

Diarrhoea is a loose consistency of stool plus increased frequency of bowel motions. It occurs when the bowel secretes increased amounts of fluid, and the speed at which contents pass through the intestines increases. The problem is usually intermittent and associated with other classic symptoms such as distension, bloating, excess wind and sensations of incomplete bowel movement.

Diarrhoea may be caused by bacterial, viral, yeast or protozoon infections, irritable bowel syndrome, overuse of laxatives, anxiety, taking antibiotics, or inflammatory bowel diseases such as Crohn's and ulcerative colitis. Diarrhoea that lasts longer than a week should always be investigated to find out its cause. Severe diarrhoea is debilitating and can even be fatal – especially in infants for whom medical advice should be sought straight away. Large amounts of electrolytes such as sodium and potassium as well as water can be washed out through the bowels, causing dehydration, low blood pressure and even shock.

Treatment

Drink plenty of fluids to counter dehydration, especially if urine production has slowed down and only small amounts of dark urine are passed. Avoid fruit juices and prunes and cut down on milk and dairy product consumption as sometimes temporary lactose intolerance (to milk sugar) can occur.

Probiotic supplements supplying friendly digestive bacteria are essential for those with diarrhoea, especially when it is caused by infection or by taking antibiotics. Lack of probiotic bacteria in the intestines encourages abnormal bacterial overgrowth of less beneficial bacteria in the colon (gut dysbiosis) which has been linked with diarrhoea. Probiotic supplements protect against a number of intestinal infections responsible for traveller's gastroenteritis such as *Bacillus cereus*, *Salmonella typhi*, *Shigella dysenteriae*, *Escherichia coli* and *Staphylococcus aureus*.

Enteric-coated *garlic* tablets are often used to treat infective diarrhoea, wind and indigestion.

Psyllium is a soluble fibre source which helps to bulk up motions and can absorb excess fluid in diarrhoea to normalize bowel motions.

Goldenseal has a natural anti-diarrhoeal effect, helping to normalize muscular action in the bowel; it may be used to treat both constipation and diarrhoea.

Manuka honey, mastic gum, olive leaf, grapefruit seed and *lapacho* have useful anti-infective actions that may help treat infective diarrhoea. *Aloe vera* juice has a cleansing and soothing action on the intestines. *Sage* leaves are traditionally used to make an infusion (tea) that is drunk to relieve pain and spasm plus frequency of bowel movements in diarrhoea.

Slippery elm and *ginger* are used to soothe the intestinal lining and reduce inflammation, while *Echinacea* and *cat's claw* help to boost general immunity against infection.

See also: **Acai, African prune, Aloe vera, Arginine, Bilberry, Bitter melon, Blue-green algae, Brewer's yeast, Carnitine, Cat's claw, Cayenne, Chamomile, Copper, Dandelion, Fenugreek, Fibre, Flaxseed, Folic acid, Ginger, Iodine, Lapacho, Magnesium, Oregano oil, Probiotics, Raspberry leaf, Reishi, Sage, Shiitake, Vitamin B3, Vitamin B5, Vitamin B12, Vitamin C, Vitamin D, Vitamin K, Wild Yam, Zinc**.

Diverticular disease

Diverticular disease affects an estimated one in three people between the ages of 50 and 60, and becomes increasingly common over this age. It occurs when small out-pouchings form in the lining of the large bowel (colon) usually as a result of increased pressure such as when straining with constipation. These pouches may become filled with bowel contents which may trigger infection, inflammation and pain known as diverticulitis.

Do not take supplements if you are pregnant, breast-feeding, or taking prescribed drugs without first seeking advice from a pharmacist about possible interactions or adverse effects.

Treatment

The best defence against diverticular disease is to follow a high-fibre diet to reduce constipation, and reduce the chance of the pouches forming or of becoming infected. Fibre aids the digestion and absorption of foods, promotes a healthy bacterial balance and provides important bulk to stimulate peristalsis – the muscular, wave-like motion which transports digested food through the intestines. For every 1 gram of fibre you eat, bowel motions increase by an estimated 5 grams in weight.

Fibre from different plants varies widely in its composition. Bowel bacteria quickly adapt to the types of fibre eaten: after a few weeks of eating a fibre-rich diet, they release more of the enzymes needed to break down the different fibre types. This means that some of the benefits are lost unless the types of fibre that are eaten are regularly varied. As wide a range of fibre-rich foods as possible should be eaten from wholegrain sources, fruit and vegetables, increasing intakes slowly to avoid wind and bloating from an initial fibre overload.

Similarly, *fibre supplements* (e.g. bran, psyllium/ispaghula, sterculia, inulin) should also be varied every month or so. A very good fluid intake is also essential as this helps fibre to swell and work effectively.

Probiotic supplements containing bowel-friendly bacteria help to maintain optimum bowel function, while *aloe vera* has a useful cleansing and soothing action on the intestines.

See also: **Flaxseed**.

Dupuytren's contracture

Dupuytren's contracture is a painless thickening of fibrous tissues which cause gradual puckering of the skin and flexion of digits. In the hand, the ring and little fingers are usually affected, and may be drawn down onto the palm. The exact cause is unknown but abnormal activity of cell growth factors may be involved.

Do not take supplements if you are pregnant, breast-feeding, or taking prescribed drugs without first seeking advice from a pharmacist about possible interactions or adverse effects.

Treatment

Unfortunately, cortisone injections and physiotherapy do not help and surgery is the treatment of choice for advanced lesions, although recurrences are common.

Some researchers have claimed that high-dose *vitamin E* can improve contracture by damping down oxidative damage in affected tissues.

Other antioxidants such as *vitamin C, Pycnogenol®, grapeseed extract, green tea extract* and *co-enzyme Q10* have also been used, but there is little research into their effectiveness for this condition.

Dyslexia

Dyslexia is a condition in which there is a considerable discrepancy between intellectual ability and written language skills. There is:

- An unexpected failure in learning to read and write
- An unusual anatomical symmetry in language areas of the brain, which are normally larger in the dominant cerebral hemisphere (the left side in right-handed individuals)
- Microscopic differences in the way cells are organized during development in the language areas of the brain
- Difficulty in processing rapid changes in visual stimulation (e.g. flicker, motion)
- Impaired night vision (dark adaptation)
- Poor peripheral vision
- Difficulty in processing rapid changes in the sounds involved in speech.

It is now thought that dyslexia is a brain development disorder linked with deficiency of omega-3 essential fatty acids during early life. This leads to mild abnormalities in the membranes of synapses in the foetal brain that are less fluid than normal, and which transmit

---

Do not take supplements if you are pregnant, breast-feeding, or taking prescribed drugs without first seeking advice from a pharmacist about possible interactions or adverse effects.

information more slowly. This may help to explain why dyslexia is more common in males, who have a higher requirement for omega-3s than females.

Treatment

The *omega-3* fatty acid, docosahexaenoic acid (DHA) found in oily fish and some algae is important for visual perception and has shown some benefit in improving dyslexia. Those with higher omega-3 levels have better word reading skills whether or not they have been diagnosed with dyslexia.

Preliminary research involving 15 children suggests that *ginkgo biloba* extracts can improve results from standardized tests for dyslexia.

See also: **Essential Fatty Acids, Fish oils**.

Eczema

Eczema is an inflammatory skin disease that affects as many as one in ten people. It most commonly appears on the hands, inside the elbows or behind the knees but may be found anywhere on the body. In severe cases, it may spread to affect skin covering most of the body. There are several different types of eczema, including:

- Atopic – mainly affects the face, neck and inner creases of the elbows and knees; it is linked with an increased risk of asthma and allergic rhinitis and tends to run in families
- Seborrhoeic – greasy crusts on the face or in the scalp (e.g. cradle cap, dandruff)
- Discoid – round lesions on the legs and trunk
- Asteatotic – dry, crazy-paving skin patterns in older people, often on the legs
- Stasis – eczema of the lower legs due to varicose veins and poor local circulation
- Pompholyx – small, itchy vesicles on the fingers, palms or soles

---

- Lichen simplex (or neurodermatitis) due to rubbing or irritation of the skin
- Allergic (contact dermatitis, e.g. due to contact with nickel)
- Photoallergic – due to the action of sunlight on skin sensitized by absorbed drugs or chemicals.

Eczema symptoms vary from mild to severe and can include dry, scaly, thickened skin, redness, itching with excoriation, blisters, weeping sores which may become infected, crusting and flaky scalp.

Worsening eczema is sometimes associated with colonization of skin by a bacterium, *Staphylococcus aureus*, even in areas that do not look obviously infected. The reason why *S. aureus* colonizes skin in atopic eczema is not known, but one suggestion is that levels of essential fatty acids (EFA) are reduced in cell membranes which might make it easier for bacteria to adhere. One study found that 95 per cent of people with moderate eczema were colonized, with 90 per cent showing a heavy growth. This bacterium secretes super-antigens that activate inflammatory cells and worsen skin inflammation. They are also thought to induce steroid insensitivity making treatment less effective, although a cream that combines steroid with a topical antibiotic (e.g. fusidic acid plus hydrocortisone or the stronger betametasone cream) may help.

Treatment
Cut right back on your intake of omega-6 oils (sunflower oil, safflower oil, corn oil, processed foods) and increase your intakes of omega-3s (oily fish, flaxseed oil, walnut oil, hempseed oil) and monounsaturates (olive oil, rapeseed oil, almonds, macadamias, hazelnuts).

Evening primrose oil contains essential fatty acids (e.g. gamma-linolenic acid also known as GLA) which can moisturize the skin from the inside. GLA is important for the formation of healthy skin cell membranes and helps to reduce itching and dryness in people with essential fatty acid deficiency – at least 80 per cent of the population. Evening primrose oil needs to be taken in large doses of around 3 g daily for at least three months before fairly evaluating the

Do not take supplements if you are pregnant, breast-feeding, or taking prescribed drugs without first seeking advice from a pharmacist about possible interactions or adverse effects.

response to treatment. Pure evening primrose oil can also be rubbed directly on to affected skin.

Omega-3 fish oils also have an anti-inflammatory action that is helpful for improving conditions such as eczema. These oils can certainly reduce itching and inflammation but may take a few months to have maximum effect.

If oral antibiotics are needed, a *probiotic* supplement will reduce intestinal side effects. Probiotic supplements taken during pregnancy and in infancy may reduce the chance of eczema developing in children through a beneficial effect on immunity.

Aloe vera gel is often very effective for treating eczema when applied twice a day. It may also be taken by mouth.

A *multivitamin and mineral supplement* is worth considering as lack of some vitamins and minerals (especially antioxidants and zinc) have been linked with scaly skin rashes.

Treatment of eczema should also include liberal application of emollient creams and soothing (non-perfumed) bath additives to soothe and moisturize the skin from the outside.

See also: **Aloe vera, Bee products, Boswellia, Brewer's yeast, Chamomile, Echinacea, Essential Fatty Acids, Evening primrose oil, Hempseed oil, Oregano oil, Probiotics, Sarsaparilla, Schisandra, Vitamin B2**.

Emphysema

Emphysema is a disease affecting the tiny air sacs (alveoli) of the lungs which become overstretched, damaged and rupture. As a result, the small sacs merge to form fewer, larger sacs with a significantly reduced surface area. This makes gas exchange less efficient and the lungs may become over-inflated.

Treatment
Almost all cases of emphysema result from smoking cigarettes, so stopping smoking is vital. Antioxidant supplements (e.g. *vitamin A,*

vitamin C, vitamin E, selenium, pine bark or grapeseed extracts) help to neutralize the free radicals (*see* **Antioxidants**) that have been implicated in emphysema.

A trial involving over 2,500 patients with respiratory illnesses found that taking the amino acid *N-actylcysteine* (which makes mucus less viscid) improved symptoms.

Garlic tablets help to loosen mucus and protect against respiratory infections.

If a chest infection starts, *Echinacea* may help, while *omega-3 fish oils* may reduce wheezing.

See also: **N-acetyl cysteine, Pomegranate, Selenium**.

Endometriosis

Endometriosis is one of the most common gynaecological conditions, with as many as one in ten women affected, although not all have troublesome symptoms. It is the only known condition in which apparently normal, non-cancerous cells spread from one part of the body (the womb lining or endometrium) to another, take root and continue to grow – most commonly in the pelvic and abdominal cavities. Because these cells remain sensitive to the monthly hormone cycle, they may swell and bleed into surrounding tissues during each menstrual period to produce pain, inflammation and scarring. As the condition progresses, fluid-filled hollow cysts or solid nodules can develop especially on the ovaries. The four classic symptoms are painful periods that may be heavy, deep pain during sex, deep pelvic pain and subfertility.

Adenomyosis is similar to endometriosis, in that ectopic endometrial deposits are found outside their normal position, within the muscular wall of the womb itself, nestled between the muscle fibres to form diffuse patches, or a larger lump similar to a fibroid.

Treatment
Self help for both conditions includes eating a healthy, wholefood

---

diet and avoiding salt, caffeine, sugar, fried and processed foods. Some nutritionists suggest avoiding meat and dairy products because of the potentially high level of animal oestrogens they contain, although it is important to seek dietary advice to ensure correct intakes of important nutrients such as iron or vitamin B12.

Essential fatty acid intake should be increased (e.g. linseed, sunflower, walnut oils and oily fish) and 3 g *evening primrose oil* daily is recommended for those essential fatty acids that help to overcome hormone imbalances and damp down inflammation.

Studies suggest that women who obtain the most fish oils in their diet have the least painful menstruation (see painful periods).

Lack of *iodine* has been linked with hormonal imbalances that may lead to endometriosis, so it is a good idea to take a multivitamin and mineral supplement that includes iodine (150 mcg). Also ensure a good intake of antioxidants – at least five servings of fruit or vegetables a day – and consider supplements such as *vitamin C*, *vitamin E*, pine bark or grapeseed extracts to reduce inflammation.

Calcium and *magnesium* will help to reduce any associated uterine muscle spasm and pain.

Agnus castus has a progesterone-like action in the body and may also help. Some practitioners also recommend using progesterone cream and/or isoflavones to balance the oestrogen dominance that is linked with endometriosis.

See also: **Black cohosh, Dandelion, Dong quai, Liquorice, Milk Thistle, Pfaffia, Raspberry leaf, Wild yam**.

Energy – lack of

A number of conditions can reduce energy levels and, if symptoms persist, it is important to consult a doctor to identify treatable conditions such as an underactive thyroid gland, anaemia, diabetes or depression.

See also: **Chronic Fatigue Syndrome**.

Do not take supplements if you are pregnant, breast-feeding, or taking prescribed drugs without first seeking advice from a pharmacist about possible interactions or adverse effects.

Treatment

Assuming that nothing requiring medical intervention is identified, treatments that might help to correct a lack of energy include a *multivitamin and mineral supplement* to safeguard against any micro-nutrient deficiencies. Additional *B group vitamins* may be helpful to optimize energy production in cells.

Kelp supplements are popular as a source of *iodine* which is needed to make thyroid hormones.

Co-enzyme Q10 is often helpful in overcoming fatigue, as are *omega-3* and *evening primrose oil* supplements.

Guarana contains a complex of natural stimulants, including a form of caffeine known as guaranine. These components are slowly absorbed to provide a stimulant action for up to six hours creating more energy without producing over-stimulation or irritability. Most people find it more gentle and calming than caffeine. A good energizing pick-me-up can be made by mixing 5 ml each of guarana powder, brewer's yeast and wheatgerm with 15 ml pure honey and topping up to a glass with mineral water and blending thoroughly. This should be drunk every morning before breakfast.

Panax ginseng is a useful energy booster – Korean ginseng is often recommended for males and American ginseng for women. *Siberian ginseng* is a good alternative if you find Panax ginseng too stimulating.

Antioxidants such as vitamin C, vitamin E, carotenoids, grape-seed or pine bark extracts will help to damp down any inflammatory processes contributing to lack of energy.

See also: **Adaptogens, Alpha-lipoic acid, Carnitine, Co-enzyme Q10, Ginseng, Goji, Goldenseal, Gotu kola, Guarana, Hawthorn, 5-HTP, Iodine, Iron, Liquorice, Kelp, Magnesium, Maiitake, Olive leaf, Pfaffia, Reishi, Rhodiola, St John's Wort, Schisandra, Shiitake, Tribulus terrestris, Vitamin B1, Vitamin B2, Vitamin B5, Vitamin B6, Vitamin D, Vitamin E, Yerba maté**.

Exam stress

It is important to balance time spent revising for exams with time for safety-valve activities such as relaxation and non-competitive exercise to burn off the adverse effects of stress hormones. While this may seem like time wasted as exams loom, the ability to absorb information is much improved after taking a break.

Treatment

Diet is very important – eating a cereal breakfast, for example, can improve concentration and increase the speed at which new information is recalled.

Lemon balm (*Melissa officinalis*) is known as the 'Scholar's Herb' as it was traditionally taken by students suffering from the stress of impending exams.

Ginkgo biloba extracts can improve short-term working memory.

Guarana helps you remain alert and has a more gentle action than caffeine.

Rhodiola can reduce anxiety and improve sleep.

Bach Rescue Remedy (containing flower essences) is excellent for when panic rises and can be used before exams to help steady the nerves.

See also: **Adaptogens, Ashwagandha, Astragalus, Biotin, Chamomile, Ginseng, Goji, Guarana, Holy basil, Lemon balm, Liquorice, Maitaki, Oast straw, Pfaffia, Phosphatidylserine, Pomegranate, Reishi, Rhodiola, Schisandra, Selenium, Siberian ginseng, Valerian, Yerba maté**.

Eyes – dry

Dry eyes are relatively common, especially if you forget to blink when concentrating on your work or VDU screen. Some people suffer with dry eyes all the time, however – a condition known as *keratoconjunctivitis sicca* – due to lack of tear production. Dry eyes

---

Do not take supplements if you are pregnant, breast-feeding, or taking prescribed drugs without first seeking advice from a pharmacist about possible interactions or adverse effects.

become more common with increasing age. They can also result from the production of abnormal antibodies that switch off tear production. This can happen in some auto-immune disorders such as rheumatoid arthritis, systemic lupus erythematosus and Sjögren's syndrome.

Treatment

The standard treatment for dry eyes involves lubricating drops known as artificial tears. These can be successful but may need to be used frequently to prevent burning, itching, grittiness and painful ulceration.

In some parts of the world, dry eyes are frequently due to lack of *vitamin A*. This is known as xerophthalmia. Although it is rare in the Western world, it may be worth taking a cod liver oil supplement (which contains vitamin A) to see if this helps.

Supplements containing *bilberry* extracts help to stabilize tears and are often very successful – they also contain *carotenoids* that can be converted into vitamin A where needed. Other supplements to consider include *omega-3 fish oils* and antioxidants such as *vitamin C, lutein* and *Pycnogenol®*.

See also: **Grapeseed**.

Feet – painful

A large number of conditions can cause painful feet. These include:

- Flat feet
- Arthritis
- Tarsal tunnel syndrome (the foot version of carpal tunnel syndrome)
- Plantar fasciitis (pain mainly under the heel and in the midline)
- Erythromelalgia (burning feet syndrome)
- Metatarsalgia (pain mainly in the ball of the foot)
- Conditions affecting nerve transmission (neuropathy).

Do not take supplements if you are pregnant, breast-feeding, or taking prescribed drugs without first seeking advice from a pharmacist about possible interactions or adverse effects.

Treatment

Occasionally, burning feet are due to lack of *B group vitamins* and supplements may help.

Osteoarthritis in the feet may be helped by *omega-3 fish oils*, *glucosamine sulphate* (with or without *chondroitin*), *devil's claw*, *MSM-sulphur, green-lipped mussel extracts* or antioxidants such as *vitamin C* and *Pycnogenol®*.

Related entries: **Osteoarthritis, Gout**.

Fibromyalgia

Fibromyalgia is a debilitating condition from which women are five times more likely to suffer than men. It causes widespread aches and pains plus sleep disturbance, and the pains tend to move from place to place, vary in severity and are often made worse by cold and stress. Sufferers develop localized areas of tenderness known as trigger points, especially around the lower spine, between the shoulder blades, at the base of the neck, over the sacro-iliac joints, elbows and knees. In some people, these tender spots develop fibrous nodules. Blood tests and X-rays do not show any consistent abnormalities and the condition seems to be due to reduced energy production in muscle cells and an inability of muscle fibres to relax.

Sufferers have a characteristic lack of delta wave activity (deep non-REM sleep) when brain waves are monitored during sleep, however. They therefore feel tired and exhausted much of the time as they wake unrefreshed. Interestingly, if normal volunteers are monitored during sleep and woken periodically so that they lack delta wave sleep, similar aches and pains will appear. Sleep disturbances have been linked with low levels of serotonin (a neurotransmitter) in the brain.

Treatment

Unfortunately, painkillers and anti-inflammatory drugs are usually unhelpful although anti-depressant drugs that raise brain serotonin levels (SSRIs) sometimes improve the sleep disturbance. *5-HTP* or *St John's Wort* are therefore worth trying (they must not be taken together, or in combination with prescribed antidepressant drugs).

People with fibromyalgia often have low *magnesium* levels, and supplements containing magnesium malate, *B group vitamins, manganese, alpha-lipoic acid* or *co-enzyme Q10,* which are involved in oxygen utilization in cells, may help.

Blood circulation to the peripheries may be improved with *ginkgo, garlic* or Padma 28 (a blend of over 20 different Tibetan herbs). Supplements may take up to two months to produce a beneficial effect.

Olive leaf extracts have an anti-viral action and may be helpful.

See also: **Cayenne, 5-HTP, Liquorice, Magnesium, Olive leaf**.

Fluid retention

Fluid retention may be due to a number of different problems and, if persistent or recurrent, it is important to seek medical advice to find out the cause.

Treatment

General measures to reduce fluid retention include losing excess weight, taking regular exercise, and cutting back on salt intake. Intakes should be increased of fruit, vegetables, salads and juices containing potassium that also help to flush excess sodium from the body.

Dandelion is a natural herbal diuretic that is widely used to flush excess fluid from the body. As well as having a powerful diuretic action, dandelion root extracts are also a rich source of mineral potassium. They should not be taken by anyone who is on other prescribed medications however.

If fluid retention is linked with premenstrual syndrome (PMS), supplements that include *magnesium* and *vitamin B6* are helpful.

Do not take supplements if you are pregnant, breast-feeding, or taking prescribed drugs without first seeking advice from a pharmacist about possible interactions or adverse effects.

Magnesium helps to maintain sodium and potassium balance in and out of body cells, while vitamin B6 increases cell membrane transfer and utilization of magnesium. Food sources of magnesium include fish, nuts, seeds, soy beans, wholegrains and dark green, leafy vegetables.

See also: **Anthocyanins, Bilberry, Calcium, Copper, Fish oils, Hawthorn, Magnesium, Sodium, Vitamin B1**.

Food poisoning

Food poisoning (gastro-enteritis) is usually associated with abdominal pain, vomiting and diarrhoea.

Treatment
Usual advice with prolonged gastro-enteritis is to replace lost fluids and minerals with an electrolyte solution (available from pharmacies).

Probiotic supplements containing healthy, digestive bacteria (e.g. *Lactobacilli*) help to keep the digestive system in balance, and keep harmful bacteria at bay through a number of mechanisms, including the production of natural antibiotics (bacteriocins), lowering the pH to discourage reproduction of less acid-tolerant bacteria and competing for available nutrients and attachment sites on intestinal cell walls.

Garlic, Manuka honey and *mastic gum* contain natural antibiotics which may also help. *Ginger* is used to soothe the intestinal lining and reduce inflammation, while *goldenseal, Echinacea* and *cat's claw* help to boost general immunity against infection.

Seek medical advice if problems continue for more than two or three days. One in three people with bacterial gastro-enteritis go on to develop symptoms of irritable bowel syndrome that can last for three months or longer.

See also: **Probiotics, Sage**.
Related entry: **Diarrhoea**.

Frozen shoulder

Frozen shoulder is the common name for pain, stiffness and immobility of the shoulder joint. It is due to inflammation and thickening in the lining of the capsule surrounding the joint (capsulitis). In most cases, no obvious cause is found, but it may come on after a fall, a task involving repetitive movements of the joint (e.g. painting the ceiling) or after unaccustomed exercise. Attacks have also been linked with other medical conditions such as chronic bronchitis, stroke or heart pain (angina), perhaps triggered by general immobility.

Treatment

During the initial, acutely painful stage of frozen shoulder, rest is usually advised along with non-steroidal, anti-inflammatory drugs to relieve pain and inflammation. Applying hot or cold packs can also help. After the pain starts to reduce, manipulation by a physiotherapist, osteopath or chiropractor will improve mobility, but it can take many months before the range of movement approaches normality again.

Omega-3 fish oils will reduce inflammation.

Antioxidants such as *vitamin C, vitamin E* and *Pycnogenol*® help to reduce pain and swelling. Other supplements that can reduce joint inflammation include *green-lipped mussel extracts, devil's claw* and *bromelain. Glucosamine sulphate* is useful for improving the quality and quantity of synovial fluid – the joint's oil.

Gallstones

Gallstones are solid collections of material that form in the gall bladder when ingredients that are usually dissolved in bile precipitate out to form stones. Most gallstones are made of cholesterol, although some contain high amounts of bile pigments or calcium salts such as calcium bilirubinate or calcium carbonate. They tend to

---

be round or oval in shape, and range in size from 1–25 mm across. Some people only develop one large stone, while others harbour up to 200 or more stones which resemble pieces of grit.

Gallstones are four times more common in women than men, as there seems to be a link with female hormones. They are more common in women who have taken the oral contraceptive pill while those who have used hormone replacement therapy (HRT) for two or more years are over three times more likely to develop gallstones than women who don't. Overall, it's estimated that one in five women develop gallstones at some time in their life, making them one of the most common digestive problems.

Gallstone pain begins suddenly across the upper abdomen – usually after a fatty meal – and is often difficult to locate exactly. It may settle in the upper right part of the abdomen, and may spread to between the shoulder blades or just under the right shoulder. The severe pain usually lasts less than two hours, and comes and goes in waves – this is known as biliary colic. Some people feel sick or vomit, and belching is common. If the stone blocks the flow of bile the person may become jaundiced. Gallstones can also lead to inflammation or infection of the gall bladder (acute cholecystitis) in which biliary pain is longer-lasting and there is abdominal tenderness and fever, or to inflammation or infection of the pancreas (pancreatitis). Eight out of ten people with gallstones do not develop symptoms, however.

Treatment

Stones not causing symptoms are usually left alone. Recent research suggests that having small gallstones may increase the risk of developing inflammation of the pancreas (pancreatitis), however. As this is a serious complication, some surgeons may recommend removing the gall bladder to prevent this. After the gall bladder is removed, bile trickles down from the liver into the gut on a continual basis, rather than being stored en route and only squirted out after eating a fatty meal. This may cause no digestive problems, although some people develop bowel looseness or discomfort when eating certain foods as a result.

Do not take supplements if you are pregnant, breast-feeding, or taking prescribed drugs without first seeking advice from a pharmacist about possible interactions or adverse effects.

People with gallstones are advised to follow a low-fat, high-fibre diet and to lose any excess weight. Following a low-fat diet helps as it is dietary fat that triggers contraction of the gall bladder, and this may push a gallstone into the mouth of the bile duct.

Some fats are beneficial, however. Olive oil is a rich source of oleic acid, a mono-unsaturated fat that has a beneficial effect on blood cholesterol balance. It's therefore worth using olive oil during cooking and in dressings. *Flaxseed oil, walnut oil, macadamia nut oil, omega-3 fish oils* and *garlic* tablets also have a beneficial effect on blood cholesterol balance and a diet rich in these may reduce gallstone formation.

Fibre is also important for people with gallstones as plants rich in soluble fibre such as pectins (e.g. found in apples, carrots) and gums (found in oat bran and beans) bind to cholesterol and bile salts in the gut to reduce their re-absorption. Eat at least five servings of fruit, vegetables and saladstuff per day. Have porridge or unsweetened oatmeal-based muesli for breakfast, mix rolled oats into yogurts, and eat oatcakes as a snack.

Lecithin is an essential part of bile and supplements help to keep cholesterol emulsified to reduce stone formation.

Globe artichoke stimulates bile flow and reduces gall bladder inflammation but don't take this if you have experienced gallstone pain, if gallstones are obstructing bile flow or if jaundice is present.

Milk thistle extracts have beneficial effects on the composition of bile (e.g. reduced cholesterol content) which may reduce formation of gallstones.

Vitamin C helps to prevent cholesterol from solidifying out of bile to form stones.

Drink plenty of fluids – especially water or herbal teas – to keep well hydrated; this helps to prevent sludging of bile.

Keep alcohol intake to within recommended levels (no more than 2–3 units of alcohol per day, and have several alcohol-free days per week, too).

See also: **Artichoke, Choline, Dandelion, Milk thistle, Peppermint, Shiitake, Vitamin C, Wild yam**.

Glandular fever

Glandular fever – also known as infectious mononucleosis – is caused by the Epstein-Barr virus (EBV), and mainly affects teenagers between the ages of 15 and 18. This is the time when the immune system is most vigorous and many of the symptoms are due to the body over-reacting to the infection. EBV is passed on in saliva and can be spread by coughing, spluttering, sneezing, kissing and by sharing toothbrushes. Someone who has recently had glandular fever can remain infectious for several months. Only around half the people who catch the virus develop symptoms, however. Glandular fever produces symptoms like influenza with aching, fatigue, high temperature, sore throat and swollen lymph nodes (glands) especially in the neck. The spleen and liver can also become enlarged and tender. During the infection, unusual white blood cells (mononuclear glandular fever cells) are found in the blood and antibodies against EBV appear after a few weeks which helps to confirm the diagnosis. During convalescence it is common to feel tired, depressed and lacking in energy for six months or more.

Treatment

It is important to take things easy for several months after glandular fever to allow the immune system time to recover. It is also advisable to avoid alcohol.

Co-enzyme Q10, B group vitamins and *evening primrose oil* may be helpful for fatigue. *Vitamin C* helps to reduce inflammation. Herbal remedies for glandular fever (e.g. *Echinacea, maitake*) are best prescribed individually by a qualified practitioner.

See also: **Maitake**.

Related entry: **Chronic fatigue syndrome**.

Do not take supplements if you are pregnant, breast-feeding, or taking prescribed drugs without first seeking advice from a pharmacist about possible interactions or adverse effects.

Gout

Gout is an inflammatory arthritis due to high levels of uric acid which precipitate out into joints and tissues. As most uric acid is produced in the body during the breakdown of purines released when the genetic material (DNA) of worn out cells is recycled, dietary changes can only lower uric acid levels by up to 20 per cent. Symptoms of gout include hot, red, extremely painful swelling of a joint, most commonly involving the big toe.

Treatment
Standard dietary advice is to reduce your intake of purine-rich foods such as offal, shellfish, oily fish, game, meats, yeast extracts, asparagus, and spinach. Alcohol both increases uric acid production and reduces its excretion (especially beer which is also rich in purines) and should therefore be avoided. A high-fibre, mainly vegetarian diet should be followed with plenty of fruit and vegetables. Dark blue-red pigmented fruits (e.g. cherries, grapes, blueberries, bilberries) contain antioxidants such as anthocyanidins that can lower uric acid levels and are said to prevent gout when around 250 g are eaten daily. Drink at least two litres of fluid each day.

Supplements containing extracts of *bilberry, cherry fruit, grape seed* or *pine bark* are helpful.

Vitamin C mobilizes uric acid from the tissues and increases its excretion – the pre-digested form known as ester-C is best as it is non-acidic.

Folic acid supplements inhibit uric acid synthesis, and are usually taken together with vitamin B12. Supplements containing more than the RDA (recommended daily amount) of vitamin B3 (niacin) or vitamin A should be avoided as high doses can increase uric acid levels.

Extracts of *devil's claw* (*Harpagophytum procumbens*) contain natural anti-inflammatory analgesics (e.g. harpagoside) that both reduce pain and also encourage excretion of uric acid, so reducing

Do not take supplements if you are pregnant, breast-feeding, or taking prescribed drugs without first seeking advice from a pharmacist about possible interactions or adverse effects.

the risk of recurrent gout. *Bromelain* is also useful for reducing pain and inflammation in acute attacks of gout.

See also: **Anthocyanins, Bilberry, Cat's claw, Devil's claw, Pfaffia, Sarsaparilla, Vitamin B3, Vitamin C.**

Gums – receding

Receding gums are a common occurrence in old age – so much so that older people are often described as being 'long in the tooth'. Receding gums are associated with a build-up of plaque in the pockets between the gums and teeth. This leads to inflammation known as gingivitis in which gums become red, swollen and bleed during brushing. If left untreated, gingivitis can progress to infect the tissues and bone surrounding tooth roots to cause periodontitis. Both gingivitis and periodontitis can lead to bad breath, receding gums and loosening or falling out of teeth.

Treatment

To help avoid receding gums, good dental hygiene is vital. Teeth must be brushed regularly, at least twice daily – and preferably after each meal. An electric toothbrush that helps to remove plaque is worth considering. Use dental floss or tape regularly (this needs to be done correctly as directed by a dentist). Dentists can also offer referrals to a dental hygienist for regular cleaning of gum pockets and removal of scale. Interestingly, scientists estimate that daily flossing can add over six years to your life, as people with inflamed gums (gingivitis, periodontitis) have a mortality rate that is between 23 per cent and 46 per cent greater than for those with healthy mouths. Inflamed gums allows mouth bacteria to enter the circulation which can trigger arterial disease and increase your risk of coronary heart disease and stroke. Gum disease is common among people with diabetes, and is most severe in those with poor glucose control. Some evidence even suggests that inflammatory chemicals

---

Do not take supplements if you are pregnant, breast-feeding, or taking prescribed drugs without first seeking advice from a pharmacist about possible interactions or adverse effects.

entering the circulation from inflamed gums may worsen insulin resistance and glucose control, but this is not conclusive.

Diseased areas of gum tissue have significantly lower levels of *co-enzyme Q10* and taking supplements can improve the outcome of dental hygiene treatments. A good intake of calcium is also essential as dietary deficiency can contribute to receding gums. A multi-vitamin and mineral supplement was found to improve gum health and reduce periodontal pocket size compared with placebo, after two months of treatment.

Note: Dental advice should be sought for redness or swelling of the gums around the teeth, or for gums that bleed during brushing.

See also: **Myrrh, Vitamin C**.

Haemorrhoids

Piles (haemorrhoids) are dilated varicose veins in the back passage. They often develop as a result of straining, overweight or pregnancy and can cause an unpleasant dragging sensation, itching, a mucous discharge and cause bright red bleeding from the back passage. If bleeding occurs, it is important to seek medical advice to confirm the diagnosis as more serious bowel conditions need to be ruled out.

Treatment
To reduce symptoms, follow a mild, non-spicy, high-fibre diet with plenty of fluids.

Glycerine suppositories will ease the passage of bowel motions and reduce straining.

A bath or shower should be taken every day using unperfumed soap, and finishing by spraying the area with cold water. The area must be kept scrupulously clean to help stop itching – this means washing the area with unscented soap after each bowel motion and patting dry with a soft tissue; if necessary the area may be kept dry using a hairdryer set on gentle heat.

Take steps to reduce constipation. *Psyllium* is an excellent source of fibre. *Probiotics* can also improve bowel function.

Vitamin C, red vine leaf, pine bark (Pycnogenol®), *horsechestnut* and *gotu kola* extracts help to strengthen supporting tissues around prolapsed veins (but do not take during pregnancy).

See also: **Bilberry, Gotu kola, Grapeseed, Horsechestnut, Pine bark, Red vine leaf**.

Related entry: **Constipation**.

Hair loss

Hair loss is an increasingly common problem. While it is sometimes linked with scalp skin conditions, lack of iron or an underactive thyroid gland, frequently no obvious cause is found. Hair is a good indicator of general health and nutrition, and is often the first part of the body to show signs of ill health, or a dietary lack of vitamins, minerals or essential fatty acids. This is because, although hair is often thought of as a dead structure, its root – the hair follicle – is very much alive. The rate at which new hair cells are produced is second only to the speed at which new blood cells are made in the bone marrow. Hair follicles, therefore, need a constant supply of nutrients for optimum health. Unlike the marrow, however, hair is a non-essential structure and the body preferentially diverts precious nutrient stores away from it in times of lack or stress.

Treatment

Research shows that levels of specific minerals laid down in the hair vary significantly with time – even from hour to hour. The majority of women who consult a trichologist about hair problems are found to be deficient in at least one nutrient as this fluctuation in supply can lead to weak, thinning hair unless steps are taken to improve hair health.

After the age of 25, the diameter of individual hairs naturally starts to decrease, especially in women. Although this often goes unnoticed, it can change the texture and body of the hair, so that by

---

Do not take supplements if you are pregnant, breast-feeding, or taking prescribed drugs without first seeking advice from a pharmacist about possible interactions or adverse effects.

the age of 40, most people have finer hair with less body. At the same time, more follicles stay in their resting phase so less hair grows and the rate of growth decreases, resulting in progressive thinning. This effect can be minimized by massaging the scalp regularly with the fingers every day. Underlying tightness can also be loosened by holding handfuls of hair near the roots and gently moving the scalp back and forth and from side to side. Massage and scalp movement open up the circulation and stimulate the flow of blood, oxygen and nutrients to the hair follicles.

Follow a healthy, balanced diet containing as many unrefined, wholefoods as possible. Wholegrains, fruit, vegetables and seeds are a rich source of vitamins, minerals and essential fatty acids that provide nourishment for hair roots and contribute to a healthy head of hair. Avoid eating erratically and skipping meals (especially breakfast) or the supply of nutrients to non-essential tissues such as hair follicles will be reduced. Try to eat something – for example a healthy snack such as fresh or dried fruit – at least every four hours. Try to maintain a healthy weight without strict dieting. Severe dietary restriction at any time of life, but especially middle age, can have permanent effects on hair health. Excess weight loss should be achieved slowly and sensibly as over-exercising and crash diets affect the body's hormone balance and dramatically reduces the nutrient supplies to hair follicles.

Consider taking a multivitamin and mineral supplement containing *iron* and *iodine*, too. Alternatively, choose one especially formulated for hair, skin and nails which often contains boosted amounts of B group vitamins such as biotin and B5 (pantothenic acid). Many herbal blends are also available which, for example, may contain *ginkgo* to improve circulation, or *kelp* as an iodine source. If you pull your hair out (trichotillomania), new research suggests that *N-acetyl cysteine* may reduce the urge to pull.

Essential fatty acids found in *evening primrose, flaxseed, hemp-seed* or *omega-3 fish oils* are important for hair health. Evening primrose oil supplements (1000 mg a day) can improve the hair and nail quality within three months as new cells grow down

---

Do not take supplements if you are pregnant, breast-feeding, or taking prescribed drugs without first seeking advice from a pharmacist about possible interactions or adverse effects.

(although as new hair only grows down at a rate of half an inch per month, it may take as long as a year for the overall improvement to show).

Hair has a high content of the tough, fibrous protein keratin, which is made from amino acid building blocks obtained from the diet. A source of protein, such as poultry, fish, eggs, nuts or beans, should be eaten at every meal. Vegetarians are more prone to thinning hair as some important amino acids (e.g. lysine) and micronutrients (e.g. *vitamin B12, iron*) may be lacking from their diet.

Reduce salt intake – excess salt reduces hair follicle function and research shows that reducing salt intake can reduce hair loss and thinning by as much as 60 per cent.

Avoid excess stress as stress hormones constrict blood supply to the scalp and hair follicles, reducing their supply of nutrients. This can lead to generalized hair thinning or even patchy hair loss. In times of stress use massage and scalp movement to loosen the scalp and improve circulation to hair follicles.

Regular exercise is important to burn off stress hormones, for weight maintenance and to boost circulation to hair follicles.

Avoid chemicals coming into contact with your scalp and follicles. Perms and colour treatments should be applied only to the hair shafts. Plastic caps can help to protect follicles when bleach is applied. Semi-permanent colour is kinder to hair than permanent.

Combs are generally kinder to hair than brushes. Choose a comb with widely spaced teeth and without mould lines down the centre of each tooth which can damage hair shafts. If using a brush, choose one with wide-spaced, plastic bristles that have smooth, blunt tips. Avoid metal prongs as these can damage the hair and scalp.

See also: **Arginine, Biotin, Copper, Iodine, Iron, Kelp, N-acetyl cysteine, Selenium, Silicon, Vitamin B2, Vitamin B5, Vitamin B6, Vitamin C**.

Related entry: **Alopecia**.

Do not take supplements if you are pregnant, breast-feeding, or taking prescribed drugs without first seeking advice from a pharmacist about possible interactions or adverse effects.

Halitosis

Bad breath, or halitosis, affects eight out of ten people at some time in their life. For two-thirds, it is a long-term problem. Most cases result from a build-up of bacterial plaque in the mouth or on the tongue. These bacteria produce around 300 different gases and volatile chemicals, of which over 100 smell unpleasant. Other less common causes include lack of saliva, nose problems (e.g. previous fracture, post-nasal drip, nose surgery), sinusitis and chronic lung infection. Breath odours due to eating onions and garlic, for example, are a dietary side effect and do not constitute true halitosis.

People with gum disease are four times more likely to have bad breath than others. Redness or swelling of the gums around the teeth, or gums that bleed when brushing, could be signs of gingivitis (infected gums) which, if ignored, will spread to involve the jawbone around the teeth (periodontitis) after which gums will start to recede. If this in turn is ignored, teeth will eventually be lost altogether.

Treatment

Unfortunately, twice daily cleaning of teeth is not enough to solve bad breath and gum disease and standard mouthwashes only solve the problem temporarily.

Use dental tape, floss or interdental brushes regularly to clean between teeth. In fact, scientists estimate that daily flossing can add over six years to your life. People with inflamed gums (gingivitis, periodontitis) have a mortality rate that is between 23 per cent and 46 per cent greater than for those with healthy mouths. This is because inflamed gums allow mouth bacteria to enter the circulation which can trigger arterial disease and increase your risk of coronary heart disease and stroke. Some evidence even suggests that inflammatory chemicals entering the circulation from inflamed gums may worsen insulin resistance and glucose control in people with Type 2 diabetes, but this is not conclusive.

Use a tongue scraper (or a shallow teaspoon) to remove bacterial

---

accumulations on the tongue as these contribute significantly to bad odours. Use an electric toothbrush designed to remove plaque and have your periodontal pockets (between your teeth and gums) cleaned and descaled regularly by a dental hygienist.

Stimulate saliva flow first thing each morning by drinking a glass of citrus juice and eating fruit. It is also important to drink at least two litres of fluid per day.

Co-enzyme Q10 helps to reverse gum inflammation and promote healing of gum disease. A multivitamin and minerals supplement has been show to improve gum health, too.

Green tea leaves contain polyphenols that have a natural deodorizing effect, and drinking green tea can help to reduce bad breath and suppress odours due to chemicals such as methyl mercaptan, ammonia and trimethylamine. Extracts of *blue-green algae* can also help.

See also: **Blue-green algae**.

Related entry: **Gums – receding**.

Hangover

A hangover is an unpleasant group of symptoms linked with excessive alcohol intake, which can include headache, nausea and dizziness. Hangover symptoms are partly due to the build-up of toxins produced in the liver while processing alcohol, partly due to irritation of the intestines, and partly due to dehydration of the brain. Hangover prevention and cure, therefore, depends on slowing the absorption of alcohol, regulating the production of toxins, protecting the intestines and ensuring you drink plenty of water.

Prevention
Think about how much you are likely to drink during a night out, and calculate how many units of alcohol this represents (See box.) You may be surprised at the number of units you regularly consume.

Do not take supplements if you are pregnant, breast-feeding, or taking prescribed drugs without first seeking advice from a pharmacist about possible interactions or adverse effects.

Calculating Units of Alcohol

It is both the strength and size of a drink that determines how many units it contains.

A unit of alcohol is 10 ml or 8 g of pure alcohol.

Half a pint (300 ml) of beer, lager or cider that is 3.5 per cent alcohol in strength contains one unit. But many lagers now contain 5 per cent and some versions supply as much as 9 per cent alcohol.

A 25 ml pub measure of 40 per cent spirit contains one unit. But, many pubs now serve 35 ml measures as standard, and will often serve a double unless you specifically say you want a single.

One small (100 ml) glass of wine that is 10 per cent alcohol in strength contains one unit. But most wines are now much stronger (12–15 per cent alcohol) and many pubs sell wine in 250 ml glasses. Depending on its per cent alcohol, a bottle of wine typically contains between 8–11 units of alcohol.

You can find a handy unit calculator at www.drinkaware.co.uk.

Official advice is to drink no more than 3–4 units of alcohol per day for men, and no more than 2–3 units for women. Have several alcohol-free days so that over the course of a week you drink no more than 21 units of alcohol if you are male, or 14 units if you are female.

People who regularly drink 6 or more units of alcohol per day, or who binge drink at weekends, are twice as likely to die from sudden heart rhythm abnormalities than moderate or non-drinkers.

Heavy drinkers also have an increased risk of death from road traffic accidents, suicide, homicide, certain cancers (e.g. mouth, throat), stroke, weakened heart muscle (cardiomyopathy), inflammation of the pancreas (pancreatitis) and cirrhosis of the liver.

Do not take supplements if you are pregnant, breast-feeding, or taking prescribed drugs without first seeking advice from a pharmacist about possible interactions or adverse effects.

During the weeks running up to a celebration, take *milk thistle* extracts which can protect liver cells from a number of poisons, including alcohol. Research suggests it regulates the flow of alcohol into liver cells for processing, and stimulates liver cell regeneration.

Before going out, take *globe artichoke* extracts to stimulate liver function. You may also want to take a *B group vitamin* supplement (50–100 mg) plus 1 g *vitamin C*, as these are involved in processing alcohol, and deficiency can worsen hangover symptoms.

Always drink on a full stomach; this slows alcohol absorption so the liver metabolizes it more efficiently. If you are going to a party and don't expect to eat until later, have a snack such as a sandwich or cheese and biscuits before going out.

Drink according to your size. Slender souls weighing 9-stone can handle less alcohol than someone weighing 18-stone so don't try to keep up with your mates. Women, in particular, handle alcohol less well than men so don't try to match them drink for drink.

Alternate alcohol with non-alcoholic drinks and select cocktails containing mixers, e.g. Spritzers (wine and soda water).

Don't gulp drinks quickly – sip slowly so your liver has more chance to keep pace with your alcohol intake. On average, you process alcohol at a rate of one unit per hour.

Avoid drinks containing congeners – substances that add flavour and colour while increasing the agonies of excess. Among the spirits, vodka and gin are kindest, while cognac, brandy and whisky tend to trigger the worst hangovers. Similarly, red wine contains chemicals that cause headache in some people.

Drink at least half a litre of water before going to bed to help overcome the dehydrating effects of alcohol. It's also worth taking another 1 g *vitamin C*, and another dose of *globe artichoke* if you've drunk more alcohol than you know you should have.

After an episode of heavy drinking it is advisable to refrain from drinking for 48 hours.

If you are pregnant, it is best to avoid alcohol altogether, especially during the first 12 weeks.

Do not take supplements if you are pregnant, breast-feeding, or taking prescribed drugs without first seeking advice from a pharmacist about possible interactions or adverse effects.

Why women don't handle alcohol as well as men

♥ Women tend to weigh less than men – a petite female can tolerate less alcohol than a tall, stocky male.

♥ Women have lower levels of a stomach enzyme, gastric alcohol dehydrogenase, than men, so less alcohol is deactivated before being absorbed into the circulation. A woman absorbs a third more alcohol than a man of the same size when they have consumed equal amounts.

♥ In men around 60 per cent of body weight is made up of water, compared with around 50 per cent in women, so absorbed alcohol undergoes less dilution in women than in men.

♥ Alcohol dependent drinkers tend to develop their dependence after several years of drinking; while it takes up to ten years of heavy drinking for a susceptible male to become dependent, it takes only three to four years for a susceptible woman to develop dependency.

♥ Women show significantly more interference with thought processes (cognitive impairment) than males with equivalent blood alcohol concentrations. But females subjectively feel they are less impaired and may therefore drink more.

♥ Women develop higher blood alcohol concentrations with the same level of intake as they get older. This effect is not fully explained by differences in body water volume and may be due to reduced ability to process alcohol with age.

♥ Women are more vulnerable to developing alcoholic liver disease than men, as hormone effects mean that liver cells are more likely to accumulate fat and undergo degenerative fatty changes.

Do not take supplements if you are pregnant, breast-feeding, or taking prescribed drugs without first seeking advice from a pharmacist about possible interactions or adverse effects.

Don't drink and drive. Designate a non-drinking driver, or travel by taxi/bus.

Treatment

If, despite your best efforts, you wake up wallowing in the after effects of over-indulgence, the following tips can help to reduce the severity of your symptoms and hasten recovery.

Alcohol is a diuretic, and as your pounding headache and dry, fuzzy mouth are partly due to dehydration, drinking water will help speed your recovery. If you wake with a hangover, sip water little and often all day to get at least two litres pure water on board. Don't gulp down lots in one go – it may come right back up again. To replenish potassium and other important salt levels, take electrolyte solutions (made up from sachets or effervescent tablets) available from pharmacies. If you don't have any, a good substitute is clear consommé soup (if necessary, made from stock cubes) or original coke (not diet versions – you need the sugar) mixed half-and-half with water.

Milk thistle extracts have a powerful effect to protect liver cells from the poisonous effects of excess alcohol. They contain an antioxidant complex known as silymarin which boosts levels of glutathione – a substance added to toxins in the liver to help neutralize them. Silymarin also regulates the entry of alcohol into liver cells so they are not overwhelmed, and promotes liver cell regeneration.

Globe artichoke has liver-protecting effects similar to those of *milk thistle*. It also stimulates bile production, so more toxins are flushed out of the liver and digestion improves. It is especially helpful the morning after the night-before as increased bile production reduces nausea, bloating and indigestion – often within 30 minutes. It can be taken together with milk thistle extracts for a synergistic action.

As the liver breaks down alcohol, millions of free radicals are produced which contribute to the damaging effects of excess. One of the most important antioxidants in the liver is glutathione, which can

---

Do not take supplements if you are pregnant, breast-feeding, or taking prescribed drugs without first seeking advice from a pharmacist about possible interactions or adverse effects.

quickly run low, so liver cell damage increases. Antioxidants such as *vitamin C* help to support the liver while it processes alcohol. Take 1 g vitamin C three times a day. If prone to indigestion after drinking, take the form known as ester-C which is non-acidic. It also helps to drink fresh orange juice, which provides fluid, potassium salts, vitamin C plus fructose – a sugar that accelerates the removal of any alcohol remaining in your system.

B vitamins are quickly used up as the body processes alcohol. Some people swear by toast plus yeast extract (rich in B group vitamins) while others prefer a high dose B supplement which usually comes in the form of effervescent tablets so you replenish fluids at the same time.

To help increase alertness and get those tired, aching muscles more energized, caffeine (traditionally in the form of strong, black coffee) will help clear a fuzzy head and reduce headache. Another good source of caffeine-like substances is *guarana* – extracted from the seeds of a Brazilian shrub. Caffeine is a diuretic, however, so if choosing this cure drink lots of water, too. Don't take caffeine at night as it will keep you awake and you'll wake up feeling worse.

Drinking another alcoholic drink in the morning may seem to improve a hangover, but this is just a temporary effect. You are only postponing the misery. What happens is that the new influx of ethanol briefly blocks the processing of alcohol already in your system so your level of toxins such as acetaldehyde and formic acid fall slightly – until they rise again even further as the new plus the old alcohol is processed. Don't indulge in the 'hair of the dog' remedy. Wanting to drink alcohol in the morning can be a sign of alcohol addiction – talk to your doctor.

A review of over one hundred medical studies suggests that the most effective cure for a hangover is time. Drink your fluids, take your supplements, eat a light diet and rest until the effects wear off. Then promise yourself you'll go easier next time – think of your liver!

See also: **Artichoke, Valerian**.

Do not take supplements if you are pregnant, breast-feeding, or taking prescribed drugs without first seeking advice from a pharmacist about possible interactions or adverse effects.

Hay fever

Hay fever is an allergic response triggered by sensitivity to plant pollens or fungal spores. It is the most common form of allergy, affecting at least 15 million people in the UK. Numbers are increasing year on year, with air pollution – especially inhaling minute hydrocarbon particles from diesel engine exhausts – suggested as a prime cause. Global warming, which means that summer starts earlier and may end later may be another factor. Symptoms such as itchy conjunctivitis, runny nose, stuffiness, sneezing and headache occur when pollen or spores come into contact with moist mucous membranes lining the eyes, nose and sinuses. This triggers the release of histamine and other powerful chemicals that cause inflammation and swelling. Hay fever may also make other allergic conditions such as asthma or eczema worse. Hay fever symptoms vary from month to month, and can last from February to October, depending on which pollens are causing the allergy.

February–May	Hazel, elder and birch pollen
April, May	Plane tree pollen
June–August	Grass pollens
August–October	Mould and fungal spores in damp weather

Only one in 20 hay fever sufferers escapes allergic eye problems altogether – usually it is those allergic to the pollen of oil-seed rape. Conjunctivitis tends to be worse in those allergic to tree pollens.

Hay fever seems to run in families. It tends to strike first between the ages of six and 20, with symptoms peaking in the late teens and early 20s. Symptoms often disappear after five to 15 years so have usually improved by middle age.

Do not take supplements if you are pregnant, breast-feeding, or taking prescribed drugs without first seeking advice from a pharmacist about possible interactions or adverse effects.

Prevention

According to the World Health Organization, immunotherapy is the only treatment that fights the underlying cause of allergies such as hay fever. A vaccine pill, called Grazax, is available, which you dissolve under the tongue, ideally starting about eight weeks before the hay fever season starts, and throughout the hay fever season. Grazax contains grass proteins which prime the immune system so it doesn't over-react to grass pollens. Research shows that it reduces symptoms such as itchy, streaming eyes, sneezing and runny nose by almost a third, with no serious side effects. Those receiving the immune treatment also reported a significant reduction in their need for antihistamines and steroidal nasal sprays. Grazax pollen extract is available on prescription for those who fail to respond to anti-allergy drugs, and your GP can provide further information.

There are several things sufferers can do to help prevent hay fever symptoms.

- Check pollen forecasts and stay indoors when levels are highest, as well as between 7–9 am and 3–7 pm when pollen is most likely to be just above ground level.
- Avoid city centres and other areas of high traffic density.
- When going out is unavoidable, dabbing petroleum jelly or Nasaleze (see box, page 478) just inside the nostrils to trap pollen and wearing sunglasses to protect the eyes are sensible precautions.
- When possible, change clothes and shower after going outside and wash your hands before touching your eyes.
- Avoid pets that have been outdoors and carry pollen on their fur.
- Keep house windows and doors shut, especially bedroom windows at night.
- Vacuum the home and dust regularly, and use a negative ionizer indoors to settle airborne pollen.
- Keep car windows and doors shut, and consider buying a car with an integral pollen filter.
- Avoid gardening or mowing the lawn, barbecues, picnics and cut grass.

Do not take supplements if you are pregnant, breast-feeding, or taking prescribed drugs without first seeking advice from a pharmacist about possible interactions or adverse effects.

- Avoid exposure to cigarette smoke and chemical fumes (e.g. paint, solvents).

Treatment

Conventional treatments include antihistamines, anti-inflammatory corticosteroids and decongestants that are taken as tablets/capsules or delivered as eye drops or nasal sprays. Treatments often work best if started early in the season before pollen counts become too high.

As a preventative, naturopaths recommend chewing lumps of honeycomb throughout winter and late spring, so long as you are not allergic to bee products. *B group vitamins* (e.g. brewer's yeast) may also be started in spring. High-dose *vitamin C* and bioflavonoids such as quercetin (found in citrus fruits, blackcurrants and rosehips) have a natural antihistamine action and help to damp down inflammation.

Many prescribed drugs are derived from plants, so it is not surprising there are several effective herbal remedies to help treat hay fever symptoms.

Butterbur is traditionally used to treat migraine, and research suggests it is as effective in reducing hay fever symptoms as antihistamines (cetirizine, fexofenidine) but without the drowsiness which affected two-thirds of those taking the drug.

Perilla frutescens has been found to reduce recurrent sneezing, watery or itchy nose and eyes, as well as facial itching in at least 80 per cent of people.

Luffa Complex contains extracts from seven freshly harvested herbs, including Sponge Cucumber, Heartseed, American Spikenard and Khella. One study found that it relieved hay fever symptoms in 75 per cent of cases.

Bromelain has a natural anti-inflammatory action that helps to reduce pain, swelling and inflammation – all symptoms that can be associated with hay fever. Its enzyme action also helps to break down mucus so it becomes thinner and easier to shift. In one study, 83 per cent of people taking it for sinusitis enjoyed complete resolution of nasal swelling and inflammation compared with only half of those taking placebo.

Do not take supplements if you are pregnant, breast-feeding, or taking prescribed drugs without first seeking advice from a pharmacist about possible interactions or adverse effects.

Helpful Tips

If you have sore, red eyes, lie down for 20 minutes with a cool compress over your eyes made from cotton pads soaked in rosewater, eyebright or cold camomile tea.

If nasal symptoms start, you can also try acupressure: Press on the top end of the web between your thumb and index finger – at the highest point of the muscle, just before you can feel the bones meet. Press and rub firmly for one minute, then repeat on the other side.

Nasaleze is a nasal powder that lines the nasal passages and sinuses to enhance the production of nasal mucus. This forms an invisible, gel-like filter over the lining of nasal passages that helps stop pollen triggering an allergic reaction. In most cases, hay fever symptoms are controlled within 3–10 seconds. See www.nasaleze.com.

Another approach is to overcome swelling of the nasal lining with Breathe Right nasal strips which gently open the nasal passages to relieve nasal congestion.

Pycnogenol® – an extract from the bark of the French maritime pine – is as effective in preventing release of histamine as a commonly used hay fever drug, sodium cromoglicate. In fact, laboratory studies have shown Pycnogenol can block as much as 70 per cent of histamine release from mast cells when they are exposed to airborne allergens such as pollen.

Garlic has also been used for centuries to help control the symptoms of hay fever, as well as for its antiseptic and decongestant properties due to its complex, sulphur-containing compounds.

See also: **Bee products – bee pollen, Butterbur, Essential Fatty Acids, Perilla**.

Do not take supplements if you are pregnant, breast-feeding, or taking prescribed drugs without first seeking advice from a pharmacist about possible interactions or adverse effects.

Headache

You may think a headache is just a headache but, surprisingly, twelve different types of headache have been identified, which can be further divided into around 100 different varieties of head pain.

One of the commonest forms is tension headache, which feels like a severe, continuous pressure on both sides of your head. It often resembles a tight, constricting band or a heavy weight pressing down on top of your head. The pain of tension headache may spread over the top of your skull, over the back of your head or over both eyes and you may feel tense around your neck and shoulders.

Several factors can trigger a tension headache, including excess stress and tiredness which can lead to muscle tension in neck and scalp muscle with associated changes in blood circulation to the head.

Tension headache is often brought on by feelings of excess pressure, relief of stress (e.g. at the end of a long, trying week), physical fatigue, lack of sleep, missed meals and extreme emotions such as anger and excitement.

To avoid muscle tension

- Try not to stoop when standing or sitting, concentrate on keeping your back straight, your shoulders square and your abdomen lightly pulled in

- Don't hunch your shoulders – hold shoulders straight yet relaxed – circle your shoulders from time to time

- Don't fold your arms tightly – let them hang loosely from your shoulders, and shake your arms and hands regularly

- Don't clench your fists – hold hands loosely with your palms open and your fingers curled lightly and naturally

- Don't clench or grind your teeth – keep your mouth slightly open and try to relax your upper and lower jaws.

Do not take supplements if you are pregnant, breast-feeding, or taking prescribed drugs without first seeking advice from a pharmacist about possible interactions or adverse effects.

Migraine is worse than just a headache, and is often described as a full-blown attack. Migraine is often misdiagnosed as a tension headache. It is important to consult a doctor about a recurrent headache that may be migraine.

Treatment
Massage is often effective, as gentle manipulation of muscles in the neck, shoulders and back will relax taut muscles.

Herbal remedies that help to reduce stress and promote relaxation and relief of tension include *valerian* (often combined with lemon balm and hops) and *Rhodiola*.

Feverfew is effective in reducing the frequency and severity of recurrent headaches, such as migraine.

Other supplements that may be used include *devil's claw, peppermint, yerba maté, 5-HTP, agnus castus* (to relieve menstrually related headaches), *vitamin B2* (riboflavin), *calcium* and *magnesium* which may help to reduce spasm of muscles and blood vessels.

See also: **Agnus castus, Blue-green algae, Gotu kola, 5-HTP, Isoflavones, Kudzu, Lemon balm, Magnesium, Nettle, Olive leaf, Vitamin B1, Vitamin B5, Vitamin B6, Vitamin D, Vitamin E.**

Related entry: **Migraine**.

Helicobacter pylori

Helicobacter pylori is a motile form of bacteria found in the stomachs of at least 20 per cent of 30-year-olds and 50 per cent of those over 50 in the UK. It burrows into the mucous lining of the stomach leaving a small breach in the wall through which acids can reach the stomach wall. *Helicobacter* then coats itself with a small bubble of alkaline ammonia, protecting itself from the acid attack and, at the same time, irritating and inflaming the stomach lining. Although it doesn't cause symptoms in everyone, virtually all patients with duodenal ulcers are infected, plus three-quarters of those with gastric ulcers. *H. pylori* infection is also associated with an increased risk of gastric cancer.

Treatment

Orthodox eradication usually involves a week's course of two antibiotics plus a drug that switches off acid production. Several natural treatments are used to help reduce *H. pylori* infection. *Manuka honey* made by bees feeding on nectar from the New Zealand tea tree contains a unique antibiotic that can eradicate *Helicobacter*. It is usually taken on an empty stomach at a dose of four teaspoons, four times a day, for eight weeks. Another natural approach is to take *mastic gum* derived from a pistachio-like tree grown on the Greek island of Chios.

Interesting research also provides preliminary evidence that *cranberry* extracts can help to stop *Helicobacter pylori* sticking to cells in the stomach lining due to the unique anti-adhesin compounds it contains. This may help to flush *Helicobacter* from the stomach so they are expelled more easily.

Pelargonium sidoides root extracts also have a powerful anti-adhesin effect on *Helicobacter pylori* to reduce their adherence to the stomach wall.

Probiotic yoghurt or supplements have also been shown to inhibit growth of *Helicobacter pylori* as well as maintaining overall intestinal health.

Note:

• Recurrent intestinal symptoms should always be reported to a doctor.
• People with diabetes should consult a doctor before using a honey treatment.

See also: **Bee products, Cranberry, Grapefruit seed, Mastic gum, Pelargonium sidoides, Probiotics, Vitamin B12, Vitamin C**.

Do not take supplements if you are pregnant, breast-feeding, or taking prescribed drugs without first seeking advice from a pharmacist about possible interactions or adverse effects.

Herpes simplex

Eight out of ten people show antibody evidence of infection with the *Herpes simplex* viruses that cause cold sores, but studies suggest that only 20–40 per cent of those exposed develop clinical symptoms. The virus is mainly caught during the first 18 months of life as a result of being kissed by an infected adult. The initial, or primary, infection passes unnoticed in up to 90 per cent of cases, or may only produce mild soreness. Occasionally, however, it can produce widespread, excruciatingly painful sores all over the inside of the mouth and on the gums and tongue (herpetic gingivostomatitis). During the first attack, the herpes virus travels up nerve endings to lie dormant in a nerve ganglion. It can then be re-activated by a number of triggers to travel down a nerve ending and cause recurrences in future years. Trigger factors can include frosty weather, a common cold, stress or exposure to ultraviolet light (e.g. sun beds, skiing holidays). As kissing is the main mode of infection, this should be avoided from the first sign of a cold sore appearing until it is fully healed.

Treatment

Echinacea increases the proliferation and activity of immune cells responsible for fighting infections and is often used to reduce herpes recurrences. A typical regime is to take 25 drops Echinacea tincture in water as soon as possible at the beginning of an attack. Repeat every two hours for four doses, then continue four times a day until symptoms resolve.

Taking 200 mg *vitamin C* plus bioflavonoids three to five times daily (starting within 48 hours of initial symptoms) was found to reduce blister development so that only 26 per cent of treated patients developed a sore, compared with 100 per cent in those receiving placebo. The average interval from onset to complete healing was also significantly reduced in those taking vitamin C.

Olive leaf extracts have a powerful anti-viral action, and a comparative trial of three products conducted by the Herpes Viruses

---

Do not take supplements if you are pregnant, breast-feeding, or taking prescribed drugs without first seeking advice from a pharmacist about possible interactions or adverse effects.

Association found that olive leaf extracts were the clear winner. Out of 45 members taking part, 78 per cent of those using olive leaf extracts were pleased with the results in treating and preventing attacks.

Topical salves that have been shown to reduce herpes virus replication include those containing lemon balm, and (my favourite) liquorice balm (from www.skinshop.co.uk).

See also: **Arginine, Damiana, Echinacea, Elderberry, Goldenseal, Grapefruit seed, Iron, Lapacho, Liquorice, Olive leaf, Sarsaparilla, Vitamin C, Zinc**.

Hiatus hernia

A hiatus hernia forms when part of the stomach pushes up – or herniates – into the chest through a natural weakness in the diaphragm. In many cases, it causes no problems and symptoms only occur when the hernia affects the valve mechanism between the stomach and oesophagus so that acid is regurgitated and refluxes upwards, sometimes as far as the mouth. This causes a condition known as gastrooesophageal reflux disease (GORD) whose main symptom is heartburn. Heartburn is partly due to acid irritation of delicate tissues lining the lower oesophagus, and partly to painful spasm of underlying muscles in the wall of the oesophagus. Hiatus hernia can also cause symptoms of coughing, shortness of breath, palpitations or hiccoughs due to extra pressure in the chest. In severe cases, bleeding and anaemia can occur. These symptoms often mimic those of angina or heart attack and it is estimated that 20 per cent of patients admitted to coronary care units have GORD rather than heart disease.

Treatment
To help reduce symptoms of hiatus hernia, try to lose any excess weight. Eat and drink little and often throughout the day to avoid over-filling the stomach. Try also to avoid stooping, bending, late-night eating and lying down after eating.

It helps to follow a relatively bland diet without hot, acid, spicy, fatty or pastry foods and to avoid tea, coffee, alcohol and acidic fruit juices. Wear loose clothing, especially around the waist. It might also help to elevate the head of the bed by about 15–20 cm.

Traditionally, eating bitter, green leafy vegetables such as endive, lettuce and *globe artichoke* (also available as supplements) are recommended for relieving symptoms due to hiatus hernia.

Live bio yoghurt and *probiotic* supplements containing digestive bacteria are also helpful. *Evening primrose oil, omega-3 fish oils* and *flaxseed oil* provide essential fatty acids which help to reduce inflammation, while *aloe vera gel* is widely used to relieve intestinal symptoms including dyspepsia. Start with a small dose (e.g. 1 teaspoon) and work up to around 1–2 tablespoons per day to find the ideal dose.

Colloidal silicol gel is also worth trying. Herbalists frequently recommend marshmallow root preparations to relieve hiatus hernia symptoms; however, diabetics on hypoglycaemia medication should monitor blood sugar levels closely if taking these as some studies have suggested that they may lower blood sugar levels.

Homocysteine levels – raised

Homocysteine is a sulphur-containing amino acid produced in the body during the breakdown of the essential amino acid, methionine. When homocysteine builds up in the circulation, it damages the lining of artery walls so they become narrow and inelastic. Research suggests that a raised homocysteine level is an independent risk factor for hardening and furring up of the arteries, coronary heart disease, stroke, peripheral vascular disease and other conditions associated with abnormal blood clotting. A raised homocysteine level is also linked with a number of other serious medical conditions, including osteoporosis, dementia and birth defects.

Normally, homocysteine levels are tightly controlled by three different enzymes that convert homocysteine to cysteine – a safe end product that promotes cell growth. Two of these three enzymes depend on adequate intakes of *folic acid, vitamin B6* and *vitamin B12* for optimal activity. If you obtain good amounts of these micronutrients in your diet, your homocysteine levels can improve significantly. Unfortunately, only 40–50 per cent of people following a typical Western diet obtain enough dietary folic acid to process homocysteine normally. When these nutrients are lacking, homocysteine levels rise. Genetic mutations also affect enzyme activity and an estimated one in ten people inherits levels of homocysteine that triple the risk of cardiovascular disease. One in 160,000 inherits extremely high homocysteine levels with 30 times the risk of premature heart disease. After the menopause, women seem less able to process homocysteine so levels build up to increase the risk of osteoporosis and coronary heart disease.

Treatment
High levels of homocysteine can be reduced by taking *folic acid* supplements (400–650 mcg per day) plus vitamins B6 and B12. Although diet should always come first, synthetic forms of folic acid found in supplements and fortified foods (e.g. breakfast cereals) are more bioavailable than those found in natural food sources (e.g. green leafy vegetables) which are in the less easily absorbed poly-glutamate form.

The safe, normal level of homocysteine is still uncertain. Initially, it was suggested as between 8 and 15 micromol/L. Researchers now believe it is important to maintain even tighter control as homocysteine levels above 6.9 micromol/L may be harmful for long-term health. As homocysteine levels naturally rise with age, however, a level of 12 or under may still be acceptable for those aged over 60 years.

Your doctor may be willing to measure your homocysteine levels but this is not yet routinely requested. If testing is not available on the NHS, a self-administered, pin-prick blood test is available from some pharmacies.

If you know you have a high homocysteine level, it is relatively

---

Do not take supplements if you are pregnant, breast-feeding, or taking prescribed drugs without first seeking advice from a pharmacist about possible interactions or adverse effects.

easy to lower it by making dietary and lifestyle changes – much easier, in fact, than it is to correct an abnormal cholesterol balance. These changes include eating more foods rich in folate/folic acid, vitamins B6 and B12, as well as taking vitamin supplements. Even people who have inherited an abnormal homocysteine metabolism do not necessarily develop a raised homocysteine level if they maintain a relatively high intake of folic acid.

Analysis of pooled data from 12 clinical trials suggests that taking supplements can reduce homocysteine levels by 25 per cent, while adding in vitamin B12 can lower levels by a further 7 per cent. A typical treatment regime is as follows:

Homocysteine Level (micromol/L)	Risk Level	Suggested Level Daily Supplements
6.9 or below	Optimal	400 mcg Folic acid
7–9.9	Mild	3 mg B6, 100 mcg B12, 400 mcg Folic acid
10–12.9	Moderate	10 mg B6, 100 mcg B12, 1 mg Folic acid
13–20	High	50 mg B6, 500 mcg B12, 2 mg Folic acid
Over 20	Very high	100 mg B6, 1 mg B12, 5 mg Folic acid

NB: Homocysteine levels naturally rise with age, and a level of 12 or under is acceptable for those aged over 60 years.

As homocysteine is thought to cause damage partly by triggering oxidation reactions in the body, it is also important to consider

---

Do not take supplements if you are pregnant, breast-feeding, or taking prescribed drugs without first seeking advice from a pharmacist about possible interactions or adverse effects.

taking antioxidant supplements such as *selenium, vitamins A, C* and *E, carotenoids, alpha-lipoic acid* and *green tea.*

See also: **Fish oils, Folic acid, Isoflavones, Vitamin B6, Vitamin B12**.

Hormone replacement therapy – natural

Hormone replacement therapy aims to restore oestrogen levels to the normal, pre-menopausal state. This relieves the signs and symptoms of oestrogen deficiency and postpones long-term consequences such as osteoporosis and coronary heart disease. Although hormone replacement therapy (HRT) is an accepted medical treatment to reduce menopausal symptoms and the risk of post-menopausal osteoporosis, many women are unwilling, or unable, to take it. For these, a number of alternative options are available. These include: *black cohosh* and *isoflavones.*

See also: **Agnus castus, Black cohosh, Dong quai, Flaxseed, Isoflavones, Kudzu, Liquorice, Maca, Oatstraw, Pfaffia, Sage, St John's Wort, Siberian ginseng, Wild yam**.

Related entry: **Menopause**.

Hypertension

When blood pressure (BP) is measured, two readings are taken: the higher reading is the pressure created as your heart contracts and pushes blood into your circulation. This is known as your systolic pressure. The lower reading is the background pressure in your circulation when your heart rests between beats, and is known as your diastolic pressure. These two pressures are recorded one over the other.

If your blood pressure is less than 130/80 mmHg, it is classed as normal. High blood pressure is diagnosed when your BP is consistently greater than 140/90 mmHg – even when you are asleep. Previously, it was assumed that blood pressure between these levels

---

Do not take supplements if you are pregnant, breast-feeding, or taking prescribed drugs without first seeking advice from a pharmacist about possible interactions or adverse effects.

was acceptable from a health-risk point of view. It's now recognized, however, that people with blood pressures in the continuum between 130/80 and 139/89 mmHg also have a higher risk of circulatory problems and are likely to progress to full-blown hypertension needing drug treatment. Blood pressures between these two ranges have therefore been given a new classification of *prehypertension*. This new category is designed to improve people's motivation towards adopting healthier habits as dietary and lifestyle changes can stop your blood pressure rising any further.

Once your blood pressure is persistently raised above 140/90, you have hypertension. This category is further sub-divided into mild, moderate and severe.

Hypertension Category	Systolic BP (mmHg)	Diastolic BP (mmHg)
Optimal	Less than 120	Less than 80
Normal	Less than 130	Less than 85
Pre-hypertension	130–139	85–89
Hypertension		
Stage 1 (mild)	140–159	90–99
Stage 2 (moderate)	160–179	100–109
Stage 3 (severe)	Greater than 180	Greater than 110
Isolated systolic hypertension		
Grade 1	140–159	Less than 90
Grade 2	160 or greater	Less than 90

If systolic blood pressure and diastolic blood pressure fall into different categories, the higher value is taken for classification.

One of the main causes of high blood pressure is hardening and furring up of the arteries (atherosclerosis). This naturally occurs with increasing age and comes on more quickly in those who smoke, are diabetic or overweight. Other risk factors that increase blood pressure include an abnormally raised blood cholesterol level, drinking too much alcohol, excessive *sodium* intake, stress, lack of exercise and the side effects of some drugs.

Some research suggests that high BP is linked with lack of essential fatty acids (such as those found in *evening primrose oil* and *omega-3 fish oils*), and the minerals *calcium* and *magnesium*. High blood pressure also runs in some families, so it is even more important to have regular checks if there is a family history.

Some people with hypertension feel dizzy, have throbbing sensations in parts of their body, feel tired or suffer from headaches but the majority of people feel relatively well even when their blood pressure is dangerously high. If not corrected, prolonged hypertension can damage blood vessels in the brain, heart, kidneys and eyes to cause serious complications, including kidney failure, impaired eyesight, heart attack and stroke. A man in his early 40s is 30 times more likely to have a stroke, for example, if he has hypertension than a man with normal blood pressure. For more information about my book on Overcoming Hypertension, visit my website www.naturalhealthguru.co.uk.

Treatment
The aim of blood pressure treatment is to reduce your BP to below 140/90 mmHg. If you have diabetes, kidney problems or established cardiovascular disease, the target is more strict at 130/80 mmHg or less. Sometimes two or even three different types of drug are needed to achieve this goal. New research indicates that people whose high blood pressure does not respond to multiple medications are likely to be eating too much salt (*see* **Sodium**).

Lifestyle changes that can improve high blood pressure include:

Do not take supplements if you are pregnant, breast-feeding, or taking prescribed drugs without first seeking advice from a pharmacist about possible interactions or adverse effects.

- Regular exercise (e.g. walking, cycling, swimming, gardening) for at least 30–60 minutes, five times a week and preferably every day
- Quitting smoking: cigarettes damage artery linings, cause spasm and constriction of vessels, and raise blood pressure
- Losing excess weight – just losing half a stone can significantly reduce a raised blood pressure
- Avoiding excess alcohol intake
- Avoiding stressful situations and taking time out to relax; transcendental meditation, for example, has been shown to significantly reduce blood pressure within three months.

In addition to the above, a low-salt, low-fat diet is recommended with plenty of fresh fruit and vegetables for protective vitamins, minerals, antioxidants, fibre and potassium, which helps to flush excess sodium from your body.

Not adding salt during cooking or at the table will lower systolic blood pressure significantly, and if everyone who was hypertensive did this it is estimated that the incidence of stroke would be reduced by as much as 26 per cent, and coronary heart disease by 15 per cent.

A daily dose of 100 mg *co-enzyme Q10* has been found to significantly reduce blood pressure compared with a placebo. *Garlic* tablets are widely prescribed in Europe to reduce hypertension, and in one study where 600–900 mg garlic powder tablets were taken daily for up to six months, systolic blood pressure fell by an average of 8 per cent.

See also: **Alpha-lipoic acid, Arginine, Astragalus, Bilberry, Calcium, Carnitine, Carotenoids, Co-enzyme Q10, Copper, Evening primrose oil, Fish oils, Folic acid, Garlic, Ginger, Ginseng, Green tea, Hawthorn, Liquorice, Magnesium, Maitake, Olive leaf, Olive oil, Potassium, Probiotics, Reishi, Rhodiola, Siberian ginseng, Sodium, Vitamin B1, Vitamin B6, Vitamin C, Vitamin D**.

Related entry: **Atherosclerosis**.

Do not take supplements if you are pregnant, breast-feeding, or taking prescribed drugs without first seeking advice from a pharmacist about possible interactions or adverse effects.

Hypotension

Low blood pressure is not routinely treated in the UK unless it causes recurrent symptoms such as dizziness. A study of over 10,000 civil servants suggested that persistent low blood pressure – sometimes known as hypotension syndrome – can also be associated with tiredness, headaches, anxiety, depression and minor psychological dysfunction. This is probably related to reduced blood circulation and supply of oxygen, glucose and other nutrients to the brain.

Treatment
Ginkgo supplements would be expected to reduce the above symptoms but would not raise the underlying blood pressure. Increasing intake of dietary table salt (sodium chloride) is the approach most usually suggested as this encourages fluid accumulation in the circulation. *Panax ginseng*, butcher's broom and liquorice can raise blood pressure but should not be taken long term except under the supervision of a medical herbalist.

In older people, low blood pressure can occur when getting up quickly from a sitting or lying position. This is known as postural hypotension and may be remedied by getting up slowly and, for example, sitting on the side of the bed for a minute or two to adjust before standing.

See also: **Sodium**.

Immunity

Your immune system is made up of millions of cells that patrol the body to protect against disease. Each cell has a different function – some absorb and destroy bacteria, some produce antibodies, while others make anti-viral substances such as interferon.

In order to function properly, the body's immune cells need a plentiful supply of vitamins, minerals and immune boosters. These help them to produce communication chemicals that control their

---

Do not take supplements if you are pregnant, breast-feeding, or taking prescribed drugs without first seeking advice from a pharmacist about possible interactions or adverse effects.

activity, and to make powerful disease-fighting substances. Dietary and lifestyle changes are also important to increase your natural protection against infections.

Eat a wholefood diet providing plenty of fresh fruit and vegetables – these supply vitamins, minerals, antioxidants and certain non-nutrient substances (phytochemicals) that help to prevent cancer and boost immune function.

Eat a relatively low-fat diet with fewer omega-6 polyunsaturated fatty acids (derived from some vegetable oils such as sunflower, safflower and corn oils) and more healthy fats such as monounsaturates (e.g. olive, rapeseed, macadamia, rapeseed, avocado and almond oils) and omega-3 fish oils. Ideally, a balanced intake of omega-3s and omega-6s is needed, but the average adult currently eats seven times more omega-6 fats than omega-3s. A better ratio is 5:1 and an optimum ratio is no more than 3:1. For those who don't like eating fish, taking an omega-3 supplement is recommended.

Take regular exercise which increases immune function (but avoid over-training which reduces your resistance to infection).

Get a regular, good night's sleep; this is a time of relaxation, regeneration and rejuvenation in which growth hormone and other vital substances involved in healing and fighting disease are secreted. People exposed to a common cold virus are three times more likely to develop symptoms if they get less than seven hours' sleep a night, than if they achieve eight hours or more.

Avoid excess stress which puts your body on red alert; in the long term, this depletes the adrenal glands, interferes with the body's ability to fight disease and increases susceptibility to infections.

Immune-boosting supplements
While diet should always come first, taking a good A-Z style *multivitamin and mineral supplement* acts as a nutritional safety net to guard against deficiencies. *Selenium* stimulates the production of natural killer cells which fight viral and bacterial infections and, together with *vitamin E*, is needed to make antibodies. It also reduces the virulence of influenza viruses. Iron is needed by white

---

Do not take supplements if you are pregnant, breast-feeding, or taking prescribed drugs without first seeking advice from a pharmacist about possible interactions or adverse effects.

blood cells to produce the powerful chemicals used to kill microbes, while *zinc* appears to be important for increasing natural immunity against viruses responsible for sore throats and colds. Certainly for older people, taking a multivitamin supplement for one year has been shown to halve the number of days ill with infections compared with those not taking multivitamin supplements (23 days in the year versus 48).

Sucking *zinc* lozenges boosts the action of white blood cells in the throat and can reduce a sore throat. It seems to be important to start treatment within 48 hours of symptoms, and to suck zinc lozenges every two hours while awake.

Vitamin C boosts immunity against cold viruses, which cannot reproduce properly in cells containing high levels of vitamin C. Studies suggest that a dose of 600 mg to 1 g per day can reduce the duration of a common cold by 20 per cent and, if symptoms do occur, they are likely to be less severe. Higher doses of vitamin C can cause indigestion – either reduce the dose or select a supplement that is buffered to make it non-acidic.

Probiotics contain 'friendly' digestive bacteria which have a number of actions in the intestines to boost immunity. As well as maintaining the correct acidity in the gut which prevents less acid-tolerant, harmful bacteria from multiplying, they also produce natural antibiotics (bacteriocins such as acidophiline and bulgarican) and increase production of anti-viral substances such as interferon. Probiotic bacteria are also believed to prime the immune system against other bacterial infections by encouraging production of anti-bacterial antibodies.

Pelargonium sidoides boosts immunity against infections and is a popular treatment to prevent or treat colds, bronchitis, sinusitis and influenza.

Echinacea is one of the most popular immune boosters. It contains several unique substances known as echinacins that stimulate immunity by increasing the number and activity of white blood cells needed to attack infections. In particular, it stimulates phagocytosis – the process in which white blood cells ingest bacteria and

---

Do not take supplements if you are pregnant, breast-feeding, or taking prescribed drugs without first seeking advice from a pharmacist about possible interactions or adverse effects.

viruses before destroying them – and also boosts production of a natural anti-viral substance called interferon. Studies suggest that, overall, Echinacea can reduce your susceptibility to a cold by around a third.

Garlic has natural antiseptic, antibacterial and anti-viral actions. While garlic in meals offers some benefit, select a supplement supplying a standardized amount of the main active ingredient, allicin, for optimum protection. As a bonus, garlic extracts also have beneficial effects on blood pressure, cholesterol levels and help to maintain a healthy heart and circulation.

Grapefruit seed extracts were first investigated when it was noted that they did not rot when thrown onto a compost heap. They have a natural anti-bacterial, anti-fungal, anti-viral and anti-parasitic action that helps to reduce the risk of infection.

Olive leaf extracts have powerful antibacterial and anti-viral actions which help stop infecting organisms from multiplying. Olive leaf extracts are especially helpful against the herpes cold sore virus.

Elderberry juice contains anti-viral compounds and can reduce the severity and duration of common cold and influenza infections. In one study, those taking elderberry extracts showed significant improvement within two days, compared with six days for those not taking elderberry extracts. Elderberry extracts also seem to increase levels of antibodies.

Siberian ginseng is widely used as an adaptogen to help the body adapt to stress. It also boosts immunity against infections and Russian researchers have found that it can reduce susceptibility to cold or flu by 40 per cent.

Reishi has antibacterial and anti-viral actions, enhances energy levels and gives a more restful night's sleep. It is traditionally used to strengthen the immune system and to promote vitality and longevity. Chinese studies involving over 2,000 people have found that reishi extracts are helpful in treating bronchitis.

Where low immunity is linked with excess stress, an adaptogenic supplement such as Siberian or Korean ginseng will help to boost general resistance.

Do not take supplements if you are pregnant, breast-feeding, or taking prescribed drugs without first seeking advice from a pharmacist about possible interactions or adverse effects.

See also: **Adaptogens, Aloe vera, Antioxidants, Arginine, Ashwagandha, Astragalus, Bee products – propolis, Cat's claw, Co-enzyme Q10, Echinacea, Elderberry, Garlic, Goldenseal, Gotu kola, Green tea, Lapacho, Maitake, Pelargonium sidoides, Probiotics, Reishi, Schisandra, Selenium, Shiitake, Wheatgrass, Zinc.**

Impotence

Impotence – known medically as erectile dysfunction – affects an estimated one in 10 men at any one time. Although it can affect men of all ages it becomes increasingly common in later life so that 40 per cent of men aged 40 and almost 70 per cent of those aged 70 years are affected.

Erectile dysfunction is defined as the persistent failure to develop erections that are firm enough for satisfactory sexual intercourse. Erections occur when physical or psychological stimulation cause smooth muscle fibres in the penis to relax, and arteries bringing blood into the area dilate. This results in a massive six-fold increase in blood flow into the penis and the three cylinders of spongy tissue running along its length become engorged. This, in turn, compresses the veins that normally drain blood away so blood remains trapped to maintain the erection. An erect penis contains up to eight times more blood than when it is flaccid.

Eighty per cent of all cases of impotence have an underlying physical cause. The most common physical causes of impotence include:

* Diabetes – which can affect both the local circulation and nerve supply to the penis
* Hardening and furring up of the arteries (atherosclerosis)
* Smoking indirectly causes impotence by increasing the effects of other risk factors such as high blood pressure and atherosclerosis
* Long-term abuse of alcohol or drugs such as marijuana, codeine, amphetamines and heroin

---

Do not take supplements if you are pregnant, breast-feeding, or taking prescribed drugs without first seeking advice from a pharmacist about possible interactions or adverse effects.

- Prescription drugs – especially those used to treat high blood pressure, depression, heart disease, gastric ulcers and cancer
- Leaky veins in the penis
- Hormone imbalances
- Previous surgery that may have affected local blood circulation or nerve supply
- Spinal cord injury
- Some nervous system diseases such as multiple sclerosis, Parkinsonism, Alzheimer's disease and epilepsy.

Treatment

Stress, overwork and tiredness are among the commonest causes of loss of sex drive and impotence. Taking time out for rest, relaxation and plenty of sleep are important. Reducing alcohol intake to no more than one or two units per day and making an effort to cut back or quit smoking are also important. Smoking cigarettes lowers sex hormone levels and can also reduce rigidity of erections. A regular exercise programme is also recommended because brisk physical activity increases secretion of hormones important for sexual function.

A number of conventional treatments are available, including oral drugs that dilate blood vessels and increase blood flow to the penis during sexual arousal. A number of herbal supplements can also help.

Catuaba bark is widely used to maintain potency and fertility in older males. A Brazilian saying states: 'Until a father reaches 60, the son is his; after that the son is Catuaba's'. It is said to stimulate erotic dreams, improve erections and stamina to overcome exhaustion.

Garlic has beneficial effects on the circulation and improves circulation to all parts of the body, including the penis.

Korean ginseng is widely used in the East to improve male potency. Research suggests that ginseng increases levels of nitric oxide (NO) in the spongy tissue of the penis. NO is a nerve communication chemical (neurotransmitter) that is essential for a number of

---

Do not take supplements if you are pregnant, breast-feeding, or taking prescribed drugs without first seeking advice from a pharmacist about possible interactions or adverse effects.

physiological processes, including increasing blood flow to the penis for normal erectile function and sexual arousal. This action is similar in effect to that of the anti-impotence drug, sildenafil.

Maca is used to increase energy and stamina and it has long been reputed to act as an aphrodisiac for men and women. It is widely used to treat male impotence and some researchers believe maca is superior to red Korean ginseng.

Muira puama contains hormone like substances that may increase sexual desire and improve impotence.

Saw palmetto can improve symptoms due to an enlarged prostate gland, and is widely used to improve impotence and low sex drive in men with prostate problems.

Tribulus terrestris is used to treat impotence in Ayurvedic medicine.

Damiana is reputed to have a powerful aphrodisiac action.

If erectile problems continue, always seek medical advice.

See also: **Agnus castus, Arginine, Ashwagandha, Carnitine, Cayenne, Damiana, Ginseng, Maca, Muira puama, Nettle, Pfaffia, Pomegranate, Sarsaparilla, Saw palmetto, Tribulus terrestris**.

Indigestion

Indigestion (or dyspepsia) is a general term used to describe any discomfort, felt centrally in the upper abdomen, as a result of eating. This includes feelings of distension from swallowing air, flatulence, nausea, heartburn, acidity, abdominal pain and sensations of burning. Heartburn is a more specific term referring to hot, burning sensations, felt behind the chest bone, which may spread upwards toward the throat.

One of the commonest causes of heartburn is acid reflux, in which stomach contents reflux up into the oesophagus – the tube connecting the mouth and stomach. This brings stomach acids and enzymes into contact with the sensitive lining of the oesophagus,

---

Do not take supplements if you are pregnant, breast-feeding, or taking prescribed drugs without first seeking advice from a pharmacist about possible interactions or adverse effects.

and can also trigger painful spasm of muscles lining this part of the gut. In severe cases, heartburn can mimic the chest pain of a heart attack, and it has been estimated that 20 per cent of cases admitted to coronary care units may actually have gastro-oesophageal reflux disease, or GORD, rather than a heart problem.

Normally, excessive reflux is prevented by downward contractions of muscles in the oesophageal wall, by a special valve-like mechanism, and by contraction of the diaphragm which pinches the lower oesophagus closed. GORD only develops when these anti-reflux mechanisms fail. This may develop due to poor muscle co-ordination, weakness of the valves, a hiatus hernia (in which part of the stomach slips up through the diaphragm into the chest) or increased pressure on the stomach, e.g. overweight, pregnancy and tight clothes.

Don't ignore recurrent heartburn, as this can lead to inflammation of the oesophagus which can lead to scarring and permanent damage. In some people, it can lead to cell changes that might increase the risk of eventually developing oesophageal cancer. Seek medical advice if symptoms continue.

Treatment
Several self-help measures will help to control your symptoms:

* Lose any excess weight
* Wear lose clothing, especially around the waist
* Avoid smoking cigarettes
* Avoid aspirin and related drugs (e.g. ibuprofen) which can irritate the stomach lining
* Eat little and often throughout the day, rather than having three large meals
* Drink fluids little and often, rather than large quantities at a time
* Avoid hot, acid, spicy, fatty foods
* Avoid tea, coffee and acidic fruit juices
* Cut back on alcohol intake
* Avoid stooping, bending or lying down after eating

Do not take supplements if you are pregnant, breast-feeding, or taking prescribed drugs without first seeking advice from a pharmacist about possible interactions or adverse effects.

- Avoid late-night eating
- Elevate the head of the bed about 15–20 cm (e.g. put books under the top two legs) if symptoms come on at night when lying down
- Try to stay calm. Stress is thought to be a major cause of indigestion – so try and give yourself time to enjoy your food.

Short-term symptoms of heartburn may be treated with antacids (containing calcium carbonate) available over the counter. More powerful drugs that temporarily switch off stomach acid production (e.g. cimetidine, ranitidine, famotidine) are also available over the counter but should not be used long term without seeking medical advice.

Liquorice (DGL form) is widely used to soothe indigestion. Other supplements that many people find helpful include *probiotics* and *aloe vera*.

See also: **Aloe vera, Black cohosh, Calcium, Cayenne, Choline, Devil's claw, Digestive enzymes, Ginger, Horsechestnut, Iron, Liquorice, Mastic gum, Peppermint, Sage, St John's Wort, Sarsaparilla, Turmeric, Vitamin B1, Vitamin B5, Vitamin C**.

Related entry: **Helicobacter pylori**.

Infertility

See: **Conception, Sperm count – low**.

Inflammatory bowel disease

See: **Crohn's disease, Ulcerative colitis**.

Do not take supplements if you are pregnant, breast-feeding, or taking prescribed drugs without first seeking advice from a pharmacist about possible interactions or adverse effects.

Influenza

Influenza is a viral disease that attacks the respiratory system. There are two main strains of the virus: Type A and Type B, of which Type A tends to be most severe. Influenza viruses are among the most primitive 'life' forms on the planet, and the replication of their genetic material (single-stranded RNA) lacks the proof-reading enzymes needed to correct errors in gene copying. As a result, newly-copied viral genes frequently contain genetic mutations. In fact, populations of influenza virus contain so many closely related mutants, that scientists refer to them as a 'quasispecies' rather than a true biological species which, by definition, must share a more or less distinctive form. This biodiversity allows influenza viruses to rapidly adapt to changing host environments, so that new, more virulent subtypes quickly arise, especially when the body's nutritional status is poor and selenium deficiency is present (see below).

The immune system makes antibodies directed at two proteins (antigens) on the surface of the virus: haemagglutinin (H) and neuraminidase (N). Mutations that change the shape of these two proteins frequently occur, so that antibodies made against previous types are less likely to lock on and neutralize a new infection. The world therefore experiences new strains of influenza virus relatively frequently. The World Health Organization monitors global patterns of influenza infection and decides, year on year, which strains are needed in the vaccine programme to provide optimum protection for the forthcoming winter.

Flu is highly contagious and spreads rapidly through airborne droplets produced by coughing and sneezing. The virus can also survive on hands, door knobs, telephones and used tissues for up to 24 hours. Touching contaminated surfaces and then touching your eyes, nose or mouth can also transmit the infection. The incubation period is short (one to three days) and it strikes quickly. Symptoms start off similar to those of a cold with cough, sore throat and runny nose, which quickly become significantly worse. Chills, fever, headache, loss of appetite, fatigue and muscle aches and pains set in,

---

often lasting for seven to ten days. All you will want to do is lie in bed without wanting to eat or move. If you can get up and potter throughout the illness, then it is unlikely that you have flu. The following may help you decide which it is:

Symptom	Common Cold	Influenza
Headache	Rare	Pronounced
Blocked nose	Usual	Sometimes
Sneezing	Usual	Sometimes
Sore throat	Common	Sometimes
Cough	Mild to moderate	Mild to severe
General aches & pains	Slight	Severe
Extreme exhaustion	Never	Pronounced
Weakness	Mild	Severe and can last 2–3 weeks
Fever	Usually absent or low grade (e.g. 37.5°C)	Usually 39°C or higher for 3–4 days

For most healthy people, flu is a nasty experience but is not life-threatening. Sometimes, however, complications – including pneumonia, inflammation of the heart (myocarditis) and febrile fits – can occur. Some people are more at risk of complications than others and are advised to have annual influenza vaccination.

Prevention
Good hygiene is vital. Wash your hands regularly with soap and water, and dry with a clean towel. If you don't have access to soap and water use an alcohol-based hand cleaner. Wipe down surfaces with an antibacterial spray/wipes, especially door handles, light switches and telephones. Use a tissue when coughing and sneezing (not your hand) and bin the tissue immediately before washing your hands again. Try to avoid touching your nose, mouth and eyes.

Do not take supplements if you are pregnant, breast-feeding, or taking prescribed drugs without first seeking advice from a pharmacist about possible interactions or adverse effects.

Always carry tissues with you so you have them to hand – anti-viral tissues are now available.

Consider taking a *selenium* supplement. Selenium is an antioxidant that reduces the formation of free radicals that damage the genetic material of primitive influenza viruses. As well as changing the H and N proteins so pre-existing antibodies no longer recognize them, selenium deficiency promotes more rapid uncoating of the viral RNA from its associated nucleoproteins – the faster the genes are uncoated, the quicker the virus can start replicating, and the rate of viral production increases. Lack of selenium is now recognized as a 'driving force' for viral mutations. Symptoms of influenza are also more severe in selenium deficient hosts and lung damage persists for longer.

Siberian ginseng may, according to Russian research, reduce the incidence of colds, flu and other respiratory infections by 40 per cent in those taking it regularly.

Treatment

Rest in bed and stay warm, but ensure your room is well ventilated. Don't let anyone smoke near you. Those who live alone should arrange for someone to check on them regularly and do any essential shopping. Painkillers such as ibuprofen or paracetamol help to relieve the aching and also keep a fever down. Drink plenty of warm fluids and eat simple, soothing foods such as soup, yoghurt or scrambled eggs on bread. Sucking ice cubes is cooling and will also relieve a sore throat. Steam inhalations with added essential oils, such as Olbas Oil or Karvol, can ease congestion.

Supplements to consider include high-dose *vitamin C* plus other antioxidants such as *vitamin E* and *selenium* (which together increase antibody production), *grapeseed* or *pine bark* extracts. Sucking lozenges containing *zinc* gluconate may shorten the duration of a sore throat.

Pelargonium sidoides, *Elderberry*, *Echinacea* and *olive leaf* extracts contain anti-viral or immune-boosting compounds that can reduce the severity and duration of influenza infections.

Do not take supplements if you are pregnant, breast-feeding, or taking prescribed drugs without first seeking advice from a pharmacist about possible interactions or adverse effects.

Note: If you develop chest pain or difficulty in breathing, seek urgent medical advice. If flu symptoms develop in the elderly, or in someone with diabetes, lung, kidney, heart or other serious problems, a doctor should be contacted straight away. In some cases, an anti-viral drug may be needed to reduce the risk of complications. These ideally need to be taken within 24 hours of the onset of symptoms.

See also: **Brewer's yeast, Echinacea, Elderberry, Goldenseal, Lapacho, Olive leaf, Pelargonium sidoides, Probiotics, Reishi, Shiitake, Siberian ginseng**.

Related entry: **Immunity**.

Insect bites and stings

Biting insects are attracted to our individual body scents with some scents proving more attractive than others. The injected venom of biting and stinging insects can contain a cocktail of over 100 chemicals which trigger rapid inflammation and pain.

Prevention
- Cover up as much exposed skin as possible, especially from dusk onwards when biting insects become more active.

- Spray a repellent inside the openings of clothes for extra protection or wear impregnated wrist and ankle bands.

- If walking in long grass, always tuck trouser legs into socks and boots.

- Sunscreens containing insect repellent are worth trying for a useful double action.

- Fit muslin screens inside windows so that they can still be opened during the day without letting in flying insects.

Do not take supplements if you are pregnant, breast-feeding, or taking prescribed drugs without first seeking advice from a pharmacist about possible interactions or adverse effects.

- Scent the home with essential oils that repel insects such as lavender, peppermint and eucalyptus.

- Natural insect repellents include garlic powder tablets taken every day, and applying diluted citronella, lemon, eucalyptus or tea tree essential oils to the skin. These strong aromas make it less easy for mosquitoes and midges to find a host.

- There are claims that taking high-dose vitamin B1 (thiamin) supplements can repel biting insects, but it takes several weeks to work and is probably not that effective.

Note: If travelling to areas where malaria or other insect-borne diseases are endemic, seek medical advice about appropriate prevention and treatments.

Treatment
If a bee leaves its sting and poison sac lodged in your skin, remove it gently by scraping with a fingernail or a sterile needle – don't grasp with fingers or tweezers or you may force more poison into the wound. Wash the affected area with soap and water and, as bee stings are acid, apply a little baking soda mixed with water. Wasp stings and gnat bites are alkaline, so apply a little wine vinegar or lemon juice to relieve pain.

Treatments to reduce itching and swelling include:

- A drop of neat lavender oil applied directly to a bite or sting, and repeated every five minutes up to a maximum of ten drops
- An ice pack (e.g. bag of frozen peas) wrapped in a clean cloth and applied for two to five minutes at a time
- Arnica cream
- Antihistamine creams (consider tablets if seriously affected)
- Local anaesthetic cream or an anti-inflammatory cream (e.g. 1 per cent hydrocortisone)

Do not take supplements if you are pregnant, breast-feeding, or taking prescribed drugs without first seeking advice from a pharmacist about possible interactions or adverse effects.

- A drop of chamomile oil applied three times a day for two days
- Aloe vera gel.

Oral supplements to reduce symptoms include *bromelain, vitamin C* and bioflavonoids such as quercetin for their anti-inflammatory actions.

Note: If someone develops symptoms such as faintness, collapse, swelling or difficulty in breathing after being stung, urgent medical help must be sought immediately by dialling 999. If they have been stung in the mouth or throat, give them ice cubes to suck while waiting for help to arrive. Anyone who has a severe allergy to bites or stings may need to carry a pre-filled syringe of adrenaline with them at all times to be injected immediately if an allergic reaction occurs.

Insomnia

Insomnia is a sleep disturbance in which there is a perception of difficulty falling asleep, or in maintaining an adequate amount of sleep. You may wake up earlier than you would like, and the sleep you do achieve is not refreshing. Surveys suggest as many as one in three people is affected, around half of whom also experience mild anxiety as a result.

Most people need less sleep as they get older. People aged 60 and over tend to sleep 1.5 hours less per 24 hour period than younger adults aged 30 and below. Sleep architecture also changes, so that by the age of 70, most people get no stage 4 (really deep) sleep at all and spend more time in the shallower stages of sleep. It is therefore common for older people to wake several times during the night, although they may not recall this the following morning. Because expectations dictate that we need a certain amount of sleep, some people may think they have insomnia when, in fact, they are getting all the sleep they need. Those who feel fit and refreshed during the day are probably getting all the sleep they

---

Do not take supplements if you are pregnant, breast-feeding, or taking prescribed drugs without first seeking advice from a pharmacist about possible interactions or adverse effects.

need and should make use of the new-found hours by developing a hobby that can be indulged at any hour, such as painting, writing memoirs or online Scrabble (www.isc.ro; my handle is DrSarah if you want to challenge me).

Having said that, many elderly people do suffer from insomnia and the tell-tale signs include difficulty getting off to sleep, waking unusually early in the morning and not being able to get back to sleep at all, feeling tired and listless during the day, yawning a lot, and feeling unusually irritable or snappy. Insomnia can also occur as part of a depressive illness.

Lack of sleep has a significant effect on your quality of life. When you suffer from sleep disturbance, you wake up feeling tired and irritable, and may not feel that you are performing at your best.

Treatment
Avoid napping during the day and overindulgence in substances that interfere with sleep such as caffeine (coffee, tea, chocolate, colas), nicotine, alcohol and rich or heavy food – especially close to bedtime.

The simplest sedative is to sprinkle a few drops of lavender essential oil on a cotton wool pad near your pillow or to invest in a lavender-scented pillow.

Herbal preparations containing valerian, hops and lemon balm are helpful in promoting sleep, especially if it is an overactive mind that is causing the problem. *Valerian* root extracts are widely used to relieve anxiety, reduce muscle tension and promote sleep, taken half an hour before going to bed. If anxiety is at the root of a sleep problem *Rhodiola* may be helpful.

5-HTP, usually combined with magnesium and B vitamins, is also beneficial, and works by providing building blocks for making melatonin – our natural sleep hormone – in the brain.

Regular exercise during the day is important, but avoid vigorous exercise in the evening which will have an alerting effect.

See also: **Folic acid, Hawthorn, 5-HTP, Lemon balm, Reishi,**

Rhodiola, St John's Wort, Siberian ginseng, Valerian, Vitamin B1.

Intermittent claudication

Intermittent claudication is a pain in the calves that comes on during exercise. It is due to hardening and furring up of peripheral blood vessels which reduces blood flow to the lower limbs. As a result, muscles in the lower legs do not get all the blood and oxygen they need during exercise, which triggers muscle pain in the calves on walking.

Treatment
Ginkgo biloba supplements can help intermittent claudication as they open up small blood vessels to improve peripheral circulation. An interesting Tibetan preparation, Padma 28, contains a complex mix of 20 Tibetan medicinal herbs but surprisingly contains no ginkgo biloba.

Folic acid supplements lower homocysteine levels and may reduce the progression of atherosclerosis. A study of over 15,000 middle-aged men found that levels of homocysteine were significantly higher in those with intermittent claudication than in those without, and high homocysteine levels mainly occurred in those with low folic acid levels.

Garlic tablets can decrease blood stickiness, increase arterial elasticity and improve circulation.

See also: **Carnitine, Co-enzyme Q10, Folic acid, Garlic, Ginkgo biloba, Grapeseed, Pine bark**.

Irritable bowel syndrome

Irritable bowel syndrome is the most common condition to affect the gut. At least a third of the population are affected at some time

---

during their life, even if only mildly. Overall, 15 per cent of people are affected badly enough to consult their doctor.

According to the Rome III Criteria (2006) for diagnosing irritable bowel syndrome, there must be:

At least three months, with onset at least six months previously, of recurrent abdominal pain or discomfort, associated with two or more of the following:

• Improvement with defecation; and/or
• Onset is associated with a change in frequency of stool; and/or
• Onset is associated with a change in form (appearance) of stool.

IBS is not a condition that should be self-diagnosed, however, as similar symptoms can occur in other more serious bowel problems needing medical or surgical treatment.

Treatment
Once diagnosed with IBS, it is important to take *probiotic* supplements containing friendly digestive bacteria which replenish the bowel with healthy bacteria. This often improves symptoms dramatically by reducing abnormal fermentation in the large bowel.

Peppermint oil is one of the most effective treatments for IBS, and is even more effective than fibre supplements.

Globe artichoke supplements also improve IBS symptoms, with over two-thirds of people noticing a benefit within ten days.

Many people find *aloe vera* juice helpful, while *psyllium* fibre can improve both diarrhoea and constipation.

See also: **Aloe vera, Artichoke, Brewer's yeast, Fibre, Peppermint, Probiotics, Turmeric.**

Do not take supplements if you are pregnant, breast-feeding, or taking prescribed drugs without first seeking advice from a pharmacist about possible interactions or adverse effects.

Jet lag

Jet lag is a disturbance of the body's 24-hour sleep-wake biorhythms due to flying across several time zones, especially in an eastward direction which shortens the traveller's day.

Jet lag is most likely to affect people over 30 who normally follow an established daily routine, causing symptoms of general disorientation, fatigue, poor memory, insomnia, headaches, irritability, poor concentration, decreased mental ability and reduced immunity.

Prevention/treatment

If flying east it can help to try going to bed earlier than usual for several nights before travelling. Conversely, if flying west, staying up later than usual for several nights before leaving can help.

On the flight it is advisable to drink plenty of fluids, avoid alcohol, only eat light meals and sleep as much as possible.

Take high-dose antioxidants (*vitamin C*, 1–3 g a day; *vitamin E* 400 IU/268 mg a day) before, during and after travelling. Also, take high-strength *vitamin B* complex (50–100 mg) twice a day during the flight and for the first two days after arrival.

Guarana is widely used to reduce the effects of jet lag when it is taken before, during and after a long-haul flight.

On arrival, herbal sleep preparations containing natural extracts of *valerian*, *lemon balm* and *hops* will help. Alternatively, lavender essential oil promotes relaxation, and rosemary or lemon will stimulate and keep you awake.

See also: **Guarana, 5-HTP, Siberian ginseng**.
Related entry: **Deep vein thrombosis**.

Joint pains

Painful, inflamed joints due to sports injury or arthritis can be helped by a number of supplements.

Do not take supplements if you are pregnant, breast-feeding, or taking prescribed drugs without first seeking advice from a pharmacist about possible interactions or adverse effects.

Glucosamine sulphate improves the quality and quantity of synovial fluid – the joint's oil – for a better internal cushioning effect. It can be taken together with *chondroitin* or *vitamin C*.

Omega-3 fish oils are also important

Raw extracts of New Zealand *green-lipped mussels* contain glycoproteins that damp down inflammation in arthritic joints.

Other beneficial supplements include *MSM-sulphur*, *devil's claw*, *bromelain, ginger, rose-hip* or *boswellia*. Choose a cod liver oil product described as high strength or extra high strength for the most effective anti-inflammatory action.

See also: **Cat's claw, Chondroitin, CMO, Essential Fatty Acids, Evening primrose oil, Ginger, Glucosamine, 5-HTP, Krill oil, MSM, Nettle, Vitamin A, Vitamin B5, Vitamin C, Vitamin B**.

Related entry: **Gout, Rheumatoid arthritis, Osteoarthritis**.

Keratosis pilaris

Keratosis pilaris is a roughness of the skin, which feels like sandpaper, commonly on the upper arms and legs. It is associated with atopic eczema.

Treatment

Apply plenty of moisturizing emollients to soothe and rehydrate the skin. This works best when you apply a generous amount on affected areas at night, then cover with a bandage to improve penetration. Cleanse the skin with aqueous cream rather than soap, and wear cotton rather than woollen or nylon clothes. Try not to get too hot, and avoid scratching at all costs.

Essential fatty acids found in *omega-3 fish oils* help to reduce inflammation and can significantly improve scaling and itching. As lack of *vitamin A* can also cause scaly skin with raised, pimply hair follicles, cod liver oil is the best source of omega-3s in this case as it is also an excellent source of *vitamin A* and *vitamin D*. *Evening primrose oil* may reduce itching. Avoid cows' milk products for a

---

Do not take supplements if you are pregnant, breast-feeding, or taking prescribed drugs without first seeking advice from a pharmacist about possible interactions or adverse effects.

trial period of ten days to see if this improves symptoms. If you decide to continue avoiding dairy products for longer, seek advice from a nutritionist to avoid long-term nutrient imbalances, especially of *calcium*. Patch testing will help to identify any common allergens that may be causing a reaction.

Kidney stones

Kidney stones are due to the precipitation of insoluble salts in the urinary tract to form solid crystals or larger clumps. Nine out of ten kidney stones contain calcium, usually combined with oxalate. Vegetarians have a lower risk of kidney stones and eating meat seems to increase the risk although this can be offset by eating more fruit and vegetables.

Paradoxically, a study of over 90,000 nurses showed that women with a good dietary calcium intake of above 1100 mg from food sources had half the risk of developing kidney stones as those with intakes of less than 500 mg per day. This is because calcium-rich foods bind oxalates in the gut so that less is absorbed. Similar results were found in a study involving more than 45,000 males – those with the highest dietary intakes of calcium were a third less likely to develop kidney stones than those with lower calcium intakes. Calcium supplements are best avoided, however, except under medical supervision, as some evidence suggests they may increase the risk of kidney stones in some people.

Avoid eating oxalate-rich foods such as beans, beets, celery, blueberries, chocolate, grapes, spinach, rhubarb, parsley, beetroot, nuts and strawberries. Avoid fizzy drinks, including diet varieties, as these contain high amounts of phosphorus. Follow a low-sodium diet and maintain a good fluid intake at all times – dehydration is a major cause of urinary stone precipitation, so ensure you drink enough to produce pale coloured urine (NB: except when taking supplements containing vitamin B2, riboflavin, which will darken urine). Various studies have shown that drinking water, milk, coffee, tea, beer, wine or orange juice is associated with a reduced risk of kidney stone formation, while drinking apple and grapefruit juice significantly increases the risks for reasons that remain unclear.

Magnesium supplements can reduce stone formation, especially when taken with *vitamin B6*.

See also: **Bilberry, Calcium, Pumpkin seed, Vitamin A, Vitamin B6, Vitamin C**.

Leg ulcers

Leg ulcers are open sores on the skin that can be difficult to heal. They are a painful and unpleasant condition that greatly reduce mobility and quality of life. The usual cause is a result of poor blood supply to the area (e.g. a blocked artery) or poor drainage from it (e.g. venous statis, commonly due to varicose veins). Poor circulation results in poor healing, and an ulcer may be triggered by a mild injury or even just a scratch. Around 10 per cent of leg ulcers are arterial ulcers (due to poor arterial circulation) in which feet are cold and may have a white-blue and shiny appearance. Around 70 per cent are venous ulcers and the leg is usually swollen, congested, weeping, with dry, itchy, brown discoloration of overlying skin (varicose eczema).

Treatment
Conventional treatment includes advice to lose weight, stop smoking, and to exercise as much as possible. For venous ulcers, it helps to keep your legs elevated above the waist when sitting down to reduce fluid accumulation. The opposite is true for arterial ulcers.

The ulcer is dressed with a variety of specialized powders, granules, pastes and coverings depending on whether it is infected, wet or dry. Most dressings work by helping to separate fluid and bacteria from the ulcer surface to encourage formation of granulation (healing) tissue. Although many leg ulcers eventually heal using this approach, as many as 70 per cent recur within a year. Surgery

---

Do not take supplements if you are pregnant, breast-feeding, or taking prescribed drugs without first seeking advice from a pharmacist about possible interactions or adverse effects.

may be needed to improve blood flow in the leg. Good control of blood glucose levels is vital in those who also have diabetes.

Garlic, ginkgo biloba or a blend of over 20 Tibetan herbs (known as Padma 28) can improve circulation through tiny blood vessels in the base of the ulcer. Ginkgo should not be combined with prescription drugs or regular blood-thinning agents such as aspirin, however. Eat more oily fish, such as salmon, sardines, mackerel and herrings, take *omega-3* fish oil supplements and follow a low-fat, low-sugar diet.

Folic acid lowers homocysteine levels and may benefit those with arterial ulcers by discouraging progression of atherosclerosis.

Low *magnesium* levels are associated with an increased risk of developing diabetic foot ulcers. No trials appear to have investigated whether or not magnesium supplements can produce clinical improvement of foot ulcers, however.

Some research suggests that leg ulcers are associated with low *zinc* levels – especially if senses of taste or smell are reduced (another possible sign of zinc deficiency) – so zinc supplements may be helpful. In addition, antioxidant supplements such as *vitamin C* and *vitamin E* will help to reduce inflammation and promote healing.

Leg swelling associated with venous ulcers may improve when taking *pine bark* extracts (Pycnogenol®) or *red vine leaf* extracts which have a beneficial effect on leg capillaries to reduce leakage of fluid into the tissues.

Aloe vera gel may be used externally to improve healing of chronic ulcers; however topical treatments should only be used with the guidance of the doctor or nurse in charge of dressing the ulcer.

See also: **Horsechestnut, Pine bark**.

Leukoplakia

Leukoplakia causes areas of white, boggy skin in the mouth that resemble patches of grey-white paint. They are usually painless. As this condition is considered premalignant (can develop into a cancer) it is usually kept under close medical supervision or even removed surgically.

Treatment

Some studies have shown that *betacarotene*, an antioxidant carotenoid, can reverse oral leukoplakia lesions, although other studies have not been conclusive (and it is best to usually only take mixed *carotenoids*, especially if you are a smoker). Antioxidants in general appear to be beneficial and, in one study, *vitamin E* supplements (800 IU/536 mg a day) taken for 24 weeks caused regression of oral leukoplakia (pre-cancerous lesions) in 67 per cent of patients. In another study, a combination of 30 mg of *betacarotene*, 1 g *vitamin C* and 800 IU/536 mg of *vitamin E* taken daily for nine months helped 55 per cent of patients who experienced either complete or partial clinical resolution of lesions.

When *olive leaf* extracts (1 g, three times a day) were taken by 67 people with dental problems including leukoplakia, 60 experienced full recovery. *Spirulina* blue-green algae are also worth trying – in a study in which 44 people with leukoplakia took 1 g a day for one year, over half the lesions either vanished or significantly reduced in size while those receiving a blue-green placebo experienced no change in their lesions. Antioxidants, olive leaf and spirulina may be taken together.

See also: **Blue-green algae**.

Libido – low

Sex drive is usually the second strongest urge in humans, after sleep. Sex drive varies considerably from person to person, however, and also from time to time. Some people are driven by a powerful libido that fuels sexual activity at least once a day. For others, sex drive is satisfied by intimacy occurring less than once a month.

Loss of sex drive can occur for a number of reasons, with hormone imbalances, stress, overwork, tiredness and lack of sleep among the most common. Other causes include alcohol, drug side effects, pregnancy, menopause and depression.

Around 5 per cent of people whose sex drive fails have a raised prolactin level. Prolactin is a hormone produced by the pituitary gland in the brain. It has a powerful negative effect on libido, and switches off the sex drive as well as reducing fertility. Raised blood levels of prolactin usually indicate a benign tumour of the pituitary gland (prolactinoma) which is treated with a drug such as bromocriptine, or surgery to remove the tumour.

Treatment

A number of supplements are claimed to increase libido.

Catuaba promotes erotic dreams in both men and women, followed by increased sexual desire within five to 21 days of regular treatment. It may also improve peripheral blood flow to improve erections.

Damiana produces localized tingling and throbbing sensations in the genitals, by increasing blood flow and nerve sensitivity.

Muira puama stimulates desire through a direct action on brain chemicals.

Ginkgo biloba increases blood flow to the peripheries, to improve erectile function.

Ginseng has been associated with sexual function for centuries and veterinary studies have found that it boosts sexual activity and sperm production in rabbits, bulls and rats, stimulates ovulation in hens and prepares female rats for mating. Preliminary studies suggest it contains an enzyme known as panquilon, which increases levels of nitric oxide (NO) in the spongy tissue of the penis and clitoris. NO is a nerve chemical essential for increasing blood flow to the penis during sexual arousal. One study found that men who took Korean ginseng for two months achieved a three times greater frequency of sexual intercourse and morning erections, and significantly firmer erections than those receiving placebo.

Siberian ginseng has similar actions and is also noted for its aphrodisiac properties. Veterinary research suggests it increases

---

Do not take supplements if you are pregnant, breast-feeding, or taking prescribed drugs without first seeking advice from a pharmacist about possible interactions or adverse effects.

milk secretion in cows, honey production by bees, and semen production in bulls.

St John's Wort can significantly boost sex drive in those who are also depressed and is especially helpful for post-menopausal women with low sex drive, low mood and physical exhaustion.

Tribulus terrestris can improve male sex drive, especially that associated with lethargy and fatigue.

Oyster extracts owe their aphrodisiac reputation to their high zinc content, which is important for maintaining testosterone levels and for both male and female fertility.

Note: If profound low sex drive continues for longer than three months, seek medical advice as you may need your prolactin hormone levels investigated.

See also: **Agnus castus, Arginine, Ashwagandha, Black cohosh, Damiana, Fo-ti, Ginseng, Maca, Muira puama, Nettle, Pfaffia, St John's Wort, Sarsaparilla, Tribulis terrestris**.

Lichen planus

Lichen planus is an inflammatory skin disease associated with intensely itchy, raised, purple lesions – usually on the inside of the wrists and lower legs, although they can occur anywhere. Papules often have a fine, white, lacy pattern on the surface and, in 50 per cent of cases, painful lacy white streaks or ulcers form on mucous membranes such as the mouth or genitals. The exact cause is unknown, but it is thought to be related to an abnormality of a type of immune cell known as T-lymphocytes. A similar rash can occur as a side effect of certain drugs (e.g. gold, penicillamine, antimalarial therapy). The prognosis is good as symptoms usually clear within two years, although recurrences can appear. Mucosal lesions need regular inspection as they may be pre-malignant.

Do not take supplements if you are pregnant, breast-feeding, or taking prescribed drugs without first seeking advice from a pharmacist about possible interactions or adverse effects.

Treatment

Aloe vera is often helpful when applied to skin or vaginal lesions.

Omega-3 fish oils have a useful anti-inflammatory action. A medical herbalist might suggest herbs that support immune function such as *Echinacea* or *cat's claw*.

Lichen sclerosus et atrophicus

Lichen sclerosus et atrophicus (LSA) is an inflammatory skin condition that affects the anal and genital regions. It is thought to affect around one in 300 people, and is most common in females. Affected skin usually becomes thinned, crinkly and ivory coloured (like cigarette paper), and when active may have a purple-red border. Itching, soreness and pain are often present. Medical diagnosis is important to rule out other skin conditions with a similar appearance, and long-term lesions need regular review.

Treatment

Unfortunately, there is no cure, although symptoms often improve with time. Some researchers have had good results from treating LSA with *evening primrose oil* (applied locally and taken orally). *Aloe vera* is also worth trying.

Liver problems

For liver problems, it is always advisable to seek medical or herbal advice about appropriate supplementation. Those most likely to be recommended include antioxidants (e.g. *vitamin C, vitamin E, carotenoids, selenium, grapeseed* or *pine bark* extracts), *milk thistle, globe artichoke, dandelion root* and *liquorice*.

Do not take supplements if you are pregnant, breast-feeding, or taking prescribed drugs without first seeking advice from a pharmacist about possible interactions or adverse effects.

Lupus

Lupus is an inflammatory disorder that affects many systems in the body. The most common form, systemic lupus erythematosus (SLE), is nine times more common in women than men. Lupus is an auto-immune condition in which the immune system attacks certain parts of the body. This causes inflammation and damage that can affect many different areas, including the joints, skin, kidneys, heart, lungs, blood vessels and brain. Symptoms usually first appear between the ages of 15 and 45 years, but it can occur at any age.

People with lupus can have many different symptoms, but the most common include extreme fatigue, painful or swollen joints, unexplained fever and skin rashes. A characteristic rash may appear across the nose and cheeks, resembling a butterfly in shape. Rashes can also appear on the ears, arms, shoulders, chest and the palms of the hands. These visible changes reflect the widespread inflammation of blood vessels (vasculitis) occurring throughout the body.

Other symptoms of lupus include chest pain, hair loss, mouth ulcers, rash after exposure to sunlight, headaches, dizziness and kidney problems. Raynaud's phenomenon, in which the digits turn white, blue then red on exposure to cold is also common. Symptoms of SLE vary from mild to serious.

A form of lupus, chronic discoid lupus, can occur in which only the skin is affected. This produces a red, raised rash on the face, scalp, or elsewhere, which may last from days to years. A small number of people with discoid lupus also develop SLE.

Lupus occurs when the immune system makes antibodies targeted against parts of the body rather than against foreign proteins. These antibodies, known as auto-antibodies attack certain body tissues to produce inflammation and damage. Some auto-antibodies join with substances from the body's own cells to form particles known as immune complexes. These immune complexes can also build up in tissues such as the joints and kidneys, to cause inflammation and fatigue. As well as inflammation, researchers now realize that

---

Do not take supplements if you are pregnant, breast-feeding, or taking prescribed drugs without first seeking advice from a pharmacist about possible interactions or adverse effects.

increased blood stickiness can also occur, leading to abnormal blood clotting.

It is thought that several factors, including a variety of genes, hormones and environmental agents such as exposure to sunlight, stress, certain drugs or viruses may interact to increase a person's susceptibility to the condition. Some research suggests that auto-antibodies may be triggered by a viral infection that causes excess death of lymph cells. As these lymph cells break up, other immune cells mistake their disintegrating membranes for foreign bodies and start to attack them. Even though lupus may be triggered by the body over-reacting to a viral illness, lupus itself is not infectious, and you cannot 'catch' it from someone who has the condition.

A rare form of lupus can be caused in certain people by taking certain drugs (e.g. hydralazine to treat high blood pressure; procainamide to treat irregular heart rhythms). This produces symptoms similar to SLE (arthritis, rash, fever, and chest pain) but typically goes away when the drug is stopped.

A condition known as Hughes Syndrome, or Antiphospholipid Syndrome, affects one in five people with lupus. Excessive 'sticki-ness' of blood leads to headache, fits, memory loss, increased risk of miscarriage, multiple sclerosis and giddiness. Treatment is with blood thinning agents such as aspirin or warfarin.

Treatment

It is advisable to avoid taking the oral contraceptive pill and HRT, which can trigger flare-ups, and to reduce intake of red meat. Aim to eat a mainly vegetarian diet and avoid caffeine, alcohol, sugar and tobacco.

Milk thistle may be recommended to help support liver function. *Flaxseed, evening primrose, omega-3 fish* or *hempseed oils* containing essential fatty acids with anti-inflammatory actions are worth trying. *Vitamin C* is important as an antioxidant, to damp down inflammation and promote tissue repair. *B group vitamins, vitamin E, carotenoids* and *selenium* also help to maintain healthy tissues. For those unable to tolerate aspirin, *pine bark* extracts

(Pycnogenol®) are a useful alternative that does not irritate the stomach.

See also: **Echinacea**.

Macular degeneration

Age-related macular degeneration (AMD) is a painless, progressive disorder that is one of the commonest causes of registered blindness in older people. AMD is a deterioration of part of the retina – the macula – which breaks down to produce a widening circle of blindness. It usually affects both eyes and – because the defect is in the centre of the visual field – can obliterate two or three words when reading at a normal distance, or blank out someone's face when you look straight at them. The cause of AMD is unknown, but those who smoke, have high blood pressure, elevated cholesterol levels and poor diet lacking in antioxidants are at greatest risk.

AMD is described as 'wet' when newly formed, fragile blood vessels start to leak fluid into surrounding tissues, or 'dry' where new blood vessel formation has not occurred. Wet AMD can be treated with laser therapy to seal the leaking blood vessels. A new technique using a light activated dye is also available. People taking a statin drug to lower cholesterol levels, or who take regular aspirin, are less likely to develop wet AMD. Although both statins and aspirin are available to buy over the counter in pharmacies, it is important to talk to a doctor or pharmacist before starting to take them on a regular basis (if taking a statin, take *co-enzyme Q10* to reduce muscle-related side effects). If either drug is clinically indicated, your doctor will prescribe them for you.

Treatment

For dry AMD, the mainstay of treatment is dietary advice to improve intakes of *carotenoids* found in yellow-orange fruit and vegetables such as sweetcorn and carrots, as well as in dark-green

---

Do not take supplements if you are pregnant, breast-feeding, or taking prescribed drugs without first seeking advice from a pharmacist about possible interactions or adverse effects.

leafy vegetables, especially spinach, and egg yolk. The macula of the eye contains two protective yellow pigments, *lutein* and *zeaxanthin* (which can be made from lutein). People with macular degeneration have, on average, 70 per cent less lutein in their eyes than those with healthy vision and poor dietary intake is thought to cause breakdown of this vital part of the retina. Those who eat the most lutein-rich foods have at least a 60 per cent lower risk of developing AMD than those with low intakes, partly due to its antioxidant action, which neutralizes harmful chemical reactions involved in light detection, and partly because its yellow colour filters out potentially harmful, visible blue light. Lutein and other carotenoids are therefore sometimes referred to as 'Nature's Sunglasses'.

Until recently it was thought that damage which has already occurred through poor dietary intake of lutein could not be repaired. Latest research published in *Optometry* – the Journal of the American Optometric Association – shows that *lutein* supplements (10 mg daily – five times the average daily intake) can improve vision in people with 'dry' AMD.

Lycopene, a red carotenoid pigment found in tomatoes is also beneficial – those with the lowest intakes have more than double the risk of developing macular degeneration. Bilberry extracts contain antioxidant blue-red pigments with a similar action and can also increase blood flow to the retina.

Zinc supplements have been found to reduce visual loss in people with AMD compared with a placebo, while extracts of ginkgo biloba have been shown to produce a significant improvement in long-distance visual acuity AMD sufferers.

The fish oil, DHA, plays an important structural role in the retina. People who eat oily fish regularly, or who take *omega-3* fish oil supplements are less likely to develop late AMD than those with low fish intake.

Research suggests that, compared with placebo, people taking a supplement containing *vitamin C, vitamin E, carotenoids, zinc* and *omega-3* fish oils are less likely to see their AMD progress.

Powerful antioxidants such as *grapeseed, bilberry* and *pine bark* extracts (Pycnogenol®) are also beneficial.

See also: **Carotenoids, Fish oils, Lutein, Lycopene.**

Memory – poor

The basic biological function underpinning intelligence is that of memory, without which every new experience and item of information would have to be processed as if it were totally unique. Memory is the ability to store, retain and subsequently retrieve information. It allows you to reason by analogy – learning how to solve new problems by thinking about similar situations in which you achieved a desired outcome. Memory is poorly understood but many different areas of the brain, such as the hippocampus, amygdala and mammillary bodies are thought to be involved. Each is related to a different type of memory, such as working (short-term) memory, long-term memory, spatial memory and emotional memory.

With increasing age, it is natural for some memories to become harder to retrieve. If the mind deteriorates too quickly, however, due to excessive loss of neurons, or the connections between them, dementia can develop. The most common type of dementia is Alzheimer's disease, which affects parts of the brain involved in thought, memory and language. It starts with mild forgetfulness and becomes noticeably worse with time, until disorientation and confusion start to cause concern.

Prevention
Following a healthy diet and lifestyle is just as important to reduce hardening and furring up of the arteries supplying blood, oxygen and nutrients to your brain as it is to your heart. As well as following the heart-healthy tips on page 369, the following will help to 'exercise' your memory. Keeping mentally active is important to maintain the connections between brain cells. Those that are not used sufficiently often are automatically pruned away.

Do not take supplements if you are pregnant, breast-feeding, or taking prescribed drugs without first seeking advice from a pharmacist about possible interactions or adverse effects.

Symptoms you should never ignore

Worsening memory loss
Difficulty performing familiar tasks
Problems with language and thinking straight
Changes in mood and behaviour
Changes in personality
Disorientation in time and place
Increasingly poor judgement
Loss of initiative

If memory loss in someone you care for is accompanied by
confusion, poor concentation or a change in behaviour or
personality, it is important to seek medical advice.

- Read demanding books, tackle crosswords, Sudoku, jigsaws and other picture, word and number puzzles that need concentration.
- Games such as Scrabble or Trivial Pursuit are excellent for testing your memory skills.
- Try to learn at least one new fact, or memorize a poem or lines from a novel every day.
- When you want to remember an important fact, keep repeating it silently to yourself.
- Write yourself a memory-jogging note of things to do on a piece of paper and stick it up where you will easily see it.
- If you keep losing something (e.g. your keys), try to form a mental photograph of where they are every time you put them down.
- Associate a fact to be remembered with a visual image, e.g. when introduced to someone who is an artist, picture him holding an enormous painting brush. If his name is Baker, picture him holding a large loaf of bread. The more outrageous or unusual your images, the easier you will remember them.

Treatment
Eating a cereal breakfast has been found to improve memory in healthy adults, increasing the speed at which new information can be

---

Do not take supplements if you are pregnant, breast-feeding, or taking prescribed drugs without first seeking advice from a pharmacist about possible interactions or adverse effects.

recalled, and improving concentration and mental performance. This is partly because it boosts glucose levels at a crucial time of the day, and partly because fortified breakfast cereals are a good source of *vitamin B1* (thiamin) which improves mood and clarity of thought.

Ginkgo biloba extracts can significantly improve short-term working memory within just two days – probably by improving blood circulation to the brain.

Phosphatidylserine provides nutrients needed to synthesize brain neurotransmitters and can improve all cognitive functions, including learning, recall, recognition and concentration. It seems to work by increasing glucose metabolism within brain cells and speeding transmission of messages from one neurone to another. Ginkgo and phosphatidylserine may be taken together.

Folic acid lowers levels of homocysteine, an amino acid that can hasten narrowing of the arteries to worsen memory loss. Research from the Netherlands suggests that folic acid supplements (800 mg daily) may help to slow the decline in memory and thinking power that often goes with age. Those using the supplements during a three-year period had memory scores as good as those of people five and a half years younger than them, while in tests of thinking speed, they performed as well as people who were almost two years younger.

Isoflavones – Oestrogen is important for brain function, and supplements have been show to help memory in older women.

See also: **Choline, Essential Fatty Acids, Fish oils, Ginkgo, Gotu kola, Guarana, Isoflavones, Kelp, Manganese, Phosphatidylserine, Pine bark, Reishi, Rhodiola, Sage, Vitamin B2, Vitamin B12, Vitamin D**.

Menopause

The menopause is a natural phase in a woman's life when her fertility draws to a close. It usually occurs between the ages of 45 and 55 with an average of 51 years. The menopause is dated from a woman's last period, but the process really starts five to ten years before as the ovaries slowly run out of egg follicles. As a result, levels of oestrogen (oestradiol, oestrone oestriol) and progesterone start to fall until too little is produced to maintain the monthly menstrual cycle.

Some women quickly adapt to lower levels of oestrogen and notice few – if any – problems. Others find it harder to lose their oestrogen and experience unpleasant symptoms that last for between one and five years – occasionally longer.

The short-term symptoms of oestrogen withdrawal vary but commonly include hot flushes, night sweats, headaches, tiredness and mood swings. In time, symptoms such as vaginal dryness, urinary problems, thinning and loss of elasticity of skin occur. In the long term, oestrogen withdrawal also increases the risk of a number of potentially serious problems such as coronary heart disease, stroke and osteoporosis.

Hot flushes are experienced by around 80 per cent of women around the menopause. They can be triggered by a number of factors, including heat, increased humidity, alcohol, caffeine and spicy foods, which are best avoided.

Treatment

Oestrogen-like plant hormones are found in many plants. Although the action of these substances (isoflavones, flavonoids and lignans) is much weaker than human oestrogen, they still provide a useful natural boost when your hormone levels are low. To increase your intake of natural plant hormones, aim to eat more:

Beans: Especially chickpeas, lentils, alfalfa and mung beans, soy beans and soy products.
Vegetables: Dark green leafy vegetables (e.g. broccoli, spinach, cabbage) and exotic members of the cruciferous family (e.g. Chinese leaves, kohl rabi); celery, fennel.
Nuts: Almonds, cashew nuts, hazelnuts, peanuts, walnuts and nut oils.

Do not take supplements if you are pregnant, breast-feeding, or taking prescribed drugs without first seeking advice from a pharmacist about possible interactions or adverse effects.

Seeds: Especially flaxseed, pumpkin, sesame, sunflower and sprouted seeds.

Wholegrains: Especially corn, buckwheat, millet, oats, rye and wheat.

Fresh fruit: Including apples, avocados, bananas, mangoes, papayas and rhubarb.

Dried fruit: Especially dates, figs, prunes and raisins.

Herbs: Especially chervil, chives, garlic, ginger, parsley, rosemary and sage.

Lifestyle tips

- Wear several layers of clothes which you can peel off during a hot flush.
- Keep a fan next to your bed to help keep you cool at night.
- Drink plenty of water to help prevent dehydration.
- If you smoke, do your utmost to stop, as smoking reduces oestrogen levels further and also increases your risk of hypertension, coronary heart disease, stroke and osteoporosis. As smoking lowers oestrogen levels further, on average smokers go through the menopause two years earlier than non-smokers.
- Avoid excess stress, which drains the adrenal glands so they are unable to produce their normal tiny amounts of sex hormones to help even out menopausal symptoms.
- Use a lubricant to overcome vaginal dryness.
- Reduce your salt intake by avoiding obviously salty foods and not adding salt during cooking or at the table – use herbs for flavour instead.
- Try to lose any excess weight.
- Take regular exercise.

To reduce your risk of heart disease, you should also consider:

- Eating more fish – especially oily fish – or take omega-3 fish oil supplements
- Reducing your intake of fat and concentrating on healthy fats such as olive oil, rapeseed oil and fish oils

---

Do not take supplements if you are pregnant, breast-feeding, or taking prescribed drugs without first seeking advice from a pharmacist about possible interactions or adverse effects.

- Drinking an extra pint of semi-skimmed or skimmed milk per day for calcium
- Avoiding excess sugar, alcohol and salt.

Isoflavones can reduce hot flushes and have beneficial effects on the circulation and bones. Increasing evidence suggests they also help to protect against breast cancer.

Black cohosh helps to relieve hot flushes, vaginal dryness, depression and anxiety.

Sage leaf extracts can relieve menopausal hot flushes and night sweats. They are also used traditionally to improve memory.

Siberian ginseng helps the body adapt to physical and emotional stress and is especially helpful for women experiencing menopausal symptoms.

Evening primrose oil is a good source of GLA, an essential fatty acid that provides building block for making sex hormones. It improves dry itchy skin, can reduce breast pain, and increases the amount of calcium laid down in bones.

Calcium and vitamin D supplements help to improve bone mineral density and can reduce the risk of bone fractures.

Rhodiola helps to reduce stress and improves energy levels to help overcome anxiety and fatigue.

St John's Wort helps to lift a low mood that can occur around the time of the menopause. It is also helpful in overcoming low sex drive and physical exhaustion in menopausal women.

5-HTP provides building blocks for making serotonin in the brain which, as well as lifting mood, also improves sleep quality.

Cranberry extracts contain substances known as anti-adhesins, which help to stop bacteria from sticking to cells lining the urinary tract wall. As a result, they are more easily flushed away to reduce the incidence of urinary tract infections after the menopause.

Omega-3 fish oils can reduce the risk of heart attack. Both the American Heart Association and the European Society of Cardiology recommend a daily intake of 1 g omega-3 fish oils to prevent a heart attack.

Do not take supplements if you are pregnant, breast-feeding, or taking prescribed drugs without first seeking advice from a pharmacist about possible interactions or adverse effects.

Folic acid helps to maintain a healthy heart by lowering levels of homocysteine – an amino acid linked with an increased risk of hardening and furring up of the arteries.

NB: Before taking supplements, check with a pharmacist if you are taking other herbal or prescribed medications to rule out any interactions.

See also: **Black cohosh, Dong quai, Fibre, Flaxseed, Isoflavones, Kudzu, Maca, Oatstraw, Pine bark, Pfaffia, Pollen pistil, Sage, St John's Wort, Siberian ginseng, Wild yam**.

Related entries: **Hormone replacement therapy – natural, Osteoporosis**.

Migraine

Migraine is a severe form of headache. Unlike tension headache, which is usually felt equally on both sides of the head, migraine is generally much worse on one side. Symptoms often begin at puberty and cause recurrent attacks until middle age, when they often disappear. Migraine pain often centres around one eye and may be accompanied by abdominal symptoms such as loss of appetite, nausea, vomiting, dislike of food, constipation or diarrhoea. Between 10–30 per cent of people with migraine experience a warning 'aura' up to an hour before an attack which may include visual problems (e.g. shimmering or flashing lights, strange zig-zag shapes or blind spots), numbness or tingling on one side of the face, and sometimes speech difficulties. The exact cause of migraine is not fully understood, but symptoms are believed to be linked to a chemical (serotonin) in the brain that causes blood vessels to widen so nerve tissues become congested.

If you think you may have migraine, try to work out what factors trigger your attacks and, where possible, avoid them. Some sufferers find that symptoms are triggered by certain factors such as tiredness, fatigue, changes in stress levels and extreme emotions. Many foods have been linked with the onset of migraine. In one study, the foods most commonly implicated were: milk (43 per cent), chocolate (29

Do not take supplements if you are pregnant, breast-feeding, or taking prescribed drugs without first seeking advice from a pharmacist about possible interactions or adverse effects.

per cent), German sausages (14 per cent), cheese (14 per cent), fish (10 per cent), wine (9 per cent), coffee (9 per cent), garlic (5 per cent) and eggs (5 per cent). Other foods reported to trigger migraine in some people include: beans, beef, citrus fruits, corn, fried foods, nuts, pork, shellfish, tea, tomatoes, caffeinated fizzy drinks and artificial sweeteners. Some dietary triggers may cause migraine through an ill-defined immune/intolerance mechanism, while others contain vasoactive substances affecting blood flow within the brain such as histamine, tyramine, phenylalanine, monosodium glutamate or nitrites to name but a few. Eating very cold food (ice-cream) can also trigger migraine.

Treatment

Lack of nutrients involved in energy production within cells has been linked with migraine. After three months, almost 60 per cent of those taking *riboflavin* (400 mg vitamin B2) experienced half the normal number of headache days, compared with only 15 per cent of those taking inactive placebo. Taking *magnesium* (600 mg daily) for 12 weeks reduced the frequency of attacks by 42 per cent compared with 16 per cent in the group taking inactive placebo. *Co-enzyme Q10* (300 mg daily) was three times more effective at reducing migraine attack frequency than placebo.

Feverfew contains a substance, parthenolide, that inhibits release of serotonin in the brain to neutralize blood flow changes linked with symptoms. Clinical trials have found that, in 70 per cent of patients taking the herb, it either prevented or lessened the severity of headaches as well as related symptoms of nausea and vomiting.

Butterbur contains a number of substances, such as petasin, which are analgesic and antispasmodic. Research suggests that taking butterbur twice a day for 12 weeks can reduce the frequency of attacks by up to 60 per cent.

Some research suggests that taking magnesium or vitamin B2 (riboflavin) supplements can also reduce the frequency of attacks.

See also: **Butterbur, Feverfew, 5-HTP, Magnesium, Vitamin B2, Yerba maté**.

Do not take supplements if you are pregnant, breast-feeding, or taking prescribed drugs without first seeking advice from a pharmacist about possible interactions or adverse effects.

Miscarriage

Sadly, of all pregnancies that are advanced enough to be recognized by the mother, around one in seven fails to progress beyond the first 20 weeks. Reasons often remain unknown and a specific, recurrent abnormality is only diagnosed in 5 per cent of cases.

Prevention

The chance of successfully becoming a parent after a miscarriage is still high at 60–70 per cent. A couple who have experienced one or more miscarriages are usually advised to follow a preconceptual care programme which includes stopping smoking (if applicable), avoiding alcohol, unnecessary drugs and foods that pose a risk of *Listeria* or toxoplasmosis infection (such as unpasteurized soft cheeses, blue cheeses, pâté).

Taking a multivitamin and mineral supplement especially designed for pregnancy is also helpful. Where no specific cause for miscarriage is found, a future pregnancy may be prepared for in the normal way. Waiting at least three months before trying for pregnancy again is usually advised, in order to allow for both physical and emotional recovery.

See also: **Aloe vera, Black cohosh, Folic acid, Selenium, Vitamin D**.

Related entry: **Conception**.

Molluscum contagiosum

Molluscum contagiosum is a harmless viral infection that forms multiple, shiny, pearly, white lumps that may have a central dimple. As its name suggests, they are contagious with close contact as, when broken, an infectious, cheesy fluid is released. Many people are naturally immune, however. Lesions usually disappear within 18 months, but can be more troublesome in some children, especially those with eczema – possibly because scratching encourages their spread.

Do not take supplements if you are pregnant, breast-feeding, or taking prescribed drugs without first seeking advice from a pharmacist about possible interactions or adverse effects.

Treatment

Treatment involves disrupting the architecture of lesions – e.g. by freezing with liquid nitrogen. If freezing is not suitable, dermatologists suggest applying betadine paint daily, assuming there is no allergy to iodine.

Alternatively dilute tea tree oil may be applied to the lesions twice a day using a cotton bud to gently irritate the lesions. Emollient bath preparations can help to reduce itching. Evening primrose oil drops should be given (by mouth) and an evening primrose oil moisturizing body cream can also be used.

An *Echinacea* product designed for children may help to boost immunity against this annoying viral infection. Some doctors have started prescribing the antacid drug cimetidine to treat the infection following the observation that it disappeared quickly in those prescribed cimetidine for excess acid production.

Morning sickness

Morning sickness affects 70 per cent of pregnant women. It has been linked with a number of triggers, including raised levels of oestrogen, progesterone and hCG hormones, low blood sugar, increased secretion of bile and increased production of an intestinal hormone that causes the gall bladder to contract (cholecystokinin).

Symptoms tend to start before the sixth week of pregnancy and have usually disappeared by the fourteenth week, although a few women suffer for longer. Excessive sickness (hyperemesis) causes dehydration, salt imbalances and a harmful build-up of ketones in the blood. Signs to watch for include weakness, dizziness and passing urine that is dark and scant.

Treatment

It is important to keep sipping water and sugary drinks.

Ginger has excellent anti-emetic properties, so drinking ginger tea and ginger beer (the fizz seems to help), or chewing crystallized

---

Do not take supplements if you are pregnant, breast-feeding, or taking prescribed drugs without first seeking advice from a pharmacist about possible interactions or adverse effects.

ginger or taking ginger tablets can all be helpful.

Some practitioners recommend treatment with *vitamin B6* but this is best used under medical supervision.

Stimulation of the PC6 acupuncture point in the wrist is effective and acupressure bands available from chemists make this easier. If problems continue, regular assessment by a doctor or midwife is important.

See also: **Ginger**.

Motion sickness

Motion or travel sickness can be triggered while travelling by car, sailing at sea or riding on other forms of transport such as a horse, camel or elephant. It can also be a major problem for weightless astronauts in space. Susceptibility to travel sickness is present in everyone, but we all have a different sensitivity. One in three people is highly susceptible to motion sickness, a further third only suffer during fairly rough conditions while another third only react under prolonged, violently rough conditions. Very young children seldom suffer from motion sickness. The worst age seems to be around ten years old.

Motion sickness is caused by excessive and repetitive stimulation of motion-detecting hair cells in the inner ear. This triggers motion sickness when the brain receives conflicting messages from the eyes that do not match the degree of movement detected by the inner ears. This is especially likely to happen when travelling in a closed space such as a car, where you tend to focus on a nearby object. Your eyes tell your brain the environment is stationary, while your balance organs say it is not. If there is good visual evidence of the head's position – as in cycling or skiing for example – motion sickness does not occur.

Treatment
Ensure that children sit high enough in the car so that they can see out of the window (in an appropriate child's car seat if applicable)

and play 'I Spy' games that encourage them to look into the distance. Try to discourage them from focusing on near objects when in a car, such as reading a book. Only supply light meals, allow fresh air to circulate in the car, and stop to stretch legs frequently. A few drops of Bach rescue remedy under the tongue often work wonders if they start feeling unwell. Travel sickness tablets containing the antihistamine cinnarizine can control symptoms for at least eight hours per dose with most children remaining alert or only slightly drowsy.

Ginger can help with the symptoms of motion sickness: try drinking ginger tea or ginger beer, chewing crystallized ginger or taking ginger tablets.

Stimulation of the PC6 acupuncture point in the wrist is effective and elasticated wrist bands or the newer disposable acupressure plasters may be used on children.

See also: **Ginger**.

Mouth ulcers

Mouth ulcers linked with stress may be cold sores due to the *Herpes simplex* virus or aphthous ulcers (canker sores) which have been linked with hypersensitivity to a common mouth bacterium, haemolytic streptococcus. Recurrent mouth ulcers can also occasionally be a sign of coeliac disease (dietary sensitivity to gluten), inflammatory bowel diseases, SLE or other immune problems. It is therefore important to seek medical advice for a proper diagnosis.

Researchers in Norway have suggested that some unexplained mouth ulcers may be linked with a detergent, sodium lauryl sulphate (SLS), found in most brands of toothpaste. As it is a detergent, it is possible that SLS dries out the protective mucous membranes in the mouth so that irritants or infection can trigger ulceration. They found that when people with recurring mouth ulcers switched to using an SLS-free toothpaste, their incidence of mouth ulcers reduced by 70 per cent.

Do not take supplements if you are pregnant, breast-feeding, or taking prescribed drugs without first seeking advice from a pharmacist about possible interactions or adverse effects.

Treatment

Severe lack of vitamin C can lead to mouth ulcers as part of scurvy, although this is now rare in developed countries. Even so, a *vitamin C* supplement will help by reducing inflammation, and assisting in the formation of collagen during the healing process. Mouth ulcers have also been linked with a lack of B vitamins (*B2, B3, B6, B12, folic acid*) and *iron*, so it is worth taking a multivitamin and mineral supplement providing around 100 per cent of the RDA for as many micro-nutrients as possible. It is also advisable to avoid smoking and maintain good oral hygiene.

Applying *aloe vera* gel has been shown to reduce healing time from ten days to between five and six days, and to rapidly improve discomfort within minutes of application.

Sucking lozenges made from *liquorice* (DGL form) also has a soothing and anti-inflammatory action.

Olive leaf extracts have a powerful antibiotic effect and in one study of people with mouth problems, including ulceration, the quickest improvement was seen in those who took olive leaf extracts (1 g) three times a day.

Other natural approaches include colloidal silicic acid, or mouth-washes containing myrrh. When feeling run down, it is worth taking a herbal adaptogen such as *Siberian ginseng* or an immune stimulant such as *Echinacea*.

Note: Any mouth ulcer or area of soreness that lasts for longer than three weeks should be checked by a doctor to exclude a mouth cancer.

See also: **Aloe vera, Ashwagandha, Cayenne, Goldenseal, Holy basil, Liquorice, Mastic gum, Myrrh, Reishi, Vitamin A, Vitamin B2, Vitamin B6**.

Multiple sclerosis

Multiple sclerosis (MS) is a progressive, degenerative condition affecting the nervous system. It is the most common cause of neurological disability in young adults, with symptoms usually starting between the ages of 20–40 years. It is more common in females with three women affected for every two males. MS is an auto-immune disease, in which the immune system attacks the fatty sheaths protecting nerve fibres within the central nervous system. The demyelination of nerves is believed to occur when antibodies made against a foreign protein (e.g. part of a virus, bacterium or food) cross-react with a similar protein found within the myelin sheath. This stimulates immune cells to attack the nerve coatings, which become inflamed and start to degenerate. As a result, transmission of information through affected nerve fibres slows or even stops, and neurological symptoms develop. Initially, affected areas may heal and become re-myelinated, although the speed at which nerve signals pass through healed areas may remain slower than normal, so some residual disability remains. In other areas, damaged myelin may be converted to scar tissue – a process known as sclerosis. It is the development of several patches of scarring, or sclerosis, that gives multiple sclerosis its name. Eventually, nerve cells underlying affected myelin sheaths may also die, and persistent disability is thought to reflect increasing loss of nerve cells as the disease progresses. Many people have minimal disability, but others may develop pain, visual difficulties, clumsiness, slurred speech, problems with walking, and loss of bowel or bladder control.

Treatment

Various nutritional approaches have been suggested but current evidence to support these approaches is largely anecdotal. One theory is that MS is affected by proteins in food, and suggests restricting intakes of foodstuff that contain proteins similar to those found in myelin, e.g. dairy products (replace with rice milk or coconut milk), gluten (wheat, rye, barley), pulses (including soybeans), as well as avoiding refined sugar which is believed to have adverse effects on immunity. You may be advised to avoid foods to which you have elevated levels of IgG antibodies.

Some experts recommend *vitamin D3* supplements, as they

Do not take supplements if you are pregnant, breast-feeding, or taking prescribed drugs without first seeking advice from a pharmacist about possible interactions or adverse effects.

Types of MS

Four types of MS are recognized: benign, relapsing remitting, secondary progressive, primary progressive.

- Relapsing remitting MS (25 per cent of cases): unpredictable exacerbations that last for at least 24 hours, in which new symptoms appear or existing symptoms worsen; after a variable period of days, weeks or months, a partial or total remission occurs which can last for months or even years.
- Secondary progressive MS (40 per cent): steady progression of symptoms, for six months or more, with no episodes of relapse or remission; usually develops after several years of relapsing, remitting MS.
- Benign MS (20 per cent): less severe symptoms at onset, with complete recovery; long periods of remission and no permanent disability (diagnosed retrospectively after 10–15 years of minimal disability in someone with presumed relapsing, remitting MS).
- Primary progressive (15 per cent): slow onset of progressive, steadily worsening symptoms and disability, with no distinct episodes of relapse or remission.

---

believe MS is linked with deficiency of vitamin D3 (made in the skin on exposure to sunlight) – this might help to explain why the prevalence of MS varies across the world depending on latitude and proximity to the equator.

Some research suggests that levels of an essential fatty acid (linoleic acid) are low in people with MS, especially during a relapse, and taking high-dose *evening primrose oil* (2–3 g a day) may help.

Other supplements that are used include omega-3 fish oils, flax seed oil, antioxidants, probiotics and co-enzyme Q10.

Selenium, magnesium, manganese, vitamin B12, vitamin C and *vitamin E* may be recommended to help relieve stiffness and spasm, and to strengthen muscles while improving co-ordination. A *vitamin B* complex is generally taken to improve nerve function, and an A to

---

Do not take supplements if you are pregnant, breast-feeding, or taking prescribed drugs without first seeking advice from a pharmacist about possible interactions or adverse effects.

Z-style vitamin and mineral formula might be helpful too.

The herbs most commonly recommended include black cohosh, Echinacea, ginseng, St John's Wort and valerian.

Ginkgo opens up small blood vessels and improves circulation to muscles and nerves and is often helpful, while *Echinacea* has a beneficial effect on the immune system and may also be suggested. However, it is always advisable to consult a trained herbalist for the most appropriate treatment.

Cannabis-derived treatments can relieve pain, spasticity and other problems associated with MS and an oral spray, Sativex, is available on prescription in some countries. *Hempseed oil* products may contain small amounts of the active ingredient, TCH.

Mercury has been implicated in worsening symptoms. Chelation therapy to remove mercury from the body, plus replacement of mercury fillings is therefore advocated by some practitioners but this should only be done by a dentist who is experienced in removing mercury fillings. Blue-green algae and N-acetyl cysteine may help in the process of chelating (binding) heavy metals in the body so that they can be excreted.

See also: **Vitamin B12, Vitamin D**.

Myalgic encephalitis (ME)
See: **Chronic fatigue syndrome**.

Myasthenia gravis

Myasthenia gravis is usually considered to be an auto-immune disorder in which weakness affects a variety of muscle groups and responds to treatment with anticholinesterase drugs.

Treatment
Some doctors feel that mercury toxicity or allergy plays a role in the development of myasthenia gravis and recommend that silver/black

dental amalgams are removed from the mouth. A dentist who specializes in the removal of these fillings should be consulted, however, as special techniques are needed for their safe elimination. Blue-green algae and N-acetyl cysteine may help in the process of chelating (binding) heavy metals in the body so that they can be excreted.

Herbal remedies used to help relieve symptoms include *astragalus* (often in combination with *ginseng*) and *reishi* mushroom.

Nail problems

Nails are made of a hard, fibrous protein called keratin which is designed to strengthen the tips of fingers and toes and protect them from damage. They grow at a rate of up to 5 mm per month. Some people have strong, thick, nails which if not cut can grow up to 30 cm in length.

White patches in fingernails are common and there are many theories regarding their cause. They have been variously attributed to lack of *calcium, zinc, vitamin A* and *vitamin B6*. The most likely cause is minor damage to nail beds which affects the way in which the nail plate is laid down – perhaps nutritional deficiencies such as zinc contribute to poor healing.

It's worth trying an A to Z-style vitamin and mineral formula plus evening primrose oil to see if this helps, although it takes at least three months for fingernails to grow through completely. *Garlic* tablets have been shown to improve blood flow to capillaries at the base of the nails by 55 per cent which will improve nutrient flow to the area. *Ginkgo* also improves peripheral circulation to nails.

Soft, brittle nails are another common problem which may be hereditary or it may be linked with deficiency of certain nutrients. Avoid prolonged immersion in water. A vitamin, mineral and herbal supplement designed to strengthen hair, skin and nails is worth taking. *Ginkgo* improves circulation to nail beds, while evening primrose oil is also helpful in strengthening nails, especially when combined with *calcium*.

Do not take supplements if you are pregnant, breast-feeding, or taking prescribed drugs without first seeking advice from a pharmacist about possible interactions or adverse effects.

Ridges in nails are believed to result from fluctuating blood flow during times of physical stress or illness, and can also relate to a lack of *B group vitamins*. An adaptogen such as *ginseng* or *Rhodiola* may also helpful. *Biotin* can strengthen keratin, and studies suggest that supplements can increase nail thickness by at least a quarter.

In-growing toenails are a common problem that can be prevented: trim toenails straight across, avoid picking them, wear comfortable shoes and walk barefoot at home as much as possible. Bathe the affected foot in a warm, diluted antiseptic solution for 15–20 minutes. After softening the flesh, carefully tuck a small wisp of cotton wool under the ingrowing corner of the nail using a blunt pair of scissors, orange stick or a tiny screwdriver. This acts as a cushion which pushes the tender flesh away from the nail and allows it to grow out normally. The old piece of cotton wool should be removed each day, and another wisp tucked in, slightly larger if necessary. The cotton wool helps to lift the nail edge away from the flesh it is digging into and encourages it to grow out properly. *Echinacea* may help to reduce infection. Medical advice should be sought as soon as possible by people with diabetes (do not treat the nail yourself), or if the toe becomes infected.

See also: **Biotin, Iodine, Iron, Kelp, Manganese, Silicon**.

Nosebleeds

Nosebleeds (epistaxis) are linked with fragile, poorly supported blood vessels in the lining of the nose. These easily become damaged by picking fingers, inflammation, and vigorous blowing or sneezing, causing them to rupture and bleed.

Treatment
Most nosebleeds are easily stopped by:

1. Sitting slightly forward, mouth open (some doctors recommend leaning backwards but this means blood trickles down the throat

---

Do not take supplements if you are pregnant, breast-feeding, or taking prescribed drugs without first seeking advice from a pharmacist about possible interactions or adverse effects.

and pools in the stomach which can cause nausea and vomiting).
2. Pinching the lower (soft) part of the nose for 10–15 minutes, while breathing through the mouth; at the same time, apply an ice pack (e.g. a bag of frozen peas) to the bridge of the nose to constrict blood flow.
3. Release the nostrils slowly, to check whether bleeding has stopped.

It is best to avoid touching or blowing the nose again for a few hours.

Extracts of *horsechestnut, red vine leaf, bilberry* or *pine bark* (Pycnogenol®) help to strengthen connective tissue surrounding veins and may help to prevent recurrent nosebleeds. *Vitamin K2* may be suggested if deficiency is thought to contribute to prolonged bleeding times.

Note: If bleeding does not stop after 20 minutes, or if it seems torrential, seek medical advice.

See also: **Siberian ginseng, Vitamin K**.

Osteoarthritis

Osteoarthritis (OA) is a slowly-progressive, long-term disease that affects certain mobile joints in the body. It is most common in weight-bearing joints, such as the knees, hips and lower spine, but can also affect non-weight-bearing joints that are used repetitively, such as in the fingers and jaw.

Although traditionally thought of as a wear-and-tear disease, researchers now believe that OA results from the active repair of damaged joints, rather than from a destructive process. It develops when more cartilage is broken down than normal, but less new cartilage is made to replace it, so repair is incomplete. Early changes include fragmentation of the cartilage surface and the appearance of vertical clefts. The amount of fluid present in the cartilage matrix also increases, and the cartilage swells, disrupting the collagen fibres so they are less resilient to injury. There is progressive loss of collagen and increased formation of a substance called fibronectin, which is involved in wound repair. As a result of all these changes, cartilage becomes weaker, stiffer and less able to withstand compressive forces. As a result, the articular cartilage protecting the bone ends becomes pitted, cracked and starts to flake away to expose the underlying bone.

When articular cartilage is lost, synovial fluid leaks into the underlying bone causing mild inflammation, bone thickening, and the formation of small cysts and bony outgrowths known as osteophytes. More and more cartilage is lost and, in severe cases, very little cartilage may remain. Inflammation and increased blood flow leads to thickening of the synovial membrane and joint capsule. Eventually, all the structures associated with the joint may be affected – the articular cartilage, synovial membrane, joint capsule, bone and related muscles and ligaments.

OA causes affected joints to become increasingly painful, stiff and deformed. The muscles around affected joints may become weak and wasted from lack of use.

Prevention
It's worth taking steps to look after your joints if you notice:

- Creakiness in one or more joints
- A joint (e.g. knee, hip) is less flexible than before, or cannot be straightened fully
- Your joints are swelling or changing shape
- Your fingers and toes easily get cold and stiff
- A joint starts aching, especially after exercise
- Your knees are painful when you kneel or squat down to sit on them
- Joint pain and stiffness limit your mobility and interfere with your life
- Joint pain starts to interfere with sleep or day-to-day activities.

Do not take supplements if you are pregnant, breast-feeding, or taking prescribed drugs without first seeking advice from a pharmacist about possible interactions or adverse effects.

Treatment

One of the most important things you can do when you have osteoarthritis is to lose any excess weight. This reduces the load exerted on weight-bearing joints. Every one pound increase in weight increases the overall force across your knee joints when walking or standing by two to three pounds. So, if you are 10 pounds overweight, the force on your knees increases by up to 30 pounds. Looked at the other way round, losing 10 pounds in weight (4.5 kg) can reduce the load on your knees by as much as 30 pounds. Losing excess weight also reduces the level of inflammation in your body, especially if you tend to store excess fat around your waist. As a result, successful weight loss can help to decrease the development and progression of OA.

Omega-3 fish oils are a rich source of EPA and DHA which are processed in the body to reduce formation of inflammatory leukotrienes. Fish oils can reduce morning stiffness, swelling, the number of painful joints, and the long-term need for painkillers in people with joint pain.

Glucosamine stimulates the formation of proteoglycans that strengthen cartilage and synovial fluid to improve resistance against compressive forces. This helps to maintain the joint space so that bone ends do not rub together.

Chondroitin attracts water into joints, inhibits enzymes that break down cartilage, and stimulates production of structural proteoglycans, glycosaminoglycans and collagen. Taking chondroitin helps to maintain the joint space width and can significantly improve pain and joint function.

MSM (methyl-sulphonyl-methane) is an important building block for glycosaminoglycans, and is a key structural component of cartilage. It also reduces joint inflammation, pain and swelling by reducing the formation of harmful free radicals by white blood cells within inflamed joints.

Green-lipped mussel extracts contain an omega-3 fatty acid (eicosatetraenoic acid) that inhibits the production of inflammatory leukotrienes. This reduces the movement of activated white blood

---

Do not take supplements if you are pregnant, breast-feeding, or taking prescribed drugs without first seeking advice from a pharmacist about possible interactions or adverse effects.

cells into joints, and damps down their release of inflammatory chemicals. This allows joint pain, swelling and stiffness to settle.

Bromelain has an anti-inflammatory action, reducing the migration of white blood cells into areas of inflammation. It significantly reduces acute knee pain, stiffness and swelling.

Rose hip extracts contain a painkilling complex which reduces movement of inflammatory cells into joints, to reduce pain and stiffness.

Turmeric contains curcumin, which has a powerful anti-inflammatory action equivalent to that of some prescribed corticosteroids, which helps to ease stiff joints.

Ginger also has warming and anti-inflammatory properties.

Vitamin C is needed for collagen synthesis. Those with the highest intake of vitamin C are three times less likely to see their OA progress, compared with those having the lowest intakes. This was mostly the result of reduced cartilage loss. Those with high vitamin C intake were also three times less likely to develop knee pain.

Vitamin D3 is important for joint health. Some studies have found a three- to four-fold increase in the risk of osteoarthritis progression in those with low vitamin D intakes, compared with people obtaining high intakes.

Vitamin E taken at a dose of 400 mg per day for six weeks reduced pain at rest, pain on movement and the need for painkillers, compared with those taking inactive placebo.

Selenium is an important trace element that forms part of a number of antioxidant enzymes that help to damp down inflammation. Some of the inflammatory chemicals that are suppressed by selenium are produced in inflamed joints and reducing their formation may therefore improve joint pain. Selenium has additional, non-antioxidant effects that may also help people with osteoarthritis, such as reducing the breakdown of cartilage.

Copper and *zinc* are both present in an antioxidant enzyme (superoxide dismutase) which helps to reduce oxidation in inflamed joints. Lack of either copper or zinc significantly lowers tissue levels of this enzyme and increases the amount of inflammatory damage

---

Do not take supplements if you are pregnant, breast-feeding, or taking prescribed drugs without first seeking advice from a pharmacist about possible interactions or adverse effects.

occurring. Both are also important for a healthy balance between the production and breakdown of joint connective tissues such as collagen and elastin.

See also: **Boswellia, Bromelain, Cat's claw, Cayenne, Chondroitin, CMA, Devil's claw, Fish oils, Ginger, Glucosamine, Green-lipped mussel, Krill oil, Nettle, Pine bark, Rosehip, Vitamin B5, Vitamin C, Vitamin D, Vitamin E.**

Osteoporosis

Osteoporosis means 'porous bones' and is a disease that is largely preventable. Bone is a living tissue made up from a network of collagen fibres filled with mineral salts. These minerals – of which the most important is calcium phosphate – are constantly broken down and replaced as part of a carefully balanced remodelling process. Osteoporosis develops when the process of bone remodelling becomes unbalanced so that not enough new bone is made to replace the old worn-out bone that is naturally reabsorbed. As a result, bones start to become thin, brittle and fracture more easily.

Thanks to the female hormone, oestrogen, which stimulates formation of healthy new bone, women are relatively protected against osteoporosis until they reach the menopause. For women, the main risk factors for osteoporosis are therefore linked with lack of oestrogen, and include:

- Early menopause (before the age of 45)
- Early hysterectomy (before the age of 45), especially if both ovaries are also removed
- Loss of periods for any cause except pregnancy (e.g. excessive dieting and weight loss, excessive exercise, use of depot progestogen contraception).

Non-oestrogen-related risk factors also increase the risk of osteoporosis, such as:

Do not take supplements if you are pregnant, breast-feeding, or taking prescribed drugs without first seeking advice from a pharmacist about possible interactions or adverse effects.

- Close family history – especially if your mother or father had a hip fracture
- Long-term use of high-dose, corticosteroid tablets
- Certain medical conditions such as adrenal, liver or thyroid problems
- Being housebound with little exposure to sunlight and low dietary intakes of vitamin D, calcium magnesium and phosphorus
- Intestinal malabsorption (e.g. due to coeliac disease, Crohn's disease, gastric surgery)
- Long-term immobility, especially confinement to bed in childhood
- Heavy drinking
- Smoking.

These non-oestrogen risk factors also apply to men, who are at additional risk if they also have low levels of the male hormone, testosterone.

Prevention

Take regular exercise which stimulates formation of new bone. High impact exercise is best (e.g. aerobics, gymnastics, netball, dancing, racquet sports, jogging, skipping) but non-weight-bearing exercise such as stretching and swimming are also beneficial. You don't have to over-do it, as significant benefits have been shown from just jumping up and down 10 to 30 times per day. For older people, any form of activity is useful, including walking, climbing stairs, carrying loads, doing housework and gardening – these activities also strengthen muscles to reduce the likelihood of a fall.

Obtain good intakes of calcium which is vital for strong bones throughout life. Calcium-rich foods include dairy products, green leafy vegetables, salmon/pilchards (tinned with bones), eggs, nuts, seeds, pulses, plus white and brown bread made from fortified flour. The easiest way to boost your intake is to drink an extra pint of skimmed or semi-skimmed milk per day which provides around 720 mg calcium. Adding calcium and vitamin D supplements to the

---

Do not take supplements if you are pregnant, breast-feeding, or taking prescribed drugs without first seeking advice from a pharmacist about possible interactions or adverse effects.

diet of older people has also been shown to significantly reduce their risk of a spinal or hip fracture.

Get enough vitamin D3 which is essential for the absorption of calcium and phosphate from your diet. Just 15 minutes' exposure to bright sunshine on your face makes enough vitamin D in your skin during summer – but you need at least 30 minutes' exposure to mid-day sun for the same benefit during winter.

Eat at least five servings of fruit and veg per day as they are rich in important micronutrients for bone health such as isoflavones, carotenoids, potassium, magnesium, boron, copper, folic acid, manganese, potassium, silica, vitamin C and zinc. A multivitamin and mineral supplement is also a good idea as a nutritional safety net.

Eat oily fish which is a rich source of vitamin D. Like other sources of essential fatty acids, including evening primrose oil, fish oils also stimulate calcium uptake from the gut, decrease calcium loss in the urine and increase calcium deposition in your bones. As we are advised to limit our intake of oily fish due to marine pollutants, a daily pharmaceutical-grade fish oil supplement (screened to ensure these are absent) is an excellent idea.

Avoid canned, fizzy drinks that contain phosphoric acid as high intakes can increase loss of calcium from your bones.

Cut back on salty foods as table salt (sodium chloride) increases the loss of calcium through your kidneys. Halving average salt intakes could cut urinary calcium losses by as much as 20 per cent, as well as having beneficial effects on blood pressure.

Avoid smoking cigarettes which, for women, can lower levels of the female hormone, oestrogen enough to trigger an early menopause.

Avoid excessive alcohol which reduces absorption of calcium from your diet. Thankfully, moderate intakes of alcohol may actually increase bone density although the reason is not yet known.

Avoid aluminium-based antacids which impair absorption of phosphates from the gut – regular use for more than ten years may double the risk of a hip fracture.

Avoid excess stress which has been linked with an increased risk

---

Do not take supplements if you are pregnant, breast-feeding, or taking prescribed drugs without first seeking advice from a pharmacist about possible interactions or adverse effects.

of osteoporosis. Stress hormones have a direct harmful effect on bone – cortisol, for example, increases calcium resorption from bone and increases calcium loss in the urine – and also reduces production of sex hormones by the adrenal glands (which provide useful top-ups in later life).

Consider cutting back on caffeine if you drink lots of coffee. Some research suggests that women who drink four cups of coffee a day are three times more likely to suffer a hip fracture in later life. To offset this effect, some experts suggest obtaining an extra 40 g calcium for every 6 fl oz (178 ml) cup of caffeinated coffee consumed.

Avoid heavy consumption of red meat which may reduce absorption of dietary calcium and has been linked with low bone mass and early osteoporosis. Aim to eat meat no more than once a day and eat more vegetarian and fish dishes, instead.

Treatment
While diet should always come first, studies suggest that taking 1.2 g *calcium phosphate* plus 800 IU/20 mcg *vitamin D* daily can potentially reduce the incidence of hip and other non-vertebral fractures by up to 30 per cent.

Essential fatty acids found in *fish, evening primrose* and *flaxseed oils* help to increase calcium deposition in bone. *Isoflavones* also mimic the beneficial action of oestrogen to increase bone mineralization.

See also: **Boron, Calcium, Copper, Fluoride, Isoflavones, Magnesium, Manganese, Silicon, Vitamin C, Vitamin D, Vitamin K, Zinc**.

Palpitations

Palpitations are an unpleasant awareness of the heartbeat, or a sensation of having rapid, missed or unusually strong heartbeats. They are felt quite normally after exercise, in periods of increased stress, or

---

Do not take supplements if you are pregnant, breast-feeding, or taking prescribed drugs without first seeking advice from a pharmacist about possible interactions or adverse effects.

after a sudden scare. They can also be brought on by a high intake of caffeine. Palpitations can sometimes be a sign of an over-active thyroid gland, an abnormal heart rhythm or a chest problem (such as hiatus hernia) that needs treatment.

Treatment
Try switching to caffeine-free versions of tea, coffee and colas. Avoid excess alcohol and nicotine. Do not take over-the-counter cough and cold preparations containing theophylline or pseudoephedrine which can also trigger attacks.

If no serious medical causes are found for palpitations, it might be helpful to take *Rhodiola* if they are linked with anxiety, or *valerian* if linked with stress.

Note: If palpitations are persistent, recurrent, or are accompanied by chest pain, shortness of breath, dizziness or faintness, always seek immediate medical advice.

See also: **Calcium, Magnesium, Vitamin B3, Vitamin D**.

Panic attacks

Panic attacks affect one in 20 people on a regular basis. When feeling stressed, your breathing patterns change so you take quick, irregular, shallow breaths to draw in more oxygen. This in turn means that you blow off more carbon dioxide – a waste acidic gas. If hyperventilating continues, your blood loses acidity and becomes too alkaline. This causes symptoms of dizziness, faintness and pins and needles, which in turn heighten anxiety and can trigger a panic attack.

People who habitually hyperventilate can experience a frightening number of physical symptoms, including chest pain, palpitations, visual disturbances, numbness, severe headache, insomnia and even collapse. Medical diagnosis of these symptoms is important to avoid missing a more serious problem.

Do not take supplements if you are pregnant, breast-feeding, or taking prescribed drugs without first seeking advice from a pharmacist about possible interactions or adverse effects.

Treatment

When panic begins rising, the classic advice is to breathe in and out of a paper bag to re-inhale some of the lost carbon dioxide – alternatively, breathe in and out of cupped hands. Concentrate on breathing slowly, deeply and quietly, holding a few breaths for a count of three if possible.

Valerian is one of the most calming herbs available and can help to relieve anxiety, muscle tension and promote calmness.

Rhodiola is widely used to combat mild anxiety as it promotes feelings of relaxation and calm whilst also increasing energy.

Lemon balm is another useful supplement, especially for students whose panic attacks are associated with exam nerves.

See also: **Kelp, Rhodiola, Valerian**.
Related entry: **Stress**.

Parkinson's disease

Parkinson's is a progressive, nervous system disorder. It occurs when pigment-containing cells in a particular part of the brain, the *substantia nigra*, start to degenerate. Someone with Parkinson's may have lost 80 per cent or more of these cells and, as a result, production of an important brain communication chemical, dopamine, also falls. Dopamine is needed to communicate with the next area of the brain (the *corpus striatum*) to ensure smooth, purposeful movements in the body. If dopamine levels fall, movements become irregular and difficult to control, leading to typical symptoms of Parkinson's. Whether loss of dopamine is the cause or result of the death of cells in the substantia nigra is still unclear. Scientists are now investigating this using positron emission tomography (PET) – a form of brain scanning that can show chemical changes in the living brain as they occur.

Parkinson's can occur at any age, but most people with the condition start to develop symptoms around the age of 60 years. The onset of Parkinson's is usually slow. Someone may feel unusually tired, a

---

Do not take supplements if you are pregnant, breast-feeding, or taking prescribed drugs without first seeking advice from a pharmacist about possible interactions or adverse effects.

little shaky and have difficulty standing up from a chair. They may start to speak more softly, their handwriting may become smaller or more spidery, and they may have difficulty concentrating. Friends and family may notice the person has become expressionless, slowed up and is generally less mobile. Sometime, the first indication that someone may have Parkinson's disease is a trembling or shaking of one or more limbs – especially when the person is resting. The tremor often begins just on one side and typically affects one hand. The tremor is a rhythmic backwards-and-forwards movement of the thumb and forefinger that is sometimes referred to as 'pill rolling'. Other symptoms can include slowing of movements, difficulty starting to move, poor balance and co-ordination, stiffness, stooped posture, speech difficulties and a shuffling walk. Not surprisingly, those affected often become depressed.

Treatment

Medical treatment consists of giving an amino acid, levodopa, which is converted into dopamine within the central nervous system. A co-enzyme, NADH, is needed for levodopa to work properly, and some researchers have claimed that taking NADH supplements alone can improve Parkinson's disease in some people. In one study it was shown to help four out of five sufferers, especially those who were younger and more recently diagnosed. This remains controversial, however.

Co-enzyme Q10 is needed for energy production in cells, and low levels of this important nutrient have been linked with accelerated death of heart muscle cells, for example. The same effect may occur in brain cells, and researchers recently found that taking co-enzyme Q10 helped to slow the progression of Parkinson's disease in those taking supplements compared with those taking inactive placebo. As the study only included 80 people, however, larger clinical trials are needed.

Phosphatidylserine and *omega-3 fish oils* may help to improve brain function. B group vitamins are also important for healthy nerve function.

Do not take supplements if you are pregnant, breast-feeding, or taking prescribed drugs without first seeking advice from a pharmacist about possible interactions or adverse effects.

Antioxidants such as *vitamin C* and *vitamin E* are sometimes prescribed by physicians to reduce the free radical attack thought to be associated with neurological damage. In one study involving over 5,000 people, those with the highest intakes of vitamin E were the least likely to develop Parkinson's disease. Other powerful antioxidants that may be recommended include *alpha-lipoic acid*, *grapeseed* or *pine bark* (Pycnogenol®) extracts. Ginkgo biloba, which improves blood flow to the brain, may also help.

Probiotics and *psyllium* can help to overcome constipation which may occur.

Blue-green algae and *N-acetyl cysteine* may help in the process of chelating (binding) heavy metals in the body so that they can be excreted.

See also: **Antioxidants, Cat's claw, Manganese, Vitamin D**.

Period problems

Painful periods (dysmenorrhoea) are due to cramping of uterine muscles. Some women suffer more than others – possibly because they make more of the chemicals (prostaglandins) that trigger muscular spasm. In around one in ten women, the cause is endometriosis, in which womb lining cells are found elsewhere in the body – most usually in the abdominal cavity. Because these cells remain sensitive to the monthly hormone cycle, they swell and bleed into surrounding tissues once a month to produce pain, inflammation and scarring. Period pains can be severe in endometriosis and may be linked with nausea, vomiting and diarrhoea. Other causes include hormone imbalances, fibroids (knot-like swellings in womb muscle), some contraceptive coils and pelvic inflammatory disease (infection of the upper reproductive tract).

If you suffer from persistent heavy periods, you will usually have a blood test to ensure you have not developed iron deficiency anaemia. You may also be screened for common blood clotting disorders such as lack of clotting factor XI, or lack of a platelet clumping protein – a condition known as von Willebrand's disease, which some researchers suggest may be present in as many as one in six women with persistent heavy periods.

Treatment

Heavy and painful periods are worse in women with a low intake of fish. Taking *omega-3 fish oils* has a beneficial effect on the types of prostaglandins produced, and can significantly improve painful periods, especially in teenage girls.

Magnesium supplements taken for six cycles can reduce back pain and lower abdominal pain associated with menstruation – especially on the second and third days – probably due to its muscle relaxant effect.

A study in Japan involving women with severe menstrual pain – in some cases due to endometriosis – found that they experienced significant improvement in menstrual cramping and abdominal pain when taking 30–60 mg *pine bark* extracts (Pycnogenol®) daily, with treatment starting at least two weeks before menstruation.

Tell your doctor straight away if you notice:

- Post-menopausal bleeding
- Bleeding after intercourse
- Unexpected bleeding (spotting) in between your periods.

Heavy periods (menorrhagia) have been linked with a lack of essential fatty acids (such as those found in *evening primrose* and *flaxseed oils*) *vitamin A*, *vitamin C*, *vitamin K*, and minerals *iron* and *zinc*.

See also: **Agnus castus, Black cohosh, Dong quai, Fish oils, Ginger, Ginseng, Iron, Krill oil, Vitamin B2**.

Related entry: **Endometriosis**.

Peripheral vascular disease
See: **Intermittent claudication**.

Do not take supplements if you are pregnant, breast-feeding, or taking prescribed drugs without first seeking advice from a pharmacist about possible interactions or adverse effects.

Peyronie's disease

Peyronie's disease affects around one in 250 adult males, and occurs when some of the spongy, erectile tissues of the penis are replaced with fibrous scar tissue. Why this should happen is unknown, but as the fibrous area does not expand during erection, the penis curves – often dramatically – towards the area of rigidity during erection. This gives the erection a distinct banana shape which can be uncomfortable or even painful.

Treatment

Treatment with *vitamin E* tablets (at least 200 mg a day) is sometimes recommended as vitamin E helps to maintain tissue elasticity. This is controversial however – partly because the condition often improves on its own and it is then difficult to know whether the vitamin E has helped or not.

One study comparing *L-carnitine* to tamoxifen in 48 men with Peyronie's found that it was more effective at reducing pain during intercourse and in minimizing penile curvature. However, another study found that carnitine and/or vitamin E was no more effective than placebo.

Other supplements that are used include proteolytic digestive enzymes, alpha-lipoic acid and co-enzyme Q10.
See also: **Carnitine**.

Phlebitis

Phlebitis – more properly known as thrombophlebitis – is the inflammation of a vein with formation of a blood clot within the affected segment. It often occurs after a minor injury such as a knock, and is frequently a complication of varicose veins. Swelling, redness and tenderness are often accompanied by fever and feeling unwell.

Do not take supplements if you are pregnant, breast-feeding, or taking prescribed drugs without first seeking advice from a pharmacist about possible interactions or adverse effects.

Treatment

Usually the condition is resolved with bandaging for support, anti-inflammatory drugs and sometimes – if infection is suspected – antibiotics. Eating more oily fish (such as salmon, sardines, herrings, mackerel) or taking *omega-3 fish oils* supplements will have a thinning effect on the blood and reduce clot formation.

Garlic tablets also have beneficial effects on the circulation, and for anyone who is not taking prescribed blood-thinning agents, *ginkgo* is also worth considering, or the Tibetan herbal blend, Padma 28, which helps to improve blood flow through the peripheral circulation.

Antioxidants (e.g. *selenium, vitamin C, vitamin E, carotenoids, pine bark, grapeseed extracts*) will reduce inflammation while extracts of *horse chestnut, red vine leaf* or *Pycnogenol®* can strengthen tissues surrounding blood vessels and reduce discomfort of varicose veins.

Co-enzyme Q10 increases oxygen uptake of cells and can also reduce leg discomfort.

Applying *aloe vera* gel or *evening primrose oil* to affected skin may help to improve the cosmetic appearance.

See also: **Bilberry**.

Piles

See: **Haemorrhoids**.

Polycystic ovary syndrome

Polycystic ovary syndrome is a condition in which the ovaries enlarge to between two and four times their normal size, and are covered in multiple tiny cysts. As many as 20–30 per cent of women are thought to have polycystic ovaries, although most cases are mild. Only around 5 per cent go on to develop symptoms, in which case

---

Do not take supplements if you are pregnant, breast-feeding, or taking prescribed drugs without first seeking advice from a pharmacist about possible interactions or adverse effects.

they are diagnosed as having polycystic ovary syndrome (PCOS).

As well as producing the female hormones, oestrogen and proges-terone, the ovaries normally produce small amounts of male hormones, such as testosterone, which help to regulate your sex drive. In PCOS, the ovaries produce too many of these male hormones which block the normal monthly growth and development of egg follicles. In an attempt to kick-start the ovaries, the pituitary gland in the brain produces more and more luteinising hormone (LH) which stimulates the growth of more and more egg follicles. As a result, the ovaries enlarge and become covered with multiple small cysts which contain under-developed eggs.

Most women with PCOS also have a metabolic abnormality in which their cells become less responsive to insulin hormone. Insulin is made in the pancreas gland and is needed for glucose to enter muscle and fat cells, where it is used as a fuel. If cells don't respond to insulin properly, blood glucose levels become higher than normal and women with PCOS are seven times more likely to develop glucose intolerance and diabetes than women with normally-functioning ovaries.

Symptoms can include light, irregular or absent periods, reduced fertility, oily skin, acne, excess unwanted hair, and being overweight, with fat mainly deposited around the waist.

Treatment
Many of the symptoms of PCOS can be improved by following a low-glycaemic diet and regular exercise. Keep alcohol intake to a minimum and avoid smoking cigarettes. The anti-diabetes drug, metformin, improves insulin resistance and helps to reduce weight gain, as well as lowering testosterone levels. Taking *omega-3 fish oils* helps to reduce inflammation and may improve immune problems.

Supplements that may help include *evening primrose oil*, *isoflavones*, *liquorice*, *magnesium*, *B group vitamins*, *chromium*, *agnus castus*, *cinnamon* and *saw palmetto*. *Chromium* is involved in glucose regulation and can improve insulin resistance and glucose

---

Do not take supplements if you are pregnant, breast-feeding, or taking prescribed drugs without first seeking advice from a pharmacist about possible interactions or adverse effects.

tolerance in people who are deficient in this important mineral.

See also: **Agnus castus, Cinnamon, Liquorice, Saw palmetto**.

Polymorphic light eruption (PLE)

See: **Sun allergy**.

Postnasal drip

Postnasal drip occurs when excess nasal fluids trickle down the back of the throat and is often a sign of long-term irritation of the sinuses.

Treatment
Exposure to cigarette smoke and industrial fumes should be avoided as much as possible. Some nutritionists recommend cutting out dairy products to reduce mucus production. If this works, and a dairy-free diet is continued for more than a week or two, a calcium supplement should be taken to guard against osteoporosis. Other foods that are said to promote mucus production and which might, therefore, be worth avoiding, are red meat, wheat and excess refined carbohydrates.

Mucus dispersion can be boosted by supplements containing *N-acetyl cysteine* (NAC) – an amino acid that boosts levels of a powerful antioxidant (glutathione) in the respiratory tract. NAC has a pronounced mucus-dissolving action and studies show that it can significantly reduce mucus production and associated cough in chronic respiratory conditions such as bronchitis, emphysema and sinusitis. It may also be helpful for ear infections and glue ear. It should not be taken by anyone who has peptic ulcers.

Pelargonium sidoides extracts improve mucus dispersion by regulating the tiny hairs (cilia) that propel mucus out of the respiratory tract.

See also: **N-acetyl cysteine, Pelargonium sidoides**.
Related entry: **Catarrh – excess**.

Post-viral fatigue syndrome

See: **Chronic fatigue syndrome**.

Pre-menstrual syndrome

Pre-menstrual syndrome (PMS) is a common and distressing problem affecting as many as one in two women. More than 150 symptoms have been described as forming part of the PMS complex which, for diagnosis, should start within the two weeks before a period and cease promptly when bleeding occurs.

Four main sub-groups of PMS are recognized:

PMS-A   in which the main symptoms are Anxiety, irritability and insomnia

PMS-C   with sugar Cravings, increased appetite, headache and fatigue

PMS-D   Depression, forgetfulness and confusion

PMS-H   (for Hyper-hydration) with fluid retention, weight gain, bloating and breast tenderness.

PMS-A and PMS-H are most common and subtypes can co-exist.

Treatment

Some research suggests that progesterone can't work properly when blood sugar levels are low. Nibbling regular carbohydrate snacks every three hours can help to reduce symptoms.

Pre-menstrual syndrome (PMS) has been linked with deficiencies of calcium, magnesium and vitamin B6. Clinical trials support the use of calcium and magnesium supplements, but the evidence for B6 is weak.

Alterations in *calcium* and *magnesium* balance are associated with mood disturbances and clinical symptoms of hypocalcaemia show similarities with those of PMS. Taking calcium (1200–1600 mg per day) can improve mood, water retention and pain. Taking calcium plus *vitamin D3* enhances calcium absorption and can reduce headache, negative emotions, fluid retention and pain.

Taking magnesium supplements (150–300 mg as citrate or other organic acid salt for optimum absorption) can improve fluid

---

Do not take supplements if you are pregnant, breast-feeding, or taking prescribed drugs without first seeking advice from a pharmacist about possible interactions or adverse effects.

retention (weight gain, oedema, mastalgia, bloating, headache) but does not seem to affect depression or anxiety.

Anecdotal evidence suggests *vitamin B6* may improve PMS in some women. However, the results from meta-analyses are not promising.

Evening primrose oil provides building blocks for making sex hormones, but needs to be taken at doses of up to 3 g a day for at least three months before an effect may be noticed.

A randomized, placebo-controlled trial of 170 women found that *agnus castus* extracts significantly reduced irritability, mood changes, headache and breast fullness.

A pilot study involving 25 women with severe PMS found *St John's Wort* effective in reducing the incidence of crying, low mood and nervous tension.

See also: **Agnus castus, Calcium, Krill oil, Magnesium, Pollen pistil, St John's Wort, Vitamin B6**.

Prostate problems

The prostate is a male gland, the size and shape of a large chestnut. It lies just beneath the bladder, wrapped around the urinary tube (urethra). There are four main problems that can affect the prostate gland:

- Prostatitis, in which the gland becomes infected or inflamed
- Prostatodynia, in which prostate pain occurs with no obvious cause
- Benign prostatic hyperplasia (BPH) in which the gland slowly enlarges
- Prostate cancer.

Prostatitis
Inflammation of the prostate gland is thought to affect 30 per cent of men at some point between the ages of 20 and 40 years. Symptoms vary and may include:

- Feeling unwell, sometimes with chills or fever
- Aching around the thighs, genitals or lower back
- Deep pain between the scrotum and anus
- Pain and difficulty on passing water
- Passing water more frequently
- Pain on ejaculation
- Discharge from the penis which may be watery or stained with blood or pus.

Prostatodynia

- Prostatodynia literally means prostate pain. It is an unpleasant condition whose symptoms can include:

- Discomfort in the lower abdomen, scrotum, testicles, groin
- A urinary flow that is often abnormally slow
- Difficulty in urination.

No sign of infection or inflammation is found with prostatodynia and it is thought to be linked with spasm of the prostate gland and/or pelvic floor muscles and prostate engorgement.

BPH

After the age of 45, the number of cells in the prostate often increases and the gland starts to enlarge in what is known as benign prostatic hyperplasia (BPH). The result is that the urethral passage is squeezed, causing interference with urinary flow. Half of all 60-year-old men are affected and, by the age of 80, four out of five men have evidence of BPH. The exact cause is unknown, but it is thought to be linked with the action of a prostate enzyme, 5-alpha reductase, which converts the male hormone, testosterone, to a more powerful hormone, dihydrotestosterone (DHT). DHT seems to trigger division of prostate cells so their numbers increase. The fact that the prostate gland is wrapped round the urinary passage is something of an evolutionary design fault, as enlargement of the gland can cause:

Do not take supplements if you are pregnant, breast-feeding, or taking prescribed drugs without first seeking advice from a pharmacist about possible interactions or adverse effects.

- Straining or difficulty when starting to pass water
- A weak urinary stream which may start and stop mid-flow
- Discomfort when passing water
- Having to rush to the toilet
- Passing water more often than normal, especially at night
- Dribbling of urine or urinary incontinence
- A feeling of not emptying the bladder fully.

Prostate cancer

Prostate cancer is one of the most commonly diagnosed male malig-
nancies. Studies suggest that 10–30 per cent of men aged between
50 and 60, and 50–70 per cent of men aged 70 to 80 have evidence
of prostate cancer when cells are examined under the microscope.
Overall, however, only around one in ten men develops significant
prostate cancer symptoms. The cause of prostate cancer is unknown,
but seems to be linked with increasing age – perhaps because the
gland enlarges as the years progress. Some research suggests that
prostate cancer is linked to diet – eating green vegetables is protective, while a diet high in animal (saturated) fats and red meat
increases the risk. Unfortunately, there are few symptoms of early
prostate cancer as nine out of ten tumours arise on the outside of the
gland and do not interfere with urinary flow. If obstructive
symptoms do occur, they are similar to those caused by BPH (see
above) but tend to come on rapidly and progress quickly.

Prostate-friendly diet

Several natural treatments and dietary changes can help to maintain
prostate health and reduce the risk of prostate symptoms occurring.
The same measures can also be used to help to treat prostate
problems once they have been medically evaluated and a satisfactory diagnosis made.

- Follow a diet low in saturated (animal) fat.
- Eat at least five servings of fresh fruit or vegetables per day for
  vitamins and minerals, especially the antioxidants.

- Eat more Japanese-style foods. Weak plant hormones (phyto-oestrogens) found in soy products, rice, and green or yellow vegetables (e.g. broccoli, Chinese leaves, kohlrabi) seem to discourage prostate gland enlargement and protect against both BPH and prostate cancer.
- Eat a high-fibre diet – this binds male hormones in the gut that have been flushed out through the bile, reduces their reabsorption and may help to prevent prostate enlargement.
- Eat foods that are rich in mineral zinc (seafood – especially oysters, wholegrains, bran, pumpkin seeds, garlic and pulses). Zinc is important for prostate health and controls its sensitivity to hormones.
- Eat more tomatoes and tomato-based foods as these contain lyco-pene and other carotenoids that can protect against prostate cancer.
- Eat more nuts and seeds (including evening primrose oil, flaxseed or hempseed supplements) for essential fatty acids needed to make prostaglandins – hormone-like substances important for prostate health.

Treatment

If a diagnosis of BPH is confirmed by your doctor, *saw palmetto* berry extracts are at least as effective as medical treatments. They are often combined with *nettle root* or *pumpkin seed* extracts.

Isoflavone supplements are also beneficial for prostate health.

Consider taking supplements containing *vitamin C, vitamin E, selenium, lycopene* and *zinc*.

See also: **African prune, Chondroitin, Evening primrose oil, Fibre, Isoflavones, Lycopene, Nettle, Pomegranate, Pumpkin seed, Reishi, Saw palmetto, Selenium, Vitamin A, Vitamin C, Vitamin D, Zinc.**

Psoriasis

Psoriasis is an inflammatory disease in which new skin cells are produced at a rate of around ten times faster than normal. As a result, they push up to the surface faster than the dead cells they are designed to replace can fall away from the body. Live cells accumulate and form characteristic raised, red patches covered with dead cells forming fine, silvery scales. Psoriasis symptoms vary and can include the appearance of bright red, scaly patches that vary in size from a few millimetres to extensive plaques covering most of the body. In some cases, sterile pustules form – usually on the palms and soles – while in others, flaky scalp, thickening and pitting of the nails, and/or a form of arthritis known as psoriatic arthropathy develop.

Treatment

Psoriasis has been linked with abnormalities in essential fatty acid metabolism, and EFAs found in *omega-3 fish oils* (e.g. EPA and DHA) have an anti-inflammatory effect which has been shown to damp down psoriasis lesions, to improve itching, scaling and redness.

Aloe vera gel is also noted for its wound-healing and anti-itching properties. Taking it by mouth may be beneficial, too.

Other topical treatments that can improve psoriasis include Dead Sea mineral salts/mud, mahonia ointment (made from the Oregon grape extract), *gotu kola* and Zambesia Botanica – a cream made from the African Kigelia tree.

Some practitioners advise taking *milk thistle* and *globe artichoke* extracts to improve liver function, which seems to improve the rate at which new skin cells are produced.

It might also be worthwhile trying to avoid foods that are high in saturated fats, red meats, dairy products, cheese, eggs, gluten and refined sugars. However, if a restricted diet is to be continued for more than a few weeks, nutritional advice should be sought. Smoking and alcohol can trigger flare-ups and should be avoided.

A case control study looked at *selenium* intakes and serum selenium levels in 59 people with psoriasis and found that, compared with similar controls, selenium status was insufficient in those with psoriasis. In males with chronic disease, selenium levels were inversely correlated to the severity of disease. Increasing

Do not take supplements if you are pregnant, breast-feeding, or taking prescribed drugs without first seeking advice from a pharmacist about possible interactions or adverse effects.

selenium intake may therefore help to reduce the severity and progression of psoriasis.

See also: **Aloe vera, Boswellia, Essential Fatty Acids, Fish oils, Gotu kola, Lapacho, Milk thistle, Oregano oil, Sarsaparilla, Vitamin A, Vitamin D**.

Raynaud's syndrome

Raynaud's is a condition where small arteries in the fingers and toes are overly sensitive to cold. They respond by constricting down and cutting off blood flow to the digits. This causes the fingers to go white, along with numbness and tingling. As a sluggish blood flow returns, the digits go blue, then when circulation becomes normal they turn bright red. The condition can cause pain and burning sensations. Fingers are affected more than toes and it seems to strike more females than males. When associated with other specific diseases, it is known as Raynaud's phenomenon.

Possible causes of Raynaud's include:

- Arterial diseases (e.g. atherosclerosis, blood clotting disorders)
- Connective tissue diseases (e.g. rheumatoid arthritis, scleroderma, lupus)
- Prescribed drugs (e.g. beta-blockers, ergotamine).

Raynaud's can also be triggered by frequent use of pneumatic drills or chain saws and may be referred to as vibration white finger. Occasionally typists and pianists may suffer, too.

Treatment
General self-help measures include keeping hands and feet as warm as possible, stopping smoking (as this further constricts small arteries) and avoiding sudden or extreme changes in temperature.

Eating more oily fish or taking *omega-3 fish oil* supplements can help to reduce blood stickiness.

Do not take supplements if you are pregnant, breast-feeding, or taking prescribed drugs without first seeking advice from a pharmacist about possible interactions or adverse effects.

Garlic tablets and *ginkgo biloba* extracts can improve blood flow to the peripheries.

Ginger has a natural warming effect and recent trials suggest that a supplement combining ginkgo, ginger and garlic was helpful in relieving symptoms. It is also worth taking a vitamin and mineral supplement that includes *magnesium* which can reduce spasm of smooth muscles in artery walls.

Vitamin E is an antioxidant that helps to protect polyunsaturated fatty acids in cell membranes from free radicals – including those in the blood vessels that constrict during Raynaud's – and in one trial, around 80 per cent of sufferers taking vitamin E (400 IU/268 mg) found it helpful.

See also: **Cayenne, Co-enzyme Q10, Garlic, Ginger, Ginkgo.**

Restless legs syndrome

Restless legs, or Ekbom's syndrome, is surprisingly common and affects most people at some time in their life. Around one in 20 people experiences it on a regular basis.

Restless legs syndrome is associated with an unpleasant creeping sensation in the lower limbs, sometimes accompanied by twitching, pins and needles, burning sensations or even pain, along with an irresistible urge to move the legs. It tends to occur during periods of tiredness, and typically an hour after settling down to rest, when leg twitching or jumping can affect sleep. The exact cause is unknown but it is thought to be associated with poor oxygenation of tissues. It seems to be a form of nerve irritation linked with fatigue, anxiety, stress and smoking, but can also occur in pregnancy, diabetes, kidney problems, chronic respiratory illness and stroke. At least half of people with restless legs have a strong family history of the condition, and researchers in Iceland have recently identified a gene that increases the susceptibility to RLS.

Treatment
Eating a light snack before going to bed might help, and alcohol and

caffeine, which may worsen symptoms, should be avoided.

Supplements containing *iron* and *folic acid* will help to improve haemoglobin concentration, while *coenzyme Q10* encourages oxygen uptake in cells.

As restless legs are linked with reduced circulation of blood, extracts of *ginkgo biloba* leaves or *garlic* are often recommended to improve blood flow through small vessels in the legs. The Tibetan preparation *Padma 28*, which contains a complex mix of 20 Tibetan medicinal herbs, is also beneficial in opening up blood flow through the peripheries.

High-dose *vitamin E* helps to stabilize cell membranes and has also been suggested as a treatment, while magnesium supplements are also often effective.

Calcium and *magnesium* supplements may help to prevent twitching and cramping. Magnesium supplements have been shown to reduce periodic limb movements during sleep.

Omega-3 fish oils supply essential fatty acids that help to maintain healthy cell membranes and a healthy circulation.

Other options include *5-HTP*, *pine bark* extracts (Pycnogenol®) and *red vine leaf* extracts. Magnet therapy is also worth trying.

See also: **Valerian**.

Rheumatoid arthritis

Rheumatoid arthritis (RA) is an inflammatory disease in which the synovial membranes lining some joints become thickened, inflamed and produce excess synovial fluid leading to redness, stiffness, swelling and pain. Inflammation gradually spreads to involve the underlying bone, which becomes worn and distorted.

Usually, RA affects the smaller joints in the hands and feet but can also occur in the neck, wrists, knees and ankles. People suffering from RA often feel unwell and may notice weight loss, fever and inflammation in other parts of their body such as the eyes. RA affects around 1 per cent of the population, with three times as many

---

Do not take supplements if you are pregnant, breast-feeding, or taking prescribed drugs without first seeking advice from a pharmacist about possible interactions or adverse effects.

women affected as men. A quarter of sufferers develop symptoms before the age of 30, but most new cases occur within the 40–50 age group.

RA is an auto-immune condition in which immune cells attack the joints leading to inflammation and damage. This may be triggered by a previous infection – 80 per cent of RA patients have antibodies to the Epstein-Barr virus which causes glandular fever.

Treatment

Avoiding cold draughts and keeping as warm as possible in winter are both important. Sufferers of RA should immerse their hands in hot, soapy water first thing in the morning and throughout the day. Frequent hot baths/showers are also soothing. Some people find hot or cold compresses helpful.

Omega-3 fish oils help to relieve joint tenderness, swelling, stiffness and fatigue as well as reducing levels of neutrophil leukotriene B4 (a marker for inflammation). As a result, many people taking them are able to reduce the dose of painkillers needed.

Extracts of New Zealand *green-lipped mussel* help to reduce inflammation in joints and can reduce joint pain and swelling. They contain substances known as glycoproteins, which are thought to work by preventing white blood cells from moving into the joints, where they would release powerful chemicals making pain and swelling worse.

See also: **Aloe vera, Arginine, Boswellia, Cat's claw, CMO, Devil's claw, Essential Fatty Acids, Fish oils, Ginger, Krill oil, Maitake, Nettle, Selenium, Vitamin B5, Wild yam**.

Related entry: **Osteoarthritis**.

Rhinitis

Persistent nasal congestion is commonly due to inflammation and swelling of the mucous membrane lining the nose.

Do not take supplements if you are pregnant, breast-feeding, or taking prescribed drugs without first seeking advice from a pharmacist about possible interactions or adverse effects.

Treatment

One of the simplest and most effective ways of relieving this is with steam inhalation which loosens mucus so that it can drain away more easily. Fill a bowl with hot water, cover your head with a tea towel and lean over the bowl to trap and inhale the hot vapours (taking care not to scald yourself). Adding decongestant essential oil blends will improve efficacy.

Supplements containing the amino acid *N-acetyl cysteine* help to dissolve excess mucus but should not be taken by anyone who has peptic ulcers. *Yerba maté* and *Pelargonium sidoides* may also help.

See also: **Blue-green algae, Brewer's yeast, Butterbur, Pelargonium sidoides**.

Related entry: **Catarrh – excess; Hay fever**.

Rosacea

Rosacea (medically known as acne rosacea) is an inflammatory skin condition in which the face flushes easily and small pimples appear along with fine, dilated capillaries (telangiectasia). The cause is unknown, although it is thought to be due to abnormal sensitivity of blood capillaries. It has also been linked with overuse of corticosteroid creams in the treatment of other skin conditions and with infection of sebaceous glands with a skin mite, *Demodex folliculorum*.

Rosacea usually starts with temporary facial flushing after drinking alcohol, eating spicy food, consuming hot drinks or entering a warm room. If the condition is allowed to progress without treatment, the skin becomes permanently red and pustules start to appear. In severe cases, there is a persistent eruption on the forehead and cheeks, with redness, puffiness and prominent blood vessels. The eyes may be affected to cause conjunctivitis and inflammation of the eyelids (blepharitis). In some people – especially older males – the skin on the nose becomes thickened and red due to enlargement of sebaceous glands.

Rosacea affects around 1 per cent of the population. Symptoms

---

Do not take supplements if you are pregnant, breast-feeding, or taking prescribed drugs without first seeking advice from a pharmacist about possible interactions or adverse effects.

can occur in the teens, but most sufferers are fair-skinned females aged 30–50. Some estimates suggest as many as one in ten middle-aged women is mildly affected. It tends to recur over a five-to-ten-year period then may improve.

Treatment

Avoid factors that may trigger flare-ups of rosacea such as stress, hot liquids, spicy foods, alcohol, vigorous exercise, heat and exposure to sunlight – use a non-greasy high protection cream (SPF 15 or higher) or apply a product that reflects and blocks out ultra-violet rays with titanium dioxide or zinc oxide. Sometimes cutting out tea, chocolate, cheese, yeast extract, eggs, citrus fruits and wheat can be beneficial.

A *B vitamin* complex may be helpful, but this must contain vitamin B3 in the form of nicotinamide rather than niacin, as niacin can itself cause flushing.

Interestingly, some researchers believe that people with rosacea have a reduced production of hydrochloric acid in the stomach and that replenishing levels with supplements containing betaine hydrochloride reduces symptoms although the mechanism is unknown. *Digestive enzymes* may also help.

Vitamin C is useful for its anti-inflammatory actions as well as its beneficial effects on collagen production and, together with *zinc*, can improve skin healing.

Topical application of natural anti-parasitic agents such as oregano, lavender or tea tree oil is helpful in many cases. If stinging is severe when applying these neat, they may be diluted first with a little olive or hempseed oil. *Aloe vera* gel applied twice a day can reduce inflammation. Skin care products containing *vitamin K, Perilla and/or caper extracts* and designed for use in rosacea (e.g. Kalme) are also available.

Note: If rosacea is suspected it is important to seek medical advice as scarring can develop if the condition is left untreated.

See also: **Aloe vera, Digestive enzymes, Grapeseed, Oregano oil, Vitamin B2.**

Do not take supplements if you are pregnant, breast-feeding, or taking prescribed drugs without first seeking advice from a pharmacist about possible interactions or adverse effects.

Scars

Scars are formed as a part of the body's natural healing process in which damaged areas of skin are replaced by collagen-rich scar tissue. This is initially pink but eventually shrinks to form a much paler scar.

Treatment

Vitamin C is needed for collagen formation and will encourage scars to heal, while evening primrose oil helps to improve tissue suppleness.

Rosa mosqueta oil is an exceptionally rich source of the essential fatty acid GLA, which is also found in *evening primrose oil*. When applied to scar tissue, anecdotal evidence suggests that it is highly effective in improving the cosmetic appearance.

Vitamin E tablets help to reduce inflammation and encourage healing and vitamin E cream may be rubbed in to soften new scar tissue.

The herb *gotu kola* may also be used externally to improve healing of wounds, chronic ulcers and excess scar tissue. It seems to act directly on fibre-producing cells to improve the quality and texture of the underlying tissues.

The appearance of scars – even those that are 20 years old – can be helped by applying colloidal silicone dressings that help to flatten, soften and fade red and raised scars.

See also: **Aloe vera, Gotu kola**.

Sciatica

See: **Back pain**.

Seasonal affective disorder

Seasonal affective disorder (SAD) is a form of depression that comes on in winter months, when exposure to natural sunlight is reduced. It affects an estimated 5 per cent of the population, with another 10 per cent experiencing a milder form known as sub-syndromal SAD. Shift workers are particularly susceptible to SAD.

Symptoms include winter tearfulness and depression, lethargy, sleepiness, carbohydrate cravings and a general slowing up. SAD is diagnosed when someone has experienced three winters of symptoms (November to March), two of which are consecutive, with remission during the summer months. In sub-syndromal SAD, symptoms appear from January to March.

The exact cause of SAD is unknown, but it is linked with changes in the secretion of various hormones and brain chemicals which are triggered as the days draw in and exposure to natural sunlight is reduced. These changes may involve an increased sensitivity to a natural sedative hormone, melatonin, which is produced by the pineal gland in the brain. During daylight hours, little melatonin is made so you feel energetic and alert. During darkness, larger quantities of melatonin are made so you naturally slow down and tend to feel more sleepy. As days shorten and nights lengthen during late autumn and early winter, overall melatonin secretion tends to go up. This cannot be the sole cause of SAD, however, as symptoms do not consistently respond to drug treatment designed to suppress secretion of melatonin hormone. Seasonal variations in the secretion of the neurotransmitter, serotonin, thyroid stimulating hormone (TSH), and the get-up-and-go hormone, adrenaline, may also be involved. Recently a genetic link between the presence of a particular gene, DRD4, has also been associated with seasonal patterns of weight gain and binge eating.

Treatment

As SAD is linked with lack of sunlight, symptoms are often improved by using a special light box that emits bright, cool white fluorescent light (2500 lux) similar to natural daylight. The box can be set up near your bed and timed to come on with increasing brightness before you wake to simulate a natural dawn. This fools the pineal gland into thinking spring has arrived, so melatonin secretion goes down, your mood increases and sleepiness and lethargy improve – usually within a week or two. Try to get up early rather than lying in bed (which will increase feelings of lethargy). Get out into the open air for exercise as much as possible, and eat little and often during the day.

Follow a low-glycaemic diet concentrating on wholegrain cereals, root vegetables, legumes, fruit, vegetables, oily fish and cheese – the later two foodstuffs contain tryptophan, a substance needed to make serotonin in the brain.

Aim to drink plenty of fluids during the day – especially mineral water or herbal teas – and eat little and often rather than having three traditional large meals a day.

Reduce intakes of alcohol, salt and caffeine.

Take a multivitamin and mineral supplement plus *co-enzyme Q10* which can boost energy levels.

St John's Wort is an effective herbal treatment for mild to moderate depression. Trials involving St John's Wort found that it was just as effective in treating SAD when used alone as when combined with light box therapy. It lowers levels of stress hormones (e.g. cortisol) and increases production of melatonin hormone to improve sleep.

5-HTP provides building blocks for making serotonin (5-HT) and melatonin and can lift a low mood. It also improves the architecture of sleep, so you are more likely to wake up feeling refreshed.

Omega-3 fish oils contain long-chain polyunsaturated fatty acids (DHA and EPA) which play an important structural and functional role within the brain. Epidemiologists have found a direct relationship between the amount of fish eaten within a population and the level of depressive illness experienced. Clinical trials suggest that intakes of 2 g omega-3 fatty acids can improve symptoms of depression, prolong periods of remission from depressive episodes, and improve the short-term course of the illness in those affected.

See also: **St John's Wort**.

Do not take supplements if you are pregnant, breast-feeding, or taking prescribed drugs without first seeking advice from a pharmacist about possible interactions or adverse effects.

Shaving rash

Sycosis barbae – or barber's itch – is a bacterial infection of hair follicles. Unfortunately, shaving can perpetuate the folliculitis by nicking off the tops of healing pustules and encouraging hair to grow back into the skin. If not treated adequately it can lead to small, white scars.

Treatment
Usual advice for men with frequent recurrences is to grow a beard, clip facial hair short with nail scissors (and go for a designer look) or to use a depilatory cream designed for facial hair once the infection has cleared with antibiotics.

Soothing creams or lotions containing calendula, *evening primrose* or *aloe vera* gel applied topically can help. Tea tree oil is a useful skin antiseptic with a gentle action.

A supplement such as *Siberian ginseng, propolis* or *Echinacea* that can boost general immunity may also help, and antioxidants will reduce inflammation.

Shingles

Shingles can affect anyone who has previously been exposed to the chicken pox virus, *Varicella zoster*. During the initial attack of chickenpox, the virus enters the nervous system and lies dormant in the roots of most sensory nerves. The virus can stay in this latent state for years without causing problems, but can occasionally reactivate, travelling back down the nerve to cause an attack of shingles localized to the area of skin supplied by that nerve.

Shingles is contagious as the fluid-filled blisters are teeming with viral particles which means that other people – particularly children – who are not immune to the virus may develop chickenpox if exposed to the blister fluid. Adults who have never had chickenpox should avoid contact with anyone who has either chickenpox or

---

Do not take supplements if you are pregnant, breast-feeding, or taking prescribed drugs without first seeking advice from a pharmacist about possible interactions or adverse effects.

shingles. This is especially important for non-immune pregnant women as the chickenpox virus can cause serious birth defects known as *Varicella* syndrome particularly during the first three months of pregnancy. If a non-immune pregnant woman is exposed to chickenpox or shingles, it is vital to seek immediate medical advice as treatment with *Varicella-zoster* immunoglobulin and/or anti-viral drugs may be needed.

Treatment
Several supplements can help in the treatment of shingles. Antioxidants such as high-dose *vitamin C, vitamin E* or *olive leaf* extract are usually taken to help reduce inflammation. (Vitamin E might also help to reduce any pain – perhaps by stabilizing the nerve cell membrane – while olive leaf extracts also have a powerful anti-viral action.)

Herbal extracts that boost immunity against viral infections include *Echinacea, cat's claw, goldenseal* and *reishi*.

One in ten people with shingles subsequently develops post-herpetic neuralgia with unpleasant burning, shooting or gnawing pains for several months or even years afterwards. Axsain cream – a prescription-only treatment containing capsaicin, derived from chilli peppers (cayenne), may help. When rubbed sparingly into the skin, it sinks in to relieve post-herpetic neuralgia by blocking the passage of pain messages.

St John's Wort or *5-HTP* can help to relieve the depression that, not surprisingly, often accompanies post-herpetic neuralgia.

See also: **Aloe vera, Goldenseal, Olive leaf, Reishi, Vitamin A**.
Related entry: **Herpes simplex**.

Sinusitis

Sinusitis is an infection or inflammation of the air-filled sinus cavities surrounding the nose. There are four pairs of sinuses: the frontal sinuses over your eyes; the ethmoids between your eyes; the

---

sphenoids in the upper part of your nose behind your eyes; and the maxillary sinuses inside your cheekbones. These help to lighten the bones of the skull and improve the resonance of your voice. They also act as a safety 'crumple zone' to absorb blows to the face.

The sinuses are lined by a membrane that secretes a thin watery fluid. When this becomes inflamed, it swells and mucus production increases. The narrow drainage channels from each sinus quickly become blocked to produce a stuffed up nose and nasal voice. If secretions remain trapped, pressure will build up with throbbing pain between the eyes, in the cheeks, headache and/or pain in the upper teeth. There may be tenderness over the sinus with swelling and redness of overlying skin. You may also lose your sense of smell. If the infection is severe, pus will build up in the sinus and you will develop a fever. Some pus may drain out through the nose to cause increasing pain and a constant, nasal discharge that drips into the back of the nose. This triggers a cough and smells and tastes foul.

Sinusitis is a common complication of the common cold. Other causes of sinusitis include hay fever, facial injury, jumping feet first into water so that dirty fluids are forced up your nose, and dental abscess.

Prevention
If you are prone to recurrent sinus infections, avoid hot, dry centrally-heated atmospheres. Installing a humidifier may help.

Avoid cigarette smoke and other air pollutants.

Avoid diving in general, and swimming in chlorinated pools.

It may help to avoid alcohol which can cause sinus membranes to swell.

Use decongestant nose drops or inhalers before flying.

Treatment
Sinusitis is generally treated with antibiotics. Nasal decongestants reduce swelling and allow the trapped secretions to drain away. Fever and aching may be relieved by aspirin, paracetamol or combi-

---

nations of paracetamol, and codeine phosphate.

Nasal congestion can be relieved by plain steam inhalation, but adding essential oils such as menthol, eucalyptus, cinnamon, or pine will bring rapid relief.

Sip hot liquids and drink plenty of fluids. Warm compresses help to relieve facial pain. Stuffiness is often worse at night when lying down and you may find it easier to lie on the side that is least congested.

If congestion makes sleeping difficult, try using a nasal decongestant spray last thing at night.

One of the most effective herbal treatments for sinusitis is *Pelargonium sidoides*. Other helpful remedies include *Echinacea* and *olive leaf* extracts. *N-acetyl cysteine* helps to thin and disperse mucus.

See also: **Astragalus, Bromelain, Cat's claw, Echinacea, Goldenseal, N-acetyl cysteine, Olive leaf, Pelargonium sidoides, Schisandra**.

Smoking – quitting

Stopping smoking is one of the most powerful preventive health measures a smoker can take. Research shows that smokers are five times more likely to suffer a heart attack in their 30s and 40s than non-smokers, and that smoking related illnesses kill 40 per cent of smokers before they reach retirement. Non-smokers therefore tend to live at least six years longer than smokers.

Risks are directly related to the number of cigarettes smoked per day – for example, the increased risk of death due to carcinoma of the bronchus is approximately equal to the number of cigarettes smoked per day (i.e. two a day doubles the risk, 20 a day increases the risk 20-fold). Stopping smoking can reduce the risk of a heart attack by as much as 50–70 per cent within five years. Within ten years, quitting halves the initial risk of lung cancer and reduces the risk of a variety of other cancers (including mouth, throat, bladder)

---

to virtually normal. Twenty years after stopping smoking, the associated risks can be considered similar to those in non-smokers.

Quitting

Unfortunately, quitting smoking is easier said than done as nicotine is highly addictive, but here are some ideas.

- Nicotine replacement therapy, which helps to wean smokers off the drug slowly, can be more effective than will power alone. A controlled trial of smoking cessation involving 400 participants found that 26 per cent of those using nicotine inhalers were no longer smoking after four months compared with only 9 per cent using a placebo. After two years, the equivalent figures were 9.5 per cent and 3 per cent.
- Hypnosis helps one in three smokers to quit.
- Taking regular brisk exercise stimulates the release of brain chemicals that can also curb nicotine cravings.
- Wild oats (oatstraw, also known as *Avena sativa*) have been used to reduce cravings, and are also a good source of B group vitamins which are needed in extra amounts during times of stress.
- Sucking an artificial cigarette or herbal stick available from chemists can help when there is an urge to smoke. Alternatively, try home-made carrot and celery sticks, apple slices, sunflower seeds or liquorice roots.

St John's Wort and *Rhodiola* are both helpful for reducing cravings when giving up smoking. Antioxidants are important to help protect against the damaging effects of free radicals liberated while smoking.

See also: **N-acetyl cysteine, Pine bark**.

Sore throat

More than one in four adults develops a sore throat each year, and it is one of the most common reasons for people to visit their doctor.

Do not take supplements if you are pregnant, breast-feeding, or taking prescribed drugs without first seeking advice from a pharmacist about possible interactions or adverse effects.

At least seven out of ten sore throats are due to a viral infection, however, and as antibiotics only work against bacteria, they are ineffective for viral sore throats. Sometimes, a persistent sore throat is due to infection with haemolytic streptococcal bacteria, and a swab will identify when antibiotics are needed.

Treatment

All but the most severe sore throats can be self-treated. Medical advice is usually only needed if a sore throat has lasted for longer than five days, is severely painful or accompanied by swelling, fever, hoarse voice, or difficulty in swallowing or breathing.

In a randomized trial, over 700 patients with sore throats received either a ten-day course of antibiotics, no treatment, or an antibiotic prescription to be used only if symptoms were no better after three days. Researchers found no difference in the incidence of complications between the three groups and less than a third of those given post-dated prescriptions decided to use them. Those given antibiotics immediately were more likely to return to the surgery next time they had a sore throat, however, rather than treating themselves appropriately at home.

At the first sign of a sore throat, take 1 g *vitamin C* three times a day, and suck a lozenge containing *zinc* gluconate every two hours while awake. Products containing *Pelargonium sidoides, Echinacea, garlic* and/or *propolis* are also effective.

Slippery elm or *liquorice* (DGL form) lozenges will help to soothe a sore throat, while steam inhalations are helpful at night to ease dryness and improve sleep. *Olive leaf extracts* are also helpful.

See also: **Myrrh, Liquorice, Eucalyptus, Pelargonium sidoides, Vitamin B2, Zinc.**

Sperm count – low

There is some concern that male sperm counts are falling, possibly due to increased exposure to environmental oestrogens.

Treatment

Alcohol, even in moderate amounts, is linked with 40 per cent of male infertility, so men planning to father a child should ideally try to avoid it altogether. In one study of men with low sperm counts, half returned to normal values within three months of avoiding alcohol completely.

Wearing tight, bikini-type briefs – especially those made from man-made fibres – can reduce sperm counts by as much as 20 per cent, sperm motility by as much as 21 per cent and semen volume by up to 12 per cent due to the damaging effects of excess heat and static electricity. Wear loose, cotton boxer shorts instead.

It takes an average of 100 days for a primitive sperm cell to mature and be ejaculated. An estimated 40 per cent of sperm damage occurring during this time is due to free radicals. Antioxidants neutralize free radicals and *vitamin C* (500 mg twice a day) has been shown to increase sperm count by 34 per cent, reduce sperm clumping by 67 per cent and reduce the number of abnormal sperm by 33 per cent. High-dose *vitamin E* (600 mg a day for three months) also improves sperm function – especially the binding of sperm to egg. In one study, 21 per cent of men taking vitamin E successfully fathered a child.

Zinc (15 mg a day) seems to prevent premature release of chemicals in the sperm head needed to drill through the egg during fertilization.

Folic acid is also important for rapidly dividing cells, while *selenium* helps to reduce oxidative damage to sperm.

See also: **Arginine, Astralagus, Carnitine, Chromium, Coenzyme Q10, Ginseng, Maca, Selenium, Vitamin C, Zinc**.

Related entry: **Conception**.

Splits in fingers

Painful splits in fingers are similar to chilblains and are thought to be triggered by reduced circulation, such as when small arteries go

---

into spasm on exposure to cold. This reduces the flow of oxygen and nutrients to tissues.

Treatment

Take *evening primrose oil* supplements and apply *aloe vera* gel to help soothe itching. Hands should also be massaged with an intensive care moisturizing cream.

Supplements containing *garlic, ginkgo* and *ginger* help to improve circulation to the fingers and have a natural warming action.

Inflammation may be reduced by taking *vitamin C* with bioflavonoids, and/or *omega-3 fish oils*.

Regular exercise is important. Wear gloves when going out in cold weather. Applying 'artificial skin' type lotions that dry to cover and protect lesions will help. Some people find tissue glue (similar to superglue) helpful.

Related entry: **Chilblains**.

Stress

A certain amount of pressure is beneficial and helps to generate the energy and reserves needed to meet life's challenges. Once pressure falls outside the range with which you feel able to cope, however, it leads to the unpleasant physical and emotional symptoms associated with distress. Stress results from increased circulating levels of adrenal gland hormones: adrenaline and cortisol. These put your body on red alert so your:

- Blood glucose level rises to provide instant energy
- Pupils dilate so your field of vision increases
- Bowels, bladder (and sometimes stomach) empty so you are lighter for running
- Circulation to the gut shuts down, so more blood is diverted to your muscles

---

Do not take supplements if you are pregnant, breast-feeding, or taking prescribed drugs without first seeking advice from a pharmacist about possible interactions or adverse effects.

- Pulse and blood pressure go up, and you breathe more deeply to increase blood and oxygen supply to muscles and brain
- Memory and ability to think straight improves
- Sensitivity to pain is reduced.

This helped our ancestors to survive by preparing the body for vigorous exercise when fighting or fleeing from dangerous situations. Nowadays, we rarely need to fight or flee, and the effects of stress hormones build up inside rather than getting burned off through physical activity. Persistently raised stress hormones can cause a number of symptoms, including:

- Sweating and flushing
- Racing pulse and palpitations
- Dizziness, faintness, trembling
- Pins and needles, numbness
- Nausea, nervous diarrhoea
- Tension headache
- Insomnia, bad dreams, tiredness
- Poor concentration and inability to make decisions
- Depression, anxiety and panic attacks
- Loss of sex drive
- Reduced immunity.

This heightened state of arousal can eventually lead to physical and emotional burn out – the so-called 'nervous breakdown'. Stress also exacerbates pre-existing conditions such as asthma, eczema, psoriasis and irritable bowel syndrome, and contributes towards serious health problems such as glucose intolerance, high blood pressure, stroke, angina and heart attack. It is important to concentrate on breathing slowly and deeply when anxious to prevent over breathing (hyperventilation) which can trigger a panic attack.

Treatment
To help reduce the effects of stress, follow a low-glycaemic diet

---

Do not take supplements if you are pregnant, breast-feeding, or taking prescribed drugs without first seeking advice from a pharmacist about possible interactions or adverse effects.

supplying foods that have minimal impact on blood glucose levels. Eat little and often to help prevent blood glucose swings. Never skip meals, however busy you are – especially breakfast, which is important to replenish energy levels after your over-night fast. Try to avoid convenience foods which, although time-saving, are often nutrient-poor and contain excessive amounts of fat and sugar.

Vitamin C and *B vitamins* are rapidly used up in the metabolic reactions associated with the fight-or-flight response. Lack of B group vitamins can itself lead to anxiety and irritability, making symptoms worse. Stress also depletes the body of *calcium* and *magnesium* so a multivitamin and mineral supplement is a good idea. A *probiotic* to replenish immune-boosting bacteria in the gut is useful, too, especially when combined with a multivitamin supplement. This can reduce the chance of developing a cold during times of stress when resistance is low.

Drink plenty of water to reduce dehydration which can lead to tiredness, headache and poor concentration to make stress symptoms worse.

Limit your alcohol intake and, as the effects of caffeine mimic the stress response, have only one or two caffeinated drinks per day (switch to herbal teas such as antioxidant-rich rooibus, and to de-caffeinated coffee brands).

Omega-3 fish oils (DHA and EPA) play an important role in brain function and mood regulation. Eating fish regularly can lift a low mood and neutralize some of the effects of excessive stress by lowering stress hormone levels.

Korean ginseng supports adrenal gland function and helps you adapt to physical or emotional stress and fatigue. It is stimulating and restorative, improving physical and mental energy, stamina, strength and alertness. Ginseng combines particularly well with ginkgo biloba to improve memory and concentration.

Like ginseng, *Rhodiola* is an excellent remedy for anxiety, stress and related sleep problems as it also has an energizing action.

St John's Wort can reduce feelings of anxiety and lift mild to moderate depression.

Do not take supplements if you are pregnant, breast-feeding, or taking prescribed drugs without first seeking advice from a pharmacist about possible interactions or adverse effects.

5-HTP helps to raise a low mood, reduce anxiety and improve sleep. It may also help to control excessive food intake triggered by stress.

Valerian is one of the most relaxing natural herbs available and has significant, positive effects on stress. It helps to relieve anxiety and tension, induce sleep, ease smooth muscle spasm and promote calm. *Lemon balm* is an alternative, especially for exam-related stress in students.

Co-enzyme Q10 improves physical energy levels and endurance.

See also: **Adaptogens, Ashwagandha, Astragalus, Ginseng, Guarana, Holy basil, Lemon balm, Liquorice, Magnesium, Maitake, Muira puama, Oat straw, Pfaffia, Siberian ginseng, Reishi, Rhodiol, Schisandra, Valerian, Vitamin B1, Vitamin B5, Vitamin C, Vitamin E, Yerba maté**.

Related entry: **Panic attacks**.

Stye

A stye is a bacterial infection causing a small abscess at the edge of the eyelid. Despite its size, usually only a single sebaceous gland draining into one of the eyelash follicles is affected.

Treatment

The affected eyelash needs to be gently removed so that pus can drain away. Carefully pull it out with a pair of tweezers – don't squeeze the area or infection may spread. Then bathe the eye regularly with an infusion of chamomile, eyebright (*Euphrasia*) or marigold (*Calendula*). Applying a recently used camomile teabag as a compress works well.

An *antioxidant* supplement will help to reduce inflammation. Recurrent styes are not usually hereditary but may suggest low immunity. Taking *Echinacea* and a multivitamin and mineral supplement could help. If infection spreads or is associated with conjunctivitis, seek medical advice.

Do not take supplements if you are pregnant, breast-feeding, or taking prescribed drugs without first seeking advice from a pharmacist about possible interactions or adverse effects.

Sun allergy

Sun allergy, also known as polymorphic light eruption (PLE), affects up to 20 per cent of people and is especially common in young women. Symptoms include an itchy, raised red rash, blisters and the development of scaly plaques that appear within hours of sun exposure. Only skin directly exposed to the sun is affected, such as the backs of hands, lower arms, face and the V of the neck.

PLE is linked with sensitivity to UVA rays, rather than UVB. Some drugs and cosmetics can also sensitize skin to sunlight to trigger a light-sensitive rash. As UVA light is not filtered by glass it is still possible to develop PLE while sitting in a car or by a house window in the sun.

Treatment
Cover up with loose cotton clothes as much as possible, apply a broad-spectrum sunscreen which filters out both UVA and UVB light (check before buying as some sun blocks only filter out UVB rays and will be ineffective) and avoid, as far as possible, exposure to sunlight between 10 am and 4 pm when UVA rays are at their most intense.

Antioxidant supplements, especially those containing *selenium* and mixed *carotenoids*, may help to protect the skin. *Aloe vera* gel is soothing when applied to the skin rash.

See: **St John's Wort**

Swollen ankles

Some people find that their ankles swell in hot weather as this encourages dilation of the blood vessels under the skin as part of the body's cooling mechanism. However, this makes it easier for fluid to escape into the tissues. When the body is less active than normal (e.g. when travelling), this will contribute to swelling as the pumping action of leg muscles helps to draw fluid away from the ankles.

Do not take supplements if you are pregnant, breast-feeding, or taking prescribed drugs without first seeking advice from a pharmacist about possible interactions or adverse effects.

Treatment

Try to increase your level of physical activity wherever possible, and raise your feet up when sitting down. Light support stockings/tights can help but are uncomfortable in hot weather.

A natural approach to mild swollen ankles is to take extracts of a diuretic herb such as *dandelion*. Follow a low-fat, low-salt, high-fibre diet and drink plenty of fluids to prevent dehydration. Avoid alcohol which can dilate blood vessels to make swelling worse. Take supplements that reduce capillary swelling such as *pine bark* extracts (Pycnogenol®) or *red vine* leaf.

If swollen ankles persist, seek medical advice to rule out kidney or heart problems.

Note: Dandelion should not be taken during pregnancy or by anyone who has kidney problems.

See also: **Pine bark, Red vine leaf.**

Systemic lupus erythematosus (SLE)

See: **Lupus.**

Taste – loss of

Taste and smell sensation are closely linked. Loss of taste sensation – ageusia – is common after a bad cold when taste buds and smell receptors in the nose become blocked. Long-term problems may result from loss of taste buds with increasing age. One of the most common, reversible causes of ageusia is *zinc* deficiency. This is easily tested by obtaining a solution of zinc sulphate.

Treatment

If needed, take 10–15 mg zinc twice a day and retest after two weeks. This is best done under the supervision of a nutritionist as higher doses of zinc should ideally be taken together with other nutrients such as *vitamin E, selenium* and *copper*. Dietary sources of zinc include red meat, seafood, especially oysters, brewer's yeast, wholegrains, pulses and eggs. Smokers should do their utmost to quit.

See: **Zinc**.

Related entry: **Smoking – quitting**.

Thyroid gland – overactive

An overactive thyroid gland – known as hyperthyroidism or thyrotoxicosis – affects an estimated 2–5 per cent of women at any one time. The commonest cause is Grave's disease, an auto-immune condition in which thyroid-stimulating antibodies bind to thyroid cells and trigger over-production of thyroid hormones.

The symptoms of an overactive thyroid gland include weight loss, increased appetite, anxiety, irritability, restlessness, tiredness, weakness, rapid pulse and palpitations, sensitivity to heat, diarrhoea, period changes and loss of sex drive. The thyroid gland may also become enlarged (goitre). Extra symptoms may occur in Grave's disease due to the production of other antibodies that cause inflammation and swelling at the back of the eyes so they seem bulge, or which affect the skin to cause vitiligo in which there is a patchy loss of skin colour.

What triggers auto-antibody production in Grave's disease is unknown, but factors such as food allergy, hypersensitivity to mercury in dental fillings and stress have been suspected. Other causes of thyrotoxicosis include the development of overactive nodules in the thyroid gland, viral inflammation of the gland (thyroiditis) and excess production of thyroid stimulating hormone (TSH) from the pituitary gland in the brain.

Treatment

Several natural treatments are helpful in combination with orthodox treatment for thyrotoxicosis. These include calming herbs such as *valerian* or *Rhodiola* to help reduce the anxiety and nervousness.

Do not take supplements if you are pregnant, breast-feeding, or taking prescribed drugs without first seeking advice from a pharmacist about possible interactions or adverse effects.

Avoid iodized salt, and stimulants such as coffee, tea and other caffeinated drinks which speed up the metabolism. Try eating more cabbage-related vegetables (e.g. broccoli, Brussel sprouts, cabbage, cauliflower, kale) which suppress thyroid hormone production – they contain fluorine which blocks iodine receptors in the thyroid gland.

Because vitamins and minerals are used up more quickly by the increased metabolic rate, take a good multivitamin and mineral supplement, plus *evening primrose oil* and/or *omega-3 fish* oils.

Siberian or *Korean ginsengs* help the body adapt to stress and medical herbalists often recommend one or the other to complement thyroid treatment.

Note: Medical advice should be sought before taking supplements.

See also: **Oatstraw, Iodine, Kelp, Selenium, Vitamin B12, Vitamin B2**.

Thyroid gland – underactive

The thyroid gland in the neck produces iodine-containing hormones that help to regulate the body's metabolism. Around one in 100 people develops an underactive thyroid gland, a condition known as hypothyroidism. Symptoms include lack of energy, a general slowing down, muscle weakness, cramps, increasing weight, feeling the cold, dry skin, brittle hair, thickening of the ankles, slow pulse, heavy periods and a deepening voice which may seem slurred. Sometimes the thyroid gland enlarges to produce a swelling in the neck known as a goitre.

Most cases of hypothyroidism are due to an auto-immune condition in which the immune system makes antibodies aimed against thyroid tissues. Other cases result from treatment of an overactive thyroid gland or, in some parts of the world, from severe dietary deficiency of *iodine, selenium* or *zinc*. Smoking cigarettes has also been linked with an increased risk of developing hypothyroidism.

Do not take supplements if you are pregnant, breast-feeding, or taking prescribed drugs without first seeking advice from a pharmacist about possible interactions or adverse effects.

Treatment

Thyroxine replacement therapy is carefully titrated until blood tests result in stable thyroid function tests. The aim is to restore the level of thyroid-stimulating hormone (TSH – secreted by the pituitary gland in an attempt to kick-start the thyroid) to well within the normal range. Total thyroxine concentration is also measured although the normal range is wide (58–174 mmol/L). Some endocrinologists believe that complete well-being is only restored when thyroxine is towards the upper limit of normal, and the TSH level is slightly suppressed. However this is something that needs to be medically tailored to individual needs, minimizing the risk of side effects while at the same time optimizing the body's metabolic rate so that problems such as weight gain are reduced.

Following a diet free from sugar and refined foods can improve thyroid function. A vitamin and mineral supplement including *iodine, selenium* and *zinc* is often recommended.

Siberian or *Korean ginsengs* help the body to adapt to stress, and medical herbalists often recommend one or the other to complement thyroid treatments.

Kelp may be suggested as a naturally rich source of *iodine* where an underactive thyroid is thought to be linked with low iodine intake. Only eat small amounts of cabbage, cauliflower, spinach, Brussel sprouts, broccoli, turnips, soy and other beans as these contain substances known as goitrogens (goitre forming) that interfere with the action of iodine and can make symptoms worse.

See also: **Oatstraw, Iodine, Kelp, Selenium, Vitamin B12, Vitamin B2**.

Tinnitus

Tinnitus is a constant, unpleasant, ringing, buzzing, hissing or whistling sensation in one or both ears. Its causes are ill understood, but it may be related to abnormal blood flow to the inner ear in some cases, or to damage to the inner ear in others.

It is important to rule out treatable causes such as a build-up of wax in the ears or side effects associated with some drugs, especially high-dose aspirin or quinine.

Treatment
Unfortunately, tinnitus is often difficult to treat. Dietary changes such as reducing intakes of salt, refined sugar and carbohydrates, meats, saturated fats and increasing intakes of fruit and vegetables have helped some sufferers, as has losing excess weight. In severe cases, a specialist may recommend a tinnitus masker that plays a random mixture of sounds at differing frequencies (white noise) to help block out noise.

Extracts of *ginkgo biloba* improve circulation to the brain and have been found helpful in some cases. Some studies have found no benefits however.

Other supplements that may be suggested include *garlic, B vitamins*, especially *B12, magnesium* and *zinc* for their importance in nerve health. An acupressure technique worth trying is to massage the area one finger's width in front of the ear at the top of the cheekbone.

See also: **Ginkgo, Vitamin B12**.

Tiredness all the time

Tiredness all the time, and lack of energy, are common problems, yet only around one in five cases is linked with an identifiable medical cause such as anaemia, underactive thyroid gland, immune disorders or abnormalities of the internal organs. Many cases are undoubtedly linked with stress, overwork, lack of exercise, dietary deficiencies or mild depression.

Treatment
Ensure you obtain adequate sleep and time for rest and relaxation.

Follow a low-fat, high-fibre diet with plenty of fresh fruit and

---

Do not take supplements if you are pregnant, breast-feeding, or taking prescribed drugs without first seeking advice from a pharmacist about possible interactions or adverse effects.

vegetables. Around half your daily energy intake should ideally be in the form of unrefined carbohydrates such as wholegrain cereals, wholemeal bread, wholewheat pasta and brown rice.

While diet should always come first, also consider taking an A to Z multivitamin and mineral supplement. Preliminary evidence suggests that *B vitamin* status, especially pyridoxine (*vitamin B6*), is low in some people with chronic fatigue and it is worth adding in a vitamin B complex to see if this helps.

If lack of energy is due to stress, an adaptogen such as *Siberian* or *Korean ginseng* may be helpful in supporting adrenal gland function.

If fatigue is linked with low mood, *St John's Wort* or *5-HTP* is often effective.

Evening primrose oil has also been shown to benefit 70–80 per cent of people suffering from long-term fatigue.

As a more gentle, buffered caffeine substitute, *guarana* is useful for a short-term energy boost.

Other supplements useful for lack of energy include: *essential fatty acids* (high-dose evening primrose, omega-3 or flaxseed oils); *co-enzyme Q10; kelp* or other iodine sources (needed for production of thyroid hormones, and often lacking in the diet due to lower intakes of iodized salt, fish etc); *alpha-lipoic acid; bee products – royal jelly; biotin, gotu kola, iron, magnesium, muira puama, oatstraw, pfaffia, reishi, Rhodiola, Schisandra, wheatgrass, yerba maté.*

Lack of energy can be a presenting sign of a number of different medical conditions so if it is persistent or troublesome, always seek advice from your doctor.

See also: **Aloe vera, Alpha-lipoic acid, Carnitin, Goldenseal, 5-HTP, Liquorice, Magnesium, Maitake, Olive leaf, Oregano oil, Pfaffia, Shiitake, Vitamin B2, Vitamin B5, Vitamin B6, Vitamin D.**

Related entry: **Chronic fatigue syndrome**.

Do not take supplements if you are pregnant, breast-feeding, or taking prescribed drugs without first seeking advice from a pharmacist about possible interactions or adverse effects.

Ulcerative colitis

Ulcerative colitis is an inflammatory bowel disease in which the lining of the bowel (colon and rectum) becomes inflamed and ulcerated. It affects around one in 1,000 people and is most common in those aged between 20 and 40. Women are more frequently affected than men.

The main symptom is blood-stained diarrhoea which may also contain pus and mucus. In severe attacks fever, abdominal pain and feelings of being quite unwell can also occur. Attacks tend to come on every few months although some sufferers find that their symptoms are infrequent while others have continuous problems.

The exact cause of ulcerative colitis is unknown but hereditary factors, poor circulation of blood to the gut, abnormal bowel fermentation and abnormal immune function have been suggested. Avoiding foods that seem to provoke attacks can reduce symptoms. Some people find that they are sensitive to dairy and wheat produce, or that following a gluten-free diet is beneficial, but no foods consistently provoke symptoms in all sufferers.

Treatment

Researchers have found a way to link the food and drinks consumed by people with ulcerative colitis with the appearance of their bowel lining, using a special telescope (sigmoidoscopy). This has allowed them to pinpoint the food and drinks most likely to be associated with active symptoms. They found that foods containing sulphites (added as a preservative) or caffeine may be important triggers, as per the table opposite.

Other researchers also found that people with ulcerative colitis are most likely to relapse if they have a high intake of red and processed meat, protein, alcohol and sulphur-rich foods.

Sulphites (and caffeine) interfere with the action of *vitamin B1* (thiamin), which is an important nutrient for friendly, digestive bacteria (*probiotics*). Some sulphur compounds (e.g. hydrogen sulphide) have also been shown to damage the bowel lining and

Do not take supplements if you are pregnant, breast-feeding, or taking prescribed drugs without first seeking advice from a pharmacist about possible interactions or adverse effects.

Foods linked with active ulcerative colitis	Foods not associated with ulcerative colitis
Burgers, sausages and other preserved meats (except organic non sulphited products)	Pork, bacon
Beer (except German beer, which is sulphite free), lager	Beef, beef products
Red and white wine	Fish
Sulphite-containing soft drinks, e.g. fruit squash made from concentrates	Raw apples, pears, bananas, citrus fruits, melon
Coffee (except de-caffeinated brands)	Milk, yoghurt, cheese
Prawns, scampi, shellfish (sulphited)	Soup (home-made, not tinned or dried)
Dried fruit and vegetables (sulphited)	Breakfast cereals
Processed fruit pies and fruit cakes	Lettuce, tomatoes, potatoes, peas, beans
Foods containing sulphites (see separate sulphite box)	
Foods containing the sulphur-rich seaweed, carrageenan (Irish Moss, E407)	

Also avoid the food additives, numbered from E220 to E229, which are reserved for sulphites.

E220 sulphur dioxide
E221 sodium sulphite
E222 sodium bisulphite (sodium hydrogen sulphite)
E223 sodium metabisulphite
E224 potassium metabisulphite
E225 potassium sulphite
E226 calcium sulphite
E227 calcium hydrogen sulphite
E228 potassium hydrogen sulphite

NB: Sulphur and sulphites may be spelled as sulfur or sulfites on labels

Do not take supplements if you are pregnant, breast-feeding, or taking prescribed drugs without first seeking advice from a pharmacist about possible interactions or adverse effects.

produce changes similar to those seen in ulcerative colitis. Although the bowel is usually able to detoxify these sulphur substances, this ability may be reduced in people with ulcerative colitis, some of whom have higher than normal levels of sulphur compounds in their bowel.

Although this is by no means proven, you may benefit from reducing your intake of sulphur-rich foods to see if this helps improve your symptoms.

In addition, there may be a link between ulcerative colitis and coeliac/celiac disease – an auto-immune condition caused by a reaction to gliadin, a small protein found in wheat gluten. Similar small proteins are found in rye and barley. Although this is not proven, you may benefit from trying a gluten-free diet if other dietary approaches have not helped. A gluten-free diet is best followed under the supervision of a dietician or other healthcare professional.

Probiotic bacteria produce beneficial substances such as butyrate. Butyrate is a short fatty acid that acts as a 'food' for bowel lining cells (colonocytes). Abnormal metabolism of butyrate has been suggested as a possible cause of ulcerative colitis. Butyrate levels are reduced by the action of sulphur compounds in the bowel (one reason why sulphur-rich foods may worsen ulcerative colitis symptoms). By helping to maintain butyrate levels, probiotic bacteria may have a beneficial role to play in inflammatory bowel disease.

The number of probiotic bacteria in the bowel can be improved by eating resistant fibre, such as that found in oat bran and *psyllium* seed (Plantago ovatum, also known as ispaghula). This type of fibre (sometimes referred to as prebiotics) is not digested by humans, but can be used by probiotic bacteria to fuel their growth in the colon.

Omega-3 fish oils help to reduce inflammation in the body and may have a beneficial effect on inflammatory bowel diseases. In a small trial, those taking fish oil extracts (equivalent to EPA 3.2 g and DHA 2.4 g daily) for six months showed significant improvements compared with those taking an inactive placebo.

People with inflammatory bowel disease are at risk of a number of vitamin and mineral deficiencies. This is partly because they may follow a restricted diet, and partly because bowel inflammation can reduce absorption of some nutrients. As a result, even people with newly diagnosed IBD may have low levels of *riboflavin (B2), folate, betacarotene, vitamin B12, calcium, phosphorus, magnesium, selenium, zinc* and *vitamin D*. A multivitamin and mineral supplement is therefore important.

As well as regulating *calcium* absorption, *vitamin D* may also regulate immune responses linked with IBD making it important to avoid deficiency of this nutrient. Lack of the B vitamin, folate (*folic acid*), has also been linked with an increased risk of developing colorectal cancer in people with ulcerative colitis.

Inflammatory bowel disease has been linked with reduced activity of an enzyme, glucosamine synthetase, that is involved in bowel wall repair. Taking *N-acetyl glucosamine* supplements has shown benefit in some studies. Do not take glucosamine sulphate (the more common form) which is a sulphur source.

See also: **Aloe vera, Boswellia, Bromelain, Fibre, Probiotics, Turmeric, Vitamin B12**.

Vaginitis

Vaginitis is an inflammation of the vagina and, usually, the vulva. This may be due to a bacterial, viral or fungal infection, to allergy, a skin disease such as eczema or psoriasis, or to lack of oestrogen. Symptoms, which may include local pain, soreness, itching, discharge and painful intercourse, should be checked by a doctor – preferably in a genito-urinary medicine clinic – for a diagnosis.

Treatment
Wear cotton rather than synthetic underwear, and avoid tight clothing as becoming hot and sweaty makes itching worse. Avoid soap, shower gel and bubble bath – only use fragrance-free bath additives; those designed to treat eczema or new born babies are

---

Do not take supplements if you are pregnant, breast-feeding, or taking prescribed drugs without first seeking advice from a pharmacist about possible interactions or adverse effects.

preferable. Replenishing washes containing lactic acid (e.g. Lactacyd) are helpful and will soothe the vulval area as well as discouraging infection.

Taking *isoflavones* can improve lubrication where dryness is associated with menopause.

Evening primrose oil is helpful in reducing itching and scaling associated with eczema and may be taken by mouth and applied locally to affected areas.

Aloe vera gel is often helpful when applied to the vulva and has a soothing, anti-inflammatory action. *Omega-3 fish oils* can also help when taken by mouth.

Varicose eczema

Varicose, or stasis, eczema is usually associated with varicose veins and oedema. It occurs when blood circulation through tissues in the lower leg is compromised and may progress to venous ulceration. Varicose eczema causes dry, scaly, flaky, discoloured skin around the ankle.

Treatment
It is important to control ankle swelling by wearing elasticated support stockings or tights which must be properly fitted by a pharmacist. Stockings or tights need to be put on first thing in the morning before getting out of bed for best results.

Regular exercise, such as walking, is important. Standing still for long periods of time should be avoided, and feet should be elevated as often as possible.

Gently massage the skin daily with a moisturizing cream to help stimulate the circulation and improve scaliness. Various emollients and bath preparations are available on prescription or over the counter.

Evening primrose oil (massaged directly into affected skin) and

---

Do not take supplements if you are pregnant, breast-feeding, or taking prescribed drugs without first seeking advice from a pharmacist about possible interactions or adverse effects.

taken orally often reduces itching although it can take a few months for a noticeable improvement to occur.

Aloe vera gel applied to the skin will help to reduce inflammation. Horse chestnut preparations are also used to help to strengthen tissues surrounding blood vessels and reduce leakage of fluid.

Leg swelling associated with venous ulcers may improve when taking *pine bark* extracts (Pycnogenol®) or *red vine leaf* extracts which have a beneficial effect on leg capillaries to reduce leakage of fluid into the tissues.

Garlic, ginkgo biloba or *omega-3 fish oils* help to improve blood flow through the peripheral circulation and may help to reduce the risk of leg ulceration.

See also: **Gotu kola, Red vine leaf**.

Related entries: **Leg ulcers, Varicose veins**.

Varicose veins

Varicose veins are one of the prices we pay for walking on two legs rather than four. The long veins in the legs contain a series of valves that allow blood to flow upwards against gravity. Weak valves often give way so that blood pools in superficial veins which become dilated and twisted.

Varicose veins tend to affect more women than men. They may be hereditary or triggered by pregnancy or overweight. Symptoms include bulging, tortuous veins, aching and dragging sensations, swelling of the ankles and itching.

Treatment
Support stockings help to keep varicose veins comfortable. Other self-help measures include losing any excess weight, walking regularly and avoiding standing still for long in order to boost circulation in the legs. Elevate feet as often as possible.

The skin over leg varicose veins should be massaged daily with moisturizing cream. Extracts of *pine bark* (Pycnogenol®), *red vine*

Do not take supplements if you are pregnant, breast-feeding, or taking prescribed drugs without first seeking advice from a pharmacist about possible interactions or adverse effects.

leaf, horsechestnut or *gotu kola* can strengthen tissues surrounding blood vessels and reduce discomfort of varicose veins.

Omega-3 fish oils, garlic, ginkgo biloba extracts or a Tibetan herbal blend, Padma 28, help to improve blood flow through the peripheral circulation. *Co-enzyme Q10* increases oxygen uptake of cells and can also reduce leg discomfort.

See also: **Anthocyanins, Bilberry, Gotu kola, Grapeseed, Horsechestnut, Pine bark, Red vine leaf**.

Related entry: **Varicose eczema**.

Warts and verrucas

Common warts are caused by infection with a skin virus – human papillomavirus (HPV) – of which over 60 different types are known. Warts usually affect areas of skin prone to injury such as the hands, elbows, face, knees and scalp. Those on the soles of the feet become flattened by the weight of the body to form painful verrucas. These tend to grow quickly and can spread through wet, macerated skin to form multiple, superficial lesions known as mosaic warts. Black threads that may form in the centre of the verruca are clotted blood vessels (capillaries) not roots as commonly believed. Warts are highly contagious and often appear in crops, especially in children.

Treatment
Half of sufferers find that their warts naturally disappear on their own within a year without treatment – that's why many folk remedies (such as buying them for a penny, or rubbing with a piece of meat which is then buried in the garden) often seem to work.

Applying vitamin E oil directly to the wart and covering with a waterproof plaster (repeat twice or three times a day) often seems to work, although it may take several weeks. Alternatively, tea tree and garlic oil may be mixed together and applied regularly until the wart dries. Only a tiny amount of garlic should be used at first, as some people develop a painful reaction to this treatment. Surrounding skin should be protected with petroleum jelly and the oil applied only to the area of hardened, raised skin. Cover with a plaster for 24 hours.

Taking *Echinacea, astragalus, goldenseal* or *garlic* extracts will help to boost immunity against viral infections. High-dose anti-oxidants such as *vitamin C, vitamin E* and *carotenoids* may also help to reduce wart growth.

Warts and verrucas can be frozen at home by 'freezing' products which are available in pharmacies, or by applying wart-dissolving gels and plasters.

Note: Genital warts should never be treated at home; always seek medical advice from a doctor or genito-urinary medicine clinic.

See also: **Lapacho, Oregano oil.**

Weight gain

Middle-aged spread commonly strikes after the age of 35 due to changes in both physiology and lifestyle. The most significant change is loss of lean muscle tissue, which is mostly replaced with fat. Between the ages of 25 and 70, the average woman loses 5 kg (11 lb) of muscle and her average body fat increases from 27 to 40 per cent. Over the same period, men lose around 10 kg (22 lb) muscle and their body fat increases from 20 to 30 per cent. As muscle cells burn more energy than fat, the resting metabolic rate slows by around 5 per cent for every ten years after the age 25. By the time a woman is 75, she needs around 300 kcals less per day than when she was 18, and 130 kcals per day less than when she was 50.

Treatment
Unfortunately, cutting back on energy intake, and increasing your level of physical activity are the only ways to lose weight. Many different types of weight loss diet exist, including:

- Low-calorie diets which typically provide 1000–1500 kcals energy per day

---

Do not take supplements if you are pregnant, breast-feeding, or taking prescribed drugs without first seeking advice from a pharmacist about possible interactions or adverse effects.

- Very-low-calorie diets which provide between 400–1000 kcals per day
- Low-fat diets that typically provide less than 30 per cent or less of daily energy in the form of fat
- Low-carbohydrate diets, which tend to provide 20–120 g carbohydrate daily
- Low-glycaemic-index diets which reduce intakes of refined carbohydrate and recommend wholegrain foods that have less impact on blood glucose levels
- Mediterranean-style diets featuring fruit, vegetables, wholegrain cereals, beans, nuts, seeds, fish and olive oil.

Unfortunately, there is a lack of agreement about which is the most effective type of weight-loss diet. A recent review of the evidence found that overweight and obese people following a low-glycaemic-index diet lost more weight and had more improvement in blood cholesterol levels than those following other types of diet, whether their calorie intake was also restricted, or whether they were allowed to eat as much as they wished. The overall conclusion was that following a low-glycaemic diet is an effective method of promoting weight loss that can be simply incorporated into a person's lifestyle.

Another recent trial, involving over 300 moderately obese people compared the effects of following three different types of diet for two years: a low-fat, restricted-calorie diet, a Mediterranean-style, restricted-calorie diet or a low-carbohydrate diet in which calorie intake was not restricted. The average weight loss was 2.9 kg for the low-fat group, 4.4 kg for the Mediterranean-diet group, and 4.7 kg for the low-carbohydrate group. The researchers concluded that the Mediterranean and low-carbohydrate diets may be effective alternatives to low-fat diets.

Exercise helps by increasing your metabolic rate (as much as tenfold), mobilizing fatty acids from fat cells and increasing the burning of fatty acids as fuel in muscle cells. Exercise replaces flab with denser muscle. In one study, middle-aged people following a two-month walking programme building up from two 15-minute

Do not take supplements if you are pregnant, breast-feeding, or taking prescribed drugs without first seeking advice from a pharmacist about possible interactions or adverse effects.

sessions a week to two hours weekly lost a total of four inches off their waist, hips and thighs even though they ate the same as before.

Research has also shown that prolonged brisk walking will cause blood fat levels to rise much less than usual after eating because dietary fats are rapidly burned for fuel rather than added to fat stores. Aim to exercise briskly (e.g. brisk walking, swimming, cycling, jogging, gym work) for at least half an hour every day, starting off slowly and increasing effort as fitness levels rise.

Chromium is needed in minute amounts to form an organic complex known as Glucose Tolerance Factor (GTF). This encourages the production of energy from glucose, and lowers blood fat levels, including harmful LDL-cholesterol. It may also suppress hunger pangs through a direct effect on the satiety centre in the brain.

Conjugated linoleic acid (CLA) is a fatty acid that helps to regulate enzymes involved in the mobilization and transport of dietary fats so that less fat is laid down in fatty tissues, and more is transported to muscle cells. Because it affects the body's ratio of lean to fatty tissue, people taking it often experience a reduction in waist size (average loss of 1.6 inches in one study) even when they do not make any other changes to their diet or lifestyle.

Hydroxycitric acid (HCA) is a fruit acid originally derived from the rind of an exotic fruit (*Garcinia cambogia*) that curbs appetite and blocks an enzyme responsible for converting excess dietary carbohydrate and protein into fat. Excess carbohydrate is diverted into the production of glycogen – a starchy, muscle energy store instead. In a placebo-controlled study, 50 overweight adults took either HCA in varying doses, or a placebo, and were instructed not to change their normal dietary lifestyle. After four weeks, the body weight of those in the placebo group had increased by an average of 1.3 kg, while those taking HCA had reduced by between 2.2 and 5.5 kg directly related to the daily dose of HCA taken. Subjective evaluation of appetite levels showed considerable reduction in those taking HCA, but not in the placebo group.

Chitosan is a fibre supplement derived from shellfish (crabs,

---

Do not take supplements if you are pregnant, breast-feeding, or taking prescribed drugs without first seeking advice from a pharmacist about possible interactions or adverse effects.

shrimps) to bind 12 times its own weight of dietary fat when taken with meals, so that less is absorbed and more is excreted. Evidence that it works is contradictory, however.

A blend of three Amazonian plants, *guarana, damiana* and *yerba maté* (Zotrim), slows the rate of stomach emptying to help reduce food intake, and helps you feel full, faster and for longer. In one study, 47 overweight people were divided into two groups. Those who took Zotrim lost an average of 11 lb over 45 days, compared with under one pound in those taking a placebo.

Iodine is essential for the production of thyroxine, a hormone that regulates metabolism. The normal range for thyroxine hormone is wide, with the upper limit of normal three times greater than the lower. If iodine intakes are low (sources include iodized salt, seaweed and seafood) thyroxine levels may be in the lower normal range. Supplements providing iodine (e.g. *kelp*) act as a mild thyroid stimulant and may encourage a more efficient metabolism if your iodine intake has been sub-optimal.

An extract from *green tea* leaves (Exolise) was shown in clinical studies with healthy volunteers to boost the rate at which the body burns calories by as much as 40 per cent over a 24-hour period. This is due to its ability to inhibit a metabolic enzyme (catechol-methyl transferase) so that levels of noradrenaline increase to stimulate the amount of energy burned in body cells (thermogenesis). It also blocks the activity of intestinal enzymes (gastric and pancreatic lipases) needed to digest dietary fat, so that 30 per cent less fat is absorbed overall. Clinical trials involving 80 overweight men and women who took green tea extracts found that they lost 3.5 kg over three months, with a decrease in waist circumference of 1 cm.

Extracts from the kernels of the Korean pine tree (PinnoThin) help to suppress the urge to snack. The active ingredient, pinolenic acid, stimulates production of intestinal hormones that tell your brain when you've eaten enough. By promoting feelings of satiety, these pine kernal extracts make it easier to control your food intake.

Hoodia also acts as a natural appetite suppressant to stave off hunger pangs.

Do not take supplements if you are pregnant, breast-feeding, or taking prescribed drugs without first seeking advice from a pharmacist about possible interactions or adverse effects.

Wind – excess

Embarrassing intestinal noises – known as borborygmi – are a common feature in irritable bowel syndrome (IBS). Bowel gases come from several different sources, including fizzy drinks (which are best avoided) and swallowing air, but most derive from bacterial fermentation of dietary fibre in the large bowel. As much as 1–2.5 litres a day may be produced and expelled.

Gases seem to pass through the gut of people with IBS more slowly than normal. Some people produce insufficient amounts of an enzyme, lactase, needed to break down milk sugar (lactose), resulting in excess wind, borborygmi and loose bowels. Lactose intolerance is relatively common and it may be present from birth or develop later in life.

Treatment

Avoid all milk-based products for a few weeks. If symptoms improve dramatically, a doctor can arrange a lactose tolerance test to confirm the diagnosis, and an appointment with a dietitian. In the meantime, avoid 'windy' foods such as beans, lentils, cauliflower, cabbage, broccoli, Brussel sprouts and cucumber.

Take a *probiotic* supplement to improve intestinal health.

Related entry: **Bloating**.

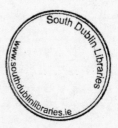

INDEX

*Note: Page numbers in **bold** refer to main discussion of a topic.*